Bridging Silos

Urban and Industrial Environments

Series editor: Robert Gottlieb, Henry R. Luce Professor of Urban and Environmental Policy, Occidental College

For a complete list of books published in this series, please see the back of the book.

Bridging Silos

Collaborating for Environmental Health and Justice in Urban Communities

Katrina Smith Korfmacher

The MIT Press
Cambridge, Massachusetts
London, England

© 2019 Massachusetts Institute of Technology

All rights reserved. No part of this book may be reproduced in any form by any electronic or mechanical means (including photocopying, recording, or information storage and retrieval) without permission in writing from the publisher.

This book was set in Stone Serif and Stone Sans by Westchester Publishing Services. Printed and bound in the United States of America.

Library of Congress Cataloging-in-Publication Data is available.

ISBN: 978-0-262-53756-8

10 9 8 7 6 5 4 3 2 1

To Karl

Contents

Contents

Foreword

The fifty American states have been termed "laboratories of democracy," places where people and communities can test and refine imaginative new laws and policies far from Washington and free of the political pressures and compromises that too often impede innovation on the national scale.

Innovation at the state and local levels is especially important in times of federal retrenchment when agencies of the national government choose not to promote public health, protect the environment, increase access to health care, or advance the common good. In these circumstances, local action can protect vulnerable populations against the consequences of ill-informed federal policy. Also local experiments can assess the feasibility of unconventional strategies and, when these strategies are found to work, pave the way for their later widescale adoption. Recent examples include Massachusetts' path-breaking creation of a universal health insurance program, a plan that became the model for the Affordable Care Act; Vermont's attempted introduction of a single-payer health care system; and courageous action by Ohio and thirty other states to expand access to Medicaid.

Hazardous environmental exposures such as air pollution, lead, toxic industrial chemicals, and pesticides are powerful determinants of health and disease in the United States, especially among disproportionately exposed minority communities, and these hazards have long been targets of state and local action. Examples of state and local interventions against environmental hazards include California's enforcement of motor vehicle emission standards much stricter than those of the federal government; New York's formation of a unique statewide network of centers of excellence in children's environmental health; Rhode Island's efforts to sue the manufacturers of lead-based paint; and actions taken by California and other states to ban brominated flame retardants and the neurotoxic insecticide chlorpyrifos.

Successful state and local initiatives in environmental public health require the formation of diverse, multisectoral collaborations whose members typically extend far beyond the "usual suspects" in the public health and environment communities. If they are to achieve their goals, these coalitions must hold together for long periods of time, sometimes for years, and persevere in the face of great opposition. The best of them are superb examples of local democracy in action.

No systematic analysis has been undertaken until now of locally based collaborations in environmental public health. What are the factors responsible for these coalitions' successes (and failures)? What are the barriers they must overcome? What are the lessons and principles that can be distilled from their work and then translated elsewhere? Such analysis is the purpose of this important new book, *Bridging Silos: Collaborating for Environmental Health and Justice in Urban Communities,* by Professor Katrina Korfmacher of the University of Rochester.

Korfmacher approaches her task by undertaking deep examinations of three local case studies in environmental public health, all of them in low-resource settings: (1) a community-based approach to lead poisoning prevention in Rochester, New York; (2) diverse efforts to promote a healthy and equitable built environment in Duluth, Minnesota; and (3) development of a systematic strategy to make protection of environmental justice communities a key planning priority for the ports of Los Angeles and Long Beach, California. Her goal is to develop a generalizable conceptual framework that assesses the key elements of successful community-based partnerships in environmental public health.

Korfmacher identifies three critical elements:

First, it is essential to properly frame the issue and precisely specify the coalition's goal. In each of the three case studies that Korfmacher examines, the local coalition framed their initiative around ending an environmental injustice. This formulation proved a powerful unifying theme. It was lofty, yet attainable. It was a target on which all could agree and few gainsay.

Second is the importance of integrating diverse systems and partners, of "bridging silos" between disparate groups, such as the public health and environment communities, local residents and academia, and community activists and government agencies. Korfmacher presents illuminating examples of how individual government officials contributed to the work of community coalitions even while their agencies sat on the sidelines. She describes how partnerships between community residents and university researchers, especially faculty and staff in university-based environmental health outreach and engagement programs, enabled communities to gain access to previously unavailable technical and intellectual resources.

Third is the need to discern the motives, professional cultures, values, goals, and constraints of each member of a coalition and to understand how these factors can either block or promote collaboration. This knowledge is critical to identifying common goals and formulating acceptable strategies. It also guides the accommodations that partner organizations may need to make to better support their members' participation in collaborative efforts.

Bridging Silos is an important and much-needed book by a scholar who has worked on the front lines of urban environmental health for more than two decades. I commend it to all who work in public health and environmental protection, and especially to my colleagues working to achieve these noble goals at the state, local, and community levels. This book presents clear guidance on how to build durable partnerships. It presents a road map on how to harness human capital—the accumulated wisdom, knowledge, and experience of communities—to advance the common good. It describes a path to attaining social justice that can successfully be followed even in times when material resources are scant and the political climate unfavorable. *Bridging Silos* sends a message of hope. It is a call to action.

Philip J. Landrigan, MD, MSc, FAAP

Director, Global Public Health Program
Schiller Institute for Integrated Science and Society
Boston College

Preface

Environmental factors significantly contribute to health inequities experienced by vulnerable populations in the United States. Environmental health injustices persist despite well-developed systems for both public health and environmental protection. The resulting health problems increase our national health care costs, and the greatest burdens are borne by lower-income communities of color.

This book integrates several important trends in community action, environmental health research, and policy approaches at a time when federal and state-level management efforts face significant challenges. Environmental advocates increasingly recognize that emphasizing public health equity benefits can broaden support for environmental protection. With the growing appreciation of environmental determinants of health, the public health community is becoming more involved in land use planning, transportation, food systems, housing, and other sectors. Local communities are more frequently highlighting how environmental injustices contribute to health disparities faced by their residents. These insights are validated by ongoing environmental health research on the lifelong, transgenerational, and cumulative impact of environmental exposures. Meanwhile, new tools are emerging that can help finance environmental public health prevention efforts, including pay for success and social impact bonds. Health care reform is contributing to the growth of value-based programs and hospital community-benefit investments in "upstream" determinants of health. Along with private and public funders' growing awareness of health-environment connections, these trends may create new opportunities for local environmental health initiatives.

In this context, collaborations of communities, governments, and researchers are working to develop and promote local solutions to environmental health problems. However, their efforts have not been systematically analyzed to distill successes, barriers, and lessons learned for future practice. This book begins to fill this gap by providing a conceptual framework, experiences of diverse initiatives, and actionable recommendations for promoting local environmental public health collaborations.

This book examines three local initiatives that aimed to alter the long-term trends, decision structures, and institutions that contributed to environmental health disparities in their communities. Although the three case studies are diverse, they share common features including strong cross-sector collaboration, community engagement, use of scientific information, and an explicit focus on health equity. None was founded with an infusion of dedicated funding, but all managed to leverage diverse resources over time. By analyzing the dynamics of these cases, the book aims to inform successful efforts in other communities.

The conceptual framework that is used to analyze these cases integrates the roles of science, multiple institutions, and community involvement in collaborative efforts. Lessons learned from these cases inform recommendations for changes in institutional structures, information systems, and resources needed to promote more effective local environmental health initiatives. The book is intended to support community members, practitioners in environmental and public health, planners, scholars, and students interested in addressing the environmental determinants of health by providing a framework for defining problems, developing collaborations, and designing solutions.

Three central themes that permeate these cases are environmental justice, integrating institutions, and systems change.

Environmental justice: All three case studies involve environmental injustices— including toxic exposures in housing, unhealthy neighborhoods, and poor air quality—that disproportionately burden historically marginalized communities. The environmental justice movement is comprised of groups that are fighting environmental threats to their communities' health and well-being. Environmental justice groups played varied roles in these cases, but none of the initiatives primarily identified itself as part of the environmental justice movement. Therefore, although these initiatives were motivated by environmental justice concerns, the term "environmental health equity" is used to describe their goal. This term clarifies that environmental justice groups may choose to join collaborative initiatives or to organize their work independently at various stages of the process.

Integrating institutions: The fields of environment and public health protection share a common origin in the sanitation efforts of cities from nearly two centuries ago. Today, however, health and environment are managed by largely separate "siloed" institutions. Solving problems of environmental health often requires finding new ways to connect or "bridge" these existing systems. This book explores how local initiatives are building bridges between these silos at the local level, where collaboration, partnerships, and resource sharing is often more feasible and decision systems are more amenable to community influence than at higher levels of government.

Systems change: In order to build robust bridges between existing institutions, it is necessary to make durable changes in the ways decisions are made, the nature of evidence that is considered, and the ways diverse community interests are engaged. To inform such changes, we first need to understand the incentives, training, motivation, professional cultures, and values of all participants, as well as how these factors can either block or promote collaboration. In-depth exploration of promising case studies can provide insight into these dynamics.

This book explores three local environmental health initiatives. These cases were selected to represent a range of locations, scales, issue-areas, and resources. Because of this diversity, the lessons learned are likely to be relevant to a wide range of urban communities. The three cases describe (1) the development of an innovative housing-based approach to lead poisoning prevention in Rochester, New York; (2) multiple efforts to promote a healthy built environment in Duluth, Minnesota; and (3) a initiative aimed at making local community health a key consideration in decisions related to goods movement around the ports of Los Angeles and Long Beach, California.

In each of these cases, government, community, and technical experts collaborated to produce significant systems changes by working outside established policy processes. They were successful in reframing long-standing problems in new ways by focusing on health equity; leveraging a variety of human, financial, and technical resources; and changing processes, practices, and policies. Their experiences suggest changes are needed in institutional structures, information systems, and resources at the state and national level to better support local innovation. The book concludes with an argument that such changes could help more effectively protect environmental public health and reduce health disparities in many communities.

Especially at times when state and federal programs are slow in addressing environmental public health problems, local collaborations hold promise for bringing attention to and helping to resolve environmental injustices. However, effective collaborations do not spontaneously arise in all settings. In fact, communities facing the most severe environmental health inequities may lack the capacity to collaborate for systems change. The experiences of these cases suggest that a better understanding of what contributes to success, more appropriately targeted resources, and changes in how governments, academia, community groups, and funders support collaboration are needed to promote expansion of promising local environmental health initiatives.

Acknowledgments

This book was sparked by a late-night conversation after a National Institute of Environmental Health Sciences Core Centers meeting in 2004. Members of four Community Outreach and Engagement Cores—Andrea Hricko, Johnnye Lewis, Fran Lynn, and myself—reflected on the impactful local collaborations taking place in our diverse communities. Although the environmental health issues, geographies, and partners differed, we noted common elements, including the involvement of multidisciplinary experts, extensive community engagement, and involvement of professionals with a sustained commitment to supporting collaboration. In each case, these collaborations were successfully changing systems to promote environmental justice. We mused that because these experiences took place in such different issue-areas, geographies, and contexts, their common themes were not widely recognized and local communities could not readily learn from one another's work. My goal in writing this book was to provide insight into the processes, successes, and challenges of local environmental health initiatives with a view toward helping diverse practitioners, community members, and scholars build on their promising potential.

For the first case study, I drew on seventeen years of direct interaction with the Coalition to Prevent Lead Poisoning in Rochester, New York. It has been an honor to work with devoted community members, health care professionals, civil servants, and researchers throughout this effort, and their contributions to telling Rochester's story were invaluable. Colleagues in the health impact assessment field pointed me toward the second case study of the policy, systems, and environmental change work in Duluth, Minnesota. In Duluth I found a rich network of people who had been promoting health equity through the regeneration of the city's built environment for over ten years. Without fail, they were generous, kind, tolerant, and patient in helping a stranger understand and recount their experiences. I hope I have done their admirable work justice. For the final case study, Andrea Hricko shared nearly two decades of experience working to address the health impacts of goods movement activities around the ports of Los Angeles and Long Beach, California. Throughout this project, she remained an active, supportive, and steadfast partner, connecting me with key resources, collaborators, and materials. For a list of case study contributors, see the methodological appendix.

To elicit common themes from these three diverse collaborations, I built on the rich social science scholarship on ecosystem management. In 2004, a group of colleagues (Koontz et al. 2004) developed a framework to identify lessons learned from in-depth case studies of diverse ecosystem management efforts (*Collaborative Environmental Management: What Roles for Government?*). One of these colleagues, Toddi Steelman, helped me adapt our framework to local environmental public health initiatives. Toddi was my constant cheerleader, supporter, and accountability partner throughout this project, and I benefited tremendously from her humor, clarity, and kindness.

The University of Rochester provided a sabbatical leave that allowed me to launch this project. Multiple funders supported my ongoing work with the Rochester Coalition to Prevent Lead Poisoning, most significantly the National Institute of Environmental Health Sciences grant P30 ES001247. Many other individuals and organizations provided logistical support. I particularly appreciate Ogonnaya Dodson-Newman's recommendation of a writing retreat. This wise suggestion led me to spend time at the Constance Saltonstall Arts Colony, Writers and Books' Gell House, and Truro Treasure, where much of the text was produced. I am grateful for the use of these lovely spaces.

I have been inspired by works in the MIT Press Urban and Industrial Environments series since graduate school and was delighted to have the opportunity to work with their excellent team. Bob Gottlieb has a special connection to this book, being both the series editor and a partner in THE Impact Project. I especially appreciate the support, advice, and assistance of Beth Clevenger and Anthony Zannino.

The themes, insights, and questions that emerged through writing this book were rich fodder for conversations with colleagues, rekindled old connections, and led me to new partners. Whether providing conceptual, substantive, or moral support, these interactions were a great source of joy. Thanks especially to Pete Andrews, Bill Ascher, Marice Ashe, Nana Bennett, Mary Jean Brown, Phil Brown, Ted Brown, Jason Corburn, Scott Cummings, Eric Faisst, Kathleen Gray, Kim Haddow, Jonathan Heller, DeWitt John, Chris Kochtitzky, Gina McCarthy, Rebecca Morley, Liam O'Fallon, Andy Sansone, Peggy Shephard, Wade Silkworth, Curt Spalding, Edwin van Wijngaarden, Steve Wing, Ben Winig, Julia Wondolleck, and Tina Yuen. In the final stages, I was fortunate to have the excellent assistance of Kara Austin, Rio Hartwell, Kate Kressmann-Kehoe, and Elizabeth Williams-Velasquez. Throughout the process, the fabulous women of the Healthy City Book Club were my muses. Their commitment to making Rochester a better place for all community members inspires me.

Finally, my family's support throughout this project was monumental. I now know that writing a book is a tremendous indulgence, and they indulged me unfailingly! Special thanks to Karl: it is indeed handy to have a mapmaker in the household, and the graphics that he created were icing on the cake.

Abbreviations

AOC	Areas of Concern
BLL	Blood lead level
CAA	Clean Air Act
CDC	Centers for Disease Control and Prevention
CEQA	California Environmental Quality Act
COEC	Community Outreach and Engagement Core
CPLP	Coalition to Prevent Lead Poisoning (Rochester, New York)
CWA	Clean Water Act (Federal Water Pollution Control Act Amendments of 1972)
EIR	Environmental impact report (under CEQA)
EIS	Environmental impact statement (under NEPA)
EPA	Environmental Protection Agency
HDAC	Healthy Duluth Area Coalition
HIA	health impact assessment
HiAP	Health in All Policies
HUD	U.S. Department of Housing and Urban Development
IOM	Institute of Medicine
MFN	Moving Forward Network
NEPA	National Environmental Policy Act
NIEHS	National Institute of Environmental Health Sciences
PSE	policies, systems, and environments
SHIP	State Health Improvement Program/Partnership

1 Changing Local Systems to Promote Environmental Health and Justice

When Hurricane Katrina devastated New Orleans in 2005, the nation witnessed environmental injustice in graphic detail. Low-income people—predominantly African Americans—suffered most from this crisis, were underserved by disaster response efforts, and recovered more slowly. Many residents were permanently displaced. As researchers, agencies, and the media searched for explanations, it became clear that historical patterns of land use had put low-income communities and people of color in harm's way (Levitt and Whitaker 2009). Lack of resources limited the ability of marginalized communities to recover. Multiple vulnerabilities including chronic disease, mental health issues, and addiction compounded the effects of the disaster on these populations. According to Bates and Swan (2010, 21), "Katrina swept away the 'traditional belief' that natural disasters are equally devastating on populations and do not discriminate in terms of what is destroyed."

Long-standing policies and practices created the environmental disparities that lay at the root of the hurricane's disproportionate impacts on these communities (Pastor et al. 2006; Levitt and Whitaker 2009; Pardee 2005; Wailoo, Dowd, and O'Neill 2010). Decades of land use and economic development decisions led to concentrated poverty in areas at high risk of flooding. Housing policies failed to provide safe housing, particularly for communities of color. Lack of transportation resources limited the mobility of poorer residents. These and other environmental conditions—such as low-income residents' lack of access to affordable and nutritious foods, preventive health care, and opportunities for physical activity—contributed to the high rates of chronic disease and the poor health status of these same communities, reducing their resilience to environmental disaster.

It is clearly better to address underlying environmental health inequities before a disaster like a hurricane, oil spill, or industrial accident reveals them through devastating impacts on disadvantaged communities. Doing so, however, requires new ways of promoting environmental health at the local level. All over the country, communities, governments, and researchers are working together to change the policies, systems, and environments that drive health inequities. This book explores the promise of these local initiatives by taking an in-depth look at three efforts to address long-standing environmental health issues: childhood lead poisoning, unhealthy built environments, and environmental hazards associated with commercial ports. These case studies all focus on urban environments and communities grappling with environmental health inequities. Environmental health collaborations also arise in rural and suburban settings; however, because the resources, community engagement approaches, and decision processes may be significantly different, this book focuses on comparative analysis of urban initiatives. The case studies explore the evolution of collaborative initiatives to reveal how they operated, what they achieved, and how it may be possible to build on their successes to promote environmental health equity in other communities.

Coalition to Prevent Lead Poisoning—Rochester, NY

The negative health effects of lead—particularly on children—have been known for centuries. Nonetheless, lead was added to gasoline and paint in the United States in the early 1900s, spreading it through homes and roadsides. Since lead was banned in the 1970s, population-wide blood lead levels have plummeted. However, children living in older housing in poor repair continue to be poisoned at alarming rates. In 1999, an elementary school principal in Rochester, New York, discovered that 41 percent of his incoming students had elevated blood lead levels—twenty times the national rate. This striking disparity galvanized diverse stakeholders including researchers, lawyers, health officials, city officials, educators, and child advocates to work together to prevent lead poisoning. The resulting coalition improved health and housing agency coordination, developed a comprehensive communications campaign, and passed a groundbreaking city lead law in 2005 (Korfmacher 2008). By 2012, the number of Rochester

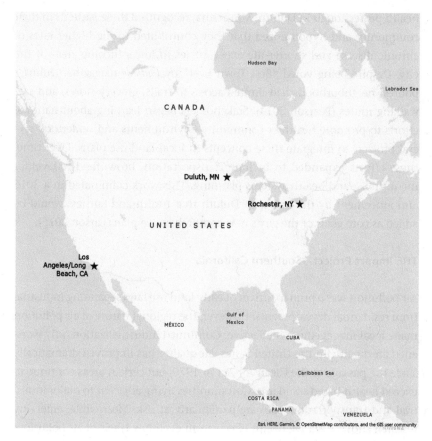

Figure 1.1
Case study locations
(Map credit: Karl Korfmacher)

children with elevated lead levels had decreased over 90 percent, 2.4 times faster than in similar upstate New York cities (Kennedy et al. 2014).

Healthy Duluth—Duluth, MN

Amid national concern over growing rates of obesity, the "healthy communities" movement has highlighted evidence that people living in poorer neighborhoods often lack access to healthy, affordable food and opportunities to be physically active in their daily lives. Community groups and public health professionals in Duluth, Minnesota, recognized these patterns in their community and hypothesized that they contributed to the higher rates of chronic disease and shorter life expectancies in lower-income areas of the city. Despite being voted "Best Town Ever" by *Outside* magazine, Duluth's poorest neighborhoods had limited access to trails, grocery stores, and safe walking routes (Pearson 2014). Stakeholders began learning about national efforts to promote healthier community environments and undertook several projects to integrate these concepts in local land-use plans. Over time, these efforts expanded to include transportation, brownfield redevelopment, trails, and health systems planning. This work culminated in a 2016 announcement by the mayor of Duluth that health and fairness would be added as core goals of the city's new comprehensive plan (Larson 2016).

THE Impact Project—Southern California

Air pollution was a primary driver of early land use laws separating industrial from residential developments. However, the regional nature of air pollution made local management ineffective. Continued industrialization only worsened air quality. In the United States, air quality has improved dramatically since the passage of the Clean Air Act in 1970, but certain areas continue to exceed health-based standards. Communities living adjacent to major industrial and transportation hubs are particularly at risk. Meanwhile, emerging research shows negative health effects from even low levels of air pollution, particularly for vulnerable populations. Southern California has been an epicenter of air quality concerns for decades. In the early 2000s, expected growth in shipping through the ports of Los Angeles and Long Beach increased community concerns about the cumulative impacts of industrial transportation. THE Impact Project was a collaborative effort by academic and local environmental justice groups to increase consideration of health effects in all decisions related to goods movement in the area (Hricko 2008). In conjunction with ongoing community efforts, THE Impact Project succeeded in attracting media attention to these issues, enhancing community participation in decision processes, and promoting analysis of health equity impacts in decisions about highway, port, and railyard expansions.

These three initiatives highlight the potential for collaborative efforts between communities, technical experts, and decision makers to make significant improvements in local environmental health problems that disproportionately impact historically marginalized populations. Although these initiatives were primarily local, their successes have national implications. Could these initiatives hold lessons for other communities about how to reduce environmental health inequities? If so, what can be done to better foster and support similar initiatives in other communities?

Answering these questions is crucial both to public health and to environmental protection in the United States. Ballooning health care costs and growing health disparities have brought renewed attention to the social determinants of health—the economic, social, and environmental factors that shape people's ability to live healthy lives. Local collaborations between community, government, and academic stakeholders can change the systems that shape environmental determinants of health and offer promising approaches to reducing health disparities. Lessons learned from these collaborations provide insights into roles, tools, processes, and institutions through which communities can support health-promoting environmental changes.

Local environmental health initiatives also hold potential for reinvigorating public support for environmental management. Although the mission of the U.S. Environmental Protection Agency (EPA) is "to protect human health and the environment," public perception and political rhetoric in recent years has increasingly painted the agency as needlessly blocking economic development to preserve narrow environmental interests. To counter this narrative, former EPA administrator Gina McCarthy embraced "Making a Visible Difference in Communities" as a top theme of the agency's 2014 strategic plan (U.S. EPA 2014a). McCarthy said, "Now that pollution is invisible, people don't actually know what EPA [Environmental Protection Agency] does and [they] don't value it. So, we tend to be more distanced from communities than state-level actions. But we need people to know what we do and why we do it" (McCarthy 2018). She initiated a series of cross-agency projects to make immediate, concrete contributions to local environmental problem-solving. Many of these efforts worked collaboratively with low-income urban communities to address environmental justice concerns (U.S. EPA 2014b). Public communications about the Making a Visible Difference initiative underscored the EPA's work with communities to solve locally identified environmental health problems. Other environmental organizations have also recognized that more explicitly connecting their work to community health can build awareness of and support for their work (Iannantuono and Eyles 2000).

Environmental health inequities exist because of the historical economic, social, and policy forces that shaped urban development. Our policies to manage environmental and public health impacts rely on technically focused, top-down management institutions separated by issue area with limited public engagement, local flexibility, and coordination. This siloed approach to addressing the environmental and public health legacies of urban development has proved insufficient to reverse unfair burdens on underserved communities. Place-based, collaborative local efforts have potential to form bridges between these silos and promote systems changes to address these intractable problems.

Environmental Health Equity and Justice

Environmental and public health stakeholders are increasingly attentive to the environmental conditions that can contribute to health inequalities in underserved communities. The terms "environmental injustice," "environmental health disparity" and "environmental health inequity," are all used to refer to the disproportionate health impacts of environmental hazards.

Environmental managers operate within legal, policy, and regulatory systems designed to protect human health. Despite this extensive system of health-based environmental laws, however, many communities remain exposed to hazards. Underserved communities are most likely to suffer from these gaps in environmental protection. As former U.S. EPA Administrator Gina McCarthy said, "Environmental protection tends to go from the grassroots up because pollution tends to go down … it hits the most vulnerable the most. There are communities that really are left behind when you do national rulemaking because you can't really get at those issues effectively through regulation … not at the national level. You have to rely on states and you have to rely on local communities" (McCarthy 2018).

Environmental justice is defined by the U.S. EPA as the "fair treatment and meaningful involvement of all people regardless of race, color, national origin, or income with respect to the development, implementation, and enforcement of environmental laws, regulations, and policies" (U.S. EPA 2018e). The environmental justice movement began with communities recognizing their excessive exposure to environmental hazards and organizing to reduce these risks. Although these concerns have existed for decades, the environmental justice movement is often traced to citizen protests of 1982 in response to a proposal to dump hazardous waste in Warren County, North Carolina, a community already burdened by multiple waste facilities (Bullard 2008). Similar stories emerged across the county of communities subjected to environmental hazards from past industrial land use or targeted for new polluting facilities (Bryant 1995; Bryant and Mohai 1992; Cole and Foster 2001; Hofrichter 2002). The environmental justice movement grew from connections between these disparate communities that organized around their experiences of unfair environmental burdens as issues of social justice and civil rights (Cole and Foster 2001; Bullard 2008; Novotny 2000). According to Bryant (1995, 9), "Environmental justice is broader in scope than environmental equity. It refers to those cultural norms and values, rules, regulations, behaviors, policies, and decisions to support sustainable communities, where people can interact with confidence that their environmental is safe, nurturing, and productive." Although the term "environmental justice" does not explicitly call out health, the movement has focused on the threats that pollution poses to community health and well-being. Environmental justice efforts have also underscored the unequal distribution of environmental benefits—like parks, urban trees, and safe, walkable streets—that can promote health.

The environmental justice movement emphasizes that current burdens of environmental exposure reflect historical patterns of development and social interaction shaped by racism, economic inequality, and the limited political power of low-income communities and people of color. These dynamics are perpetuated by the power of industry and lack of meaningful community input in public decisions. Environmental justice advocates emphasize that engagement of local communities is therefore essential to developing effective solutions. Thus, "environmental justice" can refer to a movement, an ethical principle, a process of empowerment, or an outcome.

"Health equity" is an ethical principle based on viewing health as a fundamental human right. As Braveman (2014, 7) writes, "Health equity means social justice in health (i.e., no one is denied the possibility to be healthy for belonging to a group that has historically been economically/socially disadvantaged). Health disparities are the metric we use to measure progress toward achieving health equity." By extension, environmental health equity focuses on different groups' access to environmental benefits and exposure to environmental risks. Environmental health disparities are the variations in health outcomes associated with the differing quality of people's environments. According to the National Institute of Environmental Health Sciences (NIEHS), "Environmental health disparities exist when communities exposed to a combination of poor environmental quality and social inequities have more sickness and disease than wealthier, less polluted communities" (NIEHS 2018b). Concerns about controlling health care costs, preventing disease, and reducing disparities have contributed to health professionals' growing interest in promoting environmental health equity.

This book generally uses the term "environmental health equity" to refer to patterns of environmental exposures or resources and "environmental health disparities" for associated health outcomes. To distinguish the community-based perspective of the environmental justice movement, the term "environmental justice" is generally reserved for organizing, advocacy, and policy efforts that self-identify as such. Environmental justice is also used to emphasize processes with equitable participation, community power-sharing, and a focus on fairness.

According to the NIEHS, "When environmental justice is achieved, environmental health disparities will be reduced" (NIEHS 2018b). This cause has public appeal, as evidenced by the popular press coverage of "death by zip code" maps that show striking disparities in life expectancy between adjacent urban neighborhoods (Raab 2013; Parks 2016). Public health professionals' increasing interest in environmental health equity reflects an emerging consensus that (1) environmental inequities contribute to health disparities; (2) changing these patterns requires changing the policies and systems that shape environmental quality; and (3) doing so requires new connections between community, research, environmental, and health groups.

The environmental justice movement has shown the power of local organizing, partnerships, and collaborations to address environmental health crises. There have been many individual successes—for example, pollution sources being controlled or shut down, hazardous wastes cleaned up, and destructive new developments blocked. As the impacts of Hurricane Katrina showed, it is important to proactively change the underlying systems that create environmental health inequities before crises happen. This book focuses on local environmental health initiatives that aimed to do just that.

Silos, Systems, and Boundary Spanners

The separation of policy by issue-area is often described as "siloed" management (John 1994, 5; Delreux and Happaerts 2016, 66). The image of silos evokes a lack of connection, coordination, or interaction between different areas of environmental practice (United Nations Development Program 2013). Boschken (2009, 1) defined the "silo effect" as "the dysfunctional segregation of policy disciplines often caused by differences in ideology, scientific fragmentation, and professional misunderstanding that limit the ability of one discipline to sufficiently interact with another." As examined in chapter 2, public health and environmental management agencies operate under different policy mandates, regulations, funding streams, and, often, levels of government. Silos separating different aspects of environmental health protection can both create gaps that contribute to environmental inequities and pose barriers to resolving these problems (United Nations Development Program 2013).

Siloed institutions face inherent challenges in managing complex systems. "Systems thinking" means viewing problems as interconnected webs of multiple causes, flows, and feedbacks. Originally developed in the context of ecosystem sustainability, systems thinking has also been applied to computer science, business, economic modeling, and other fields (Meadows 2008; Senge 2013). Public health scholars have increasingly promoted viewing public health as a system, particularly with regard to environmental health (Northridge, Sclar, and Biswas 2003; Trochim et al. 2006; Ashe et al. 2016). According to Ashe and colleagues (2016), "The essence of systems thinking lies in a shift of thinking to see interrelationships rather than linear cause-effect chains, and longer-term processes of change rather than simply snapshots in time. ... Through systems thinking, we know that we have to look for the fundamental causes of the problems we are trying to solve."

In this context, "systems thinking" means examining the multiple causes of environmental health problems that lie in different sectors (health or environment), levels of government (federal, state, local), or stakeholder roles (community, academic, government, private sector, etc.). It implies that effective, sustainable solutions often require multilevel changes throughout the management system. Focusing on systems change calls attention to the key role of "boundary spanning" in solving local environmental health problems (Guston 2001). A fundamental dynamic encountered in environmental health problem-solving is that health and environmental interests are not well integrated in decision-making structures. Involving individuals from various institutions in systems-change efforts requires stakeholders to form bridges between their organizations. Solutions often require individuals within existing agencies, groups, and systems to see their roles differently, act in new ways, and shift their organizations' practices. Doing so may involve stepping outside the boundaries of their normal responsibilities, disciplinary training, and professional experience. Collaboration can contribute to successful systems change, particularly when promising solutions involve multiple organizations, new roles, and diverse targets for action.

When we think about public health as a system, it is clear that poverty—ameliorated or exacerbated by social forces like racism and discrimination—is the underlying driver of health disparities, including those related to environmental determinants. Although environmental and public health professionals may recognize poverty, racism, and social discrimination as root causes, their institutions do not have the tools to directly address these underlying causes (Freudenberg 2004).

However, thinking about environmental health equity as part of a larger system can guide collaborations with other community efforts to reduce poverty. For example, working with anti-poverty efforts can ensure that environmental health activities maximize economic benefits to disadvantaged communities (e.g., workforce development, local hiring) and avoid socioeconomic hardships (e.g., gentrification and displacement). Engaging with local residents, organizations, and community groups can inform efforts that are ethically responsible, suited to local conditions, and culturally appropriate. This engagement can be done in ways that empower communities and build their capacity to self-advocate in multiple issue-areas (Freudenberg, Pastor, and Israel 2011). Highlighting environmental health inequities can justify additional environmental programs, resources, and policies devoted to assisting disproportionately burdened communities. Thus, while environmental efforts are often portrayed—especially at the national level—as threatening economic improvement, community-engaged local initiatives can complement efforts to fight poverty.

Local Environmental Health Initiatives

Many communities have undertaken efforts to address local environmental health inequities. However, most are time-limited, funded for a specific campaign, or focused on a single development project, policy, plan, or practice. This book defines local environmental health initiatives as collaborative problem-solving efforts that aim to make durable changes in systems in order to reduce environmental health disparities. Environmental health inequities persist despite existing laws, regulations, and agencies that aim to protect human health from environmental hazards. Therefore, efforts to address local environmental health inequities are likely to challenge existing systems. Multisector involvement, community engagement, and sustained collaboration are essential.

Initiatives aiming to address environmental health problems must be informed by health, environmental, and community knowledge. Public health data can help highlight the economic and social benefits of preventing disease through environmental change. Accessing public health knowledge does not necessarily require formal involvement by health systems or public health agencies. Informal relationships, internal research capacity, or consultants can also inform the effort. Public health groups may include government agencies, health care institutions, health foundations, or community health organizations. Because of rising concerns about health care costs, the ability to engage public health interests can be a powerful and sustaining source of moral, political, and financial support for environmental health equity efforts.

Local environmental health initiatives must also be able to characterize environmental health risks. In some cases, this means simply analyzing existing data and presenting it in a new light, such as estimating the economic impacts of environmental exposures, showing the geographic distribution of health outcomes, or summarizing the existing research in the context of local conditions. Other initiatives may access experts whose cutting-edge environmental health research helps them demonstrate how existing environmental standards are insufficient to protect health. Some groups conduct "citizen science" to document previously unrecognized hot spots of exposures. Local environmental health initiatives can develop credible, effective solutions if they are able to make use of high-quality, multidisciplinary information.

Meaningful engagement of communities is vital to the success of local environmental health initiatives for several reasons. First, it is ethically essential. As environmental justice advocates have long argued, communities have a right to participate in decisions that affect their health and well-being—especially communities that have not had this opportunity in the past. Second, environmental health inequities manifest at the neighborhood level. Therefore, community knowledge is critical for designing effective solutions. Third, the voice of communities that experience environmental health disparities can be a source of political power to drive systems change. Local environmental health initiatives can provide a vehicle for community influence on policies, systems, and environments that current decision processes lack.

Community engagement may take many forms. In local environmental health initiatives that arise from community-identified concerns, community members may remain active as leaders or partners throughout the collaboration. In other cases, the environmental health issue may not be a high priority for residents, in which case the initiative may work with existing community groups to raise public awareness. Or, residents may be concerned about the issue but lack the capacity to participate directly, in which case the initiative may devote resources to eliciting their input, representing their perspectives, and building their capacity to engage in the future.

Finally, collaborative initiatives must be structured in ways that allow them to influence policies, systems, and environments. Knowledge and strong community engagement contribute to the credibility of an initiative, but they must be coordinated effectively over a period of time to achieve systems change. Participants must understand *why* existing systems are failing to protect environmental health equity and whether local levers (e.g., policies, practices, funding) can be shifted to address these gaps. Stakeholders with experience in policy change may be helpful by identifying promising advocacy strategies. Involving stakeholders from multiple sectors can inform effective boundary-spanning solutions. As well, participants may influence the decisions and behaviors of their home institutions, encouraging them toward ongoing collaboration. Most environmental health problems require action in multiple sectors over a period of years. Therefore, a sustainable collaborative structure is essential for success.

This begs the question: What is a successful local environmental health equity initiative? Collaborative initiatives may have complex goals, evolving objectives, and diverse modes of action, which makes evaluating the impacts of local environmental health initiatives challenging. As well, their effects may be indirect, long term, or influenced by external factors, further complicating efforts to assess their impacts. This book takes the broad view that a successful local environmental health initiative engages community perspectives, fosters multisectoral collaboration, and contributes to systems changes that are likely to improve environmental health equity over time.

This book refers to local environmental health "initiatives," rather than calling them organizations, collaboratives, partnerships, or coalitions. The term "initiatives" emphasizes the diversity in their structures and highlights that while the individuals involved may consider themselves to be collaborators, their employers, institutions, or agencies may have no formal relationship with or commitment to the efforts. Finally, calling these efforts "initiatives" emphasizes that they are problem-oriented—the collaboration may disband or adopt a different form over time.

A number of national groups and agencies have promoted this type of local collaboration. One example is the Community Outreach and Engagement Cores (COEC) within the NIEHS environmental health research core centers (NIEHS 2018a; O'Fallon et al. 2003).[1] The twenty or so COECs across the country participate in innovative efforts to address community environmental health and justice problems. The NIEHS encourages COECs to leverage their environmental health research resources in support of partnerships that can develop solutions to address identified community needs. Another example is the Robert Wood Johnson Foundation's Active Living by Design program, which has provided funding and technical support for communities to take a data-driven "policy, systems, and environment approach" to creating healthier community environments (Sallis et al. 2006; Active Living by Design 2018). The EPA's Collaborative Problem-Solving Model was developed to guide community-based environmental justice efforts funded through its Environmental Justice Cooperative Agreement Program (U.S. EPA 2018b). Most of these EPA grant-funded partnerships focus on particular projects or facilities, rather than policy processes and systems. Nonetheless, the Collaborative Problem-Solving Model embodies many of the principles of local environmental health initiatives described here. Many other government agencies, foundations and nonprofit organizations have supported similar efforts in their sectors of interest.

Despite some isolated efforts by academics, journalists, and foundations to disseminate these experiences, local environmental health initiatives have not been comparatively analyzed across sectors, geographies, or issue-areas. To fill that gap, this book explores what gives rise to such initiatives, what resources they need to thrive, how effective they are in achieving systems change, and how to foster more effective local environmental health collaborations.

Local environmental health initiatives hold underexplored promise for promoting environmental health equity for several reasons. First, environmental injustices are most often identified at the community level. People living in disproportionately polluted neighborhoods readily perceive the unfairness of being exposed to hazards and having fewer environmental amenities than other communities. Their voices can be a powerful moral, political, and economic driver of systems change. Second, environmental disparities often result from gaps between existing federal and state regulatory systems and require locally informed solutions that are adapted to the unique resources, needs, preferences, and constraints of communities. Third, environmental health problem-solving requires coordination between sectors. Such collaboration is generally easier to initiate and sustain at the local level than between state or federal bureaucracies. Fourth, localities are an important source of innovation and new approaches to intractable problems. Cities have created, tested, and implemented many public health and environmental innovations that have eventually informed broader policy change. Fifth, many of the policies that drive environmental conditions are locally controlled, including land use, transportation, redevelopment, and housing. Finally, particularly in a time of limited budgets and gridlock within state and national legislatures, local initiatives may hold the greatest promise for effective and timely solutions to environmental health challenges.

Introduction to the Case Studies

In each of the three cases presented, local action succeeded in addressing a long-standing issue of environmental injustice: housing-based lead hazards, the built environment, and the environmental impacts of ports. The cases have common features, as well as differences. Comparing the cases provides an opportunity to identify resources, approaches, and strategies that may contribute to successful local health initiatives in other communities. Table 1.1 provides an overview of these case characteristics.

Table 1.1

Case study characteristics

	Coalition to Prevent Lead Poisoning	Healthy Duluth	THE Impact Project
Geographic target of action	Pre-1978 housing; focus on private rental housing in high-risk city neighborhoods	Streets, trails, healthy food access transportation, and land use in Duluth	Regional transportation facilities associated with ports of Los Angeles and Long Beach
Population of area (2010 Census)	City of Rochester, NY: 210,000	City of Duluth, MN: 86,000	Los Angeles County, CA: 10,000,000+
Target population	Children living in high-risk rental housing	All residents; focus on low income and residents of color	Transportation hub-adjacent communities
Environmental issue	Lead in paint and soil around pre-1978 housing	Limited access to active transportation and healthy food sources	Air pollution and other impacts from ships, trains, trucks, and port equipment
Health disparity	Elevated rates of lead poisoning among children living in high-risk neighborhoods	Lower life expectancy in low-income neighborhoods	High rates of asthma, chronic disease, risk of cancer near transportation hubs
Convening/host organization(s)	Community (United Way, Finger Lakes Health Systems Agency)	Multiple community/ government/ conveners (city, county, Healthy Duluth Area Coalition)	Academic (University of Southern California)/community (4 partner groups)
Scope of systems change	*Narrow*: city housing inspection policy (also county and housing authority inspections)	*Medium*: local decisions about roads, public transit, city planning, brownfields, data systems	*Broad*: environmental review of rail, highway, warehouse facilities; local land-use decisions; air quality policies

All three cases were "locally initiated" collaborations, meaning that the problem was identified by local stakeholders. Although all of the cases had significant interaction with national networks, funders, or technical resources, they were not primarily led or supported by a single source of external funding or part of a national program. This dynamic allowed for examination of the role of outside expertise and resources in supporting local initiatives. The process of issue framing, decisions about appropriate structures, objectives, and approaches, and leveraging resources to support the effort were part of the local initiative's work. These decisions may have been influenced by external organizations, but in general they were driven by local stakeholders.

Each initiative was sparked by a growing awareness of an environmental health inequity in the local area. The environmental issues addressed had all been long known to cause health problems, and emerging research had shown even greater reason for concern than was previously thought. Notably, these environmental health problems exist in many other areas, which suggests that the approaches used in these cases might be relevant to other contexts. Finally, there are well-developed policy systems in each of these issue-areas. Thus, rather than starting from scratch, each of these local environmental health initiatives reframed an old problem in a new way, relied primarily on existing data, and focused on shaping how decisions are made within existing policy frameworks.

The three cases differed with respect to institutional structure, decision-making process, and the roles of government, community groups, and academia in the collaboration. For example, THE Impact Project was hosted by a university, whereas the Coalition to Prevent Lead Poisoning was housed at a community health agency, and the Healthy Duluth built environment efforts were convened by a several different government and community groups over time. Although various sectors played different roles in the cases, none was dominated by a single organization. The internal decision-making processes ranged from informal consensus to specific bylaws and voting rules.

These three initiatives were active over at least ten years, and in each case there was substantial documentation that made it possible to describe the initiative's formation, evolution, the sustainability of impacts, and the likely future trajectory. Because many local collaborations are not formal, there is often limited record keeping about their formation, processes, activities, and outcomes. In these cases, however, a combination of data sources including strategic plans, project reports, funding proposals, news articles, and key informant interviews allowed for in-depth analysis of decision processes, activities, and outcomes over time (see the methodological appendix).

All of the initiatives had significant impacts on local policies, systems, and environments, but the nature of their activities and the scope of systems change varied greatly. Early on, the Coalition to Prevent Lead Poisoning in Rochester was narrowly focused on passage and implementation of a local lead law. Over time, it pursued changes in intergovernmental relationships, promoted community awareness, and facilitated broader partnerships. The Healthy Duluth efforts began by integrating health considerations into specific local area plans and brownfields redevelopment, but eventually expanded to influence the city's comprehensive plan. THE Impact Project had the broadest scope: to increase attention to health in a wide spectrum of transportation, land use, and air quality decisions related to the movement of goods in Southern California. The target of action for these initiatives ranged in scale from the household (Rochester) to neighborhood (Duluth) to regional (Southern California).

Although all are based in urban settings, these cases represent diverse geographies, scales, contexts, and issue-areas. Duluth, Minnesota, the smallest city represented, has a population of around 86,000 and is surrounded by rural areas. Rochester, New York, is a midsize city of around 210,000 within a metropolitan area of around a million people. The goods-movement case focuses on communities living adjacent to transportation hubs across Los Angeles County, which is home to over 10 million people.

In each of these cases, stakeholders responded to perceived environmental health injustices by collaborating to change the systems that allowed these inequities to persist. Each initiative leveraged diverse information sources, community connections, and cross-sector collaboration in response to a place-specific concern about environmental health inequities. They all took a broad, upstream view of what drove the distribution of environmental harms and access to benefits in their communities. Instead of targeting single decisions, developments, or projects, they addressed multiple decision sectors to reduce environmental contributors to health disparities. The phrase "policies, systems, and environmental change" is often used to describe this kind of effort (ChangeLab Solutions 2018b; Public Health Institute 2018). While these collaborations focused on local systems, in some cases state or federal strategies that impact multiple communities emerged from the local work. They all engaged in a range of education, research, projects, campaigns, and data analyses over time to support their systems change goals. Recognizing that policy systems are dynamic, they also sought to change how, by whom, and by what criteria future decisions are made. Thus, although these groups differed with respect to issue-area, structure, stakeholders, scope, and scale, they all engaged multidisciplinary stakeholders, communities, and collaborative approaches to develop new solutions to long-standing environmental justice issues.

Each of these initiatives reframed an existing issue as one of environmental health inequity. As noted previously, the identified environmental concerns were improving overall but continued to plague historically marginalized communities. These initiatives present a potential model for proactively identifying gaps in existing systems that result in environmental health disparities, filling these gaps, and reducing future health disparities. This potential is why it is important to explore their effectiveness, what contributed to their successes, and how to build on their potential in the future. In addition, it is important to consider whether these approaches—or the solutions they devised—can be replicated in other communities to leverage their impact on promoting environmental health equity throughout the country.

Chapter Overviews

Chapter 2 begins with an overview of how environmental and public health management systems in the United States began as an integrated field but evolved separately to create the current siloed system. The gaps created by these silos contribute to persistent environmental health inequities. Chapter 3 presents burgeoning efforts to rebuild bridges between environment and health to impact the social determinants that contribute to persistent health disparities. These integrative efforts parallel the development of ecosystem management in the 1990s as a way to more effectively manage natural resources. Borrowing from social science research evaluating ecosystem management, chapter 3 presents a Local Environmental Health Initiative Framework as a conceptual guide to analyzing the cases.

The three case studies comprise chapters 4 through 6. Chapter 4 traces the development of an innovative housing-based approach to lead poisoning prevention in Rochester, New York. Chapter 5 examines a diverse set of local efforts to promote a healthier built environment in Duluth, Minnesota. Chapter 6 analyzes the development and results of THE Impact Project, a systematic effort to consider community health in decisions related to goods movement from the ports of Los Angeles and Long Beach, California.

Chapter 7 analyzes the case studies using the conceptual framework laid out in chapter 3, highlighting how these initiatives reframed environmental problems as issues of health equity, what resources and approaches supported their efforts, and how they changed their communities.

Chapter 8 reflects on how such local environmental health initiatives might be expanded. It examines the initiatives' ability to address gaps in existing systems of environmental management and public health and to create sustainable solutions to problems of environmental justice. This final chapter identifies key themes and opportunities to enhance learning, dissemination, and replication of successful initiatives, and the changes in all sectors that could support future efforts.

This book intends to inform those who are doing—or hope to do—local environmental health and justice work. Community groups, government agencies, academic institutions, funders, and private-sector partners all have important roles. To maximize accessibility to those diverse audiences, each case study provides a brief overview of relevant policy structures and systems. Lessons learned from the three cases may be translated to different sectors, issue-areas, and geographic, political, and social contexts. Environmental professionals may see new ways to gain support for their efforts by connecting them to public health and equity. Public health professionals may glean insights into how they can engage in systems change to address environmental determinants of health. Community groups may identify new approaches they can use to engage government and academic institutions in addressing environmental justice problems. Finally, these initiatives suggest that academic researchers, students, and funders all play critical roles in supporting local problem-solving based on their unique skills and resources. Collaborating effectively, however, requires stakeholders to appreciate each other's diverse incentives, capacities, and constraints. For that reason, this book emphasizes the development of collaborative relationships that often had impacts beyond the scope of the local environmental health initiative.

2 Standing Silos: Public Health and Environmental Management

The connections between environment and public health have been recognized for thousands of years. Indeed, most current policies for protecting the environment evolved from concerns about human health in crowded urban environments. Every year, new research provides additional evidence that environmental degradation, exposure to toxic chemicals, and cumulative neighborhood stressors are harming people's health—particularly in low-income neighborhoods, urban areas and communities of color. The short answer to why we are not doing a better job of creating environmentally healthy communities is that there are gaps in existing systems for managing the environment. As described in chapter 1, these systems include environmental and public health laws, agencies at every level of government, and private businesses, community groups, and nongovernmental organizations. Existing management systems do not effectively account for cumulative, concentrated, or interactive effects at the local level. Public health and environmental management agencies operate under different policy mandates, regulations, funding streams, and levels of government. Siloed approaches to management of different sectors pose barriers to resolving these problems. Community-based solutions have the potential to fill these gaps by linking environment, public health, and equity concerns at the local level. Connecting environmental and public health decisions makes sense, but doing so is challenging because of disciplinary, funding, institutional, policy-making, and scientific barriers.

Throughout the country, community groups, researchers, government officials, and health professionals are working at the local level to shape environmental decisions in ways that better protect public health and promote environmental justice. These collaborations often take place outside existing institutions. Because they are initiated in response to locally identified problems, their collaborative structures, objectives, and activities are extremely diverse. Innovative local efforts have emerged to address the community health impacts of industrial air emissions, port and vehicular traffic, water contamination, the walkability of neighborhoods, ambient noise, consumption of contaminated fish, energy development, and legacy pollution from toxic waste, among many other issues. However, these local efforts are generally isolated and have not been systematically analyzed, evaluated, or disseminated to other communities.

To address problems of environmental health equity at the local level, it is necessary to understand the existing system for protecting public health from environmental harms, how it evolved, and what gaps allow some communities to continue to be disproportionately exposed. This chapter presents a brief history of the field of public health as it relates to environmental factors, tracing how environmental management functions were separated from public health protection over time, creating gaps in management that continue to create localized problems. The structure of the current U.S. environmental protection system is discussed, focusing on the relationships between local, state, and federal entities. Although a comprehensive overview of U.S. environmental policy is beyond the scope of this book, it is useful to highlight here those aspects that are most relevant to understanding the urban environmental health issues explored in the case studies. The specific policies related to each initiative are presented in greater detail in the case chapters.

Public Health and the Environment

The evolution of environmental and public health protection systems in the United States has shaped the current legal context, perspectives of diverse stakeholders, and roles of various government entities. This brief overview of the historical relationship between public health and environmental management contextualizes the scope and limitations of public health agencies' involvement in local environmental health problems.

Defining Public Health

Most people think of "public health" as describing the health status of a population, but the term also refers to society's efforts to protect the public's well-being. In 1920, Winslow defined public health as the "science and

Box 2.1
Defining Public Health

The Institute of Medicine's Committee for the Study of the Future of Public Health defined public health as having three elements (Institute of Medicine 1988):

- *The mission of public health*: the fulfillment of society's interest in ensuring the conditions in which people can be healthy.

- *The substance of public health*: organized community efforts aimed at the prevention of disease and promotion of health. It links many disciplines and rests on the scientific core of epidemiology.

- *The organizational framework of public health*: encompasses both activities undertaken within the formal structure of government and the associated efforts of private and voluntary organizations and individuals.

---

art of preventing disease, prolonging life, and promoting physical health and efficiency through organized community efforts. ..."(Winslow [1923] 1984, 30). More recent definitions of public health (see box 2.1, *Defining Public Health*) similarly encompass process, policy, practice, and outcomes related to the public's well-being (Patel and Rushefsky 2005; Dannenberg, Frumkin, and Jackson 2011).[1] Thus, public health includes not only public sector efforts but also organized community initiatives, public interest groups, and private institutions (hospitals, private businesses, etc.).

The conceptualization of public health as a multidisciplinary, applied field of practice with the goal of promoting the public good was embodied in the seminal 1988 report, *The Future of Public Health* (Institute of Medicine 1988). According to this report, government should support three "core functions": (1) assessment (monitoring of the population's health status, analyzing emerging problems, and evaluating outcomes); (2) policy development (working with stakeholders to make policy and resource allocation decisions); and (3) assurance (implementing policies, providing services, and promoting private-sector action). Public health is concerned with trends and conditions that negatively affect a community's current or future health and well-being. Thus, the focus of public health evolves as the types of problems dominating people's health concerns shift over time.

The government role in public health includes but is not limited to the work of federal, state, and local health departments. Because the U.S.

Constitution leaves the fundamental responsibility for protection of the public health to the states, most public health efforts are organized at the state or local level (Schneider 2016). At the federal level, the Centers for Disease Control and Prevention (CDC), the National Institutes of Health, and the Food and Drug Administration play important roles in researching, funding, and tracking public health (Schneider 2016). In addition, many non-health agencies ranging from agriculture to transportation are involved in managing environmental impacts on human health.

The Common History of Environmental and Public Health Policy

Western understanding of the relationship between health and environmental factors dates back at least 2,000 years to the Hippocratic book on *Airs, Waters, and Places* (Rosen 2015). The concept that environmental forces or "miasmas" affect human health guided early efforts to provide clean air, water, and sanitation services to reduce disease (Andrews 2006; Melosi 2001). Most introductory public health texts highlight the foundational importance of environmental health through the example of John Snow's efforts to address cholera epidemics in London in the 1850s (Rosen 2015; Schneider 2016; Snow 1855). Snow identified that many of those who died from cholera took their water from a single pump that was contaminated by sewage (Rosen 2015). When the pump handle was removed from that well, the rates of cholera plummeted. To this day, the "pump handle" is a common icon for public health (CDC 2004a).

Mortality from cholera and other contagious diseases in cities, health problems from industrial and domestic smoke, and the lack of decent housing for rapidly expanding urban populations gave rise to the sanitary movement, which began in England in the mid-1800s and spread to the United States (Patel and Rushefsky 2005; Melosi 2001; Duffy 1990). Although people did not understand exactly how diseases were transmitted, they made the connection between dirty water, air, or waste and health problems in crowded urban neighborhoods. This observation suggested that environmental controls could reduce disease (Corburn 2009). Thus, the origins of public health practice were grounded in environmental management (Rosen 2015, Melosi 2001).

However, progress in addressing sanitary issues in the United States was limited by a lack of government entities to implement regulations (Patel and Rushefsky 2005; Rosen 2015). Although many large U.S. cities had

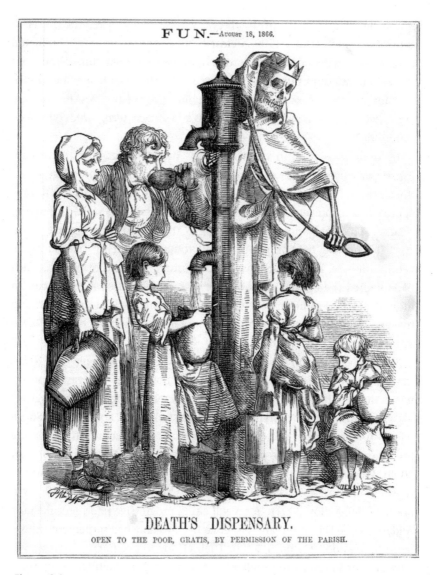

Figure 2.1
"Death's Dispensary": 1866 cartoon linking cholera and contaminated water pumps.
Source: George John Pinwell illustration, *Fun*, August 18, 1866.

established Boards of Health by the early 1880s, they lacked the power to control pollution (Duffy 1990; Melosi 1980). "Sanitary surveys" conducted in several cities delineated the burden of disease and premature death from environmental causes in poor neighborhoods. This data helped build support for stronger agencies, laws, and public investments in infrastructure (e.g., sewers and drinking water treatment) and services (e.g., waste collection) (Andrews 2006; Melosi 2001).

By the end of the nineteenth century, medical researchers had established that microbes, not general environmental miasmas, produced infectious disease (Andrews 2006; Rosen 2015). This understanding led to new approaches to preventing outbreaks, such as sterilizing milk, improving cleaning practices, and eliminating pests that could carry disease. Soon after, the growing field of immunology produced the first vaccines for preventing disease. By the early twentieth century, the field of public health had adopted the biomedical model of disease, which led it to a focus on individual-based solutions, including vaccination, medical treatment, and hygiene education rather than environmental or social change (Rosen 2015; Corburn 2002; Andrews 2006).

Urban social reform movements during this period were also key forces in the development of public health in the United States. The vast improvements in overall population health made possible through "bacteriological" interventions placed health disparities into stark relief (Rosen 2015). Social reform movements in the early twentieth century focused on alleviating the many problems of the poor, including ill health (Andrews 2006; Starr 2008). Women's civic organizations played an important role in many of these "municipal housecleaning" efforts (Hoy 1995; Sivulka 1999; Rynbrandt 1999; Melosi 2001). In several cities, progressive reformers like Jane Addams, Alice Hamilton, and Florence Kelly established settlement houses to serve the poor (Corburn 2009). Their efforts to document, address, and advocate for solutions to problems of the urban poor highlighted connections between neighborhood environments, poverty, and public health. Nevertheless, public health continued to move away from such population-based social justice efforts to focus on individual medical approaches.

At the same time, technical agencies and regulatory structures emerged to address environmental issues including air quality, water quality, and housing and neighborhood conditions (Melosi 2001). In the early 1900s, the field of planning developed to promote well-functioning urban environments through better housing, separating industries from residential areas, and public parks (Corburn 2009; Peterson 2003). Sanitation agencies run by engineers were created to manage drinking water and wastewater treatment to meet health-based standards for quality. By the 1940s, many cities had established agencies to address issues of housing quality, municipal trash collection, school health, and occupational safety (Melosi 2001; Duffy 1990). At the federal level, the U.S. Food and Drug Administration and the Department of Agriculture took on the task of setting standards for food safety, although local health departments continued to play a role in implementing these regulations (Patel and Rushefsky 2005; Andrews 2006).

The Evolution of Public Health and Health Departments

Cities' efforts to manage environmental sanitation and public health agencies' focus on clinical health services drastically reduced infectious disease during the early twentieth century (Starr 2008; Schneider 2016). As these diseases declined, chronic illnesses like heart disease, cancer, and respiratory disease emerged as the leading causes of death (CDC 2016b). Responsibility for treating these diseases fell on the health care system, which experienced rapid growth over the same time period (Starr 2008).

The role of public health agencies diminished as the health care system assumed responsibility for treating chronic disease. By the 1980s, the public health system was viewed as underfunded and ineffective (Walker 1989). The Institute of Medicine (1988) report on *The Future of Public Health* was written to inform efforts to better define, resource, and organize the field of public health. Although this framework offered general guidelines for what the public health system should do, implementation of these services was uneven and differed from place to place (Public Health Law Center 2015; NACCHO 2005).

Today, most states have a central Department of Health that oversees these core public health functions in partnership with health care providers and local health departments. The structure, authority, and responsibilities of local health departments varies by state (Association of State and Territorial Health Officials 2018; Schneider 2016). In "home rule" states, local government has more power, which can mean greater authority for local health departments (Dannenberg, Frumkin, and Jackson 2011). Many large cities have their own health departments; in other areas, public health efforts are organized at the county or regional level. Most local health departments provide some clinical preventive services, health care services (e.g., treatment for communicable disease, home visits, maternal or child health clinics for low-income residents), prevention education, and surveillance of health conditions (Salinsky 2010). They may partner with other entities to provide some of these services (Association of State and Territorial Health Officials 2018). The structure, staffing, and function of health departments has changed over time as new health challenges emerge and budget priorities shift (Madamala et al. 2011). For example, after the terrorist attacks of September 2001, infusions of federal funding significantly expanded health departments' emergency preparedness programs while resources for other programs dwindled (Schneider 2016). Overall public health funding further declined after the recession of 2008 (Mays and Hogg 2015).

Most health departments have an environmental health division that focuses on sanitary inspections, rabies control, pest management, and monitoring environmental quality (e.g., lead exposure, sanitation, water quality, waste sites) (NACCHO 2015). The Centers for Disease Control and Prevention (CDC) developed ambitious "Environmental Health Performance Standards" to encourage more comprehensive programs, but many local health departments (especially in smaller cities and rural areas) lack the funding, technical capacity, or legal mandates to carry out these functions (CDC 2014a, 2016a). Nationwide, local health departments' staff capacity in environmental health shrank from 15,300 in 2008 to 13,000 in 2016 (NACCHO 2016). The technical focus of many local environmental health departments means that staff may have little training or experience in the broader environmental determinants of public health such as built environment, food access, and housing quality, policy work, or community partnerships (McGinty, Castrucci, and Rios 2018). Thus, in the context of health departments, "environmental health" usually refers to core functions like monitoring and sanitary inspections (National Environmental Health Association 2018). Outside of health department contexts, however, the definition of "environmental health" varies greatly (See box 2.2, *Defining Environmental Health*). In this book, the term "environmental health" is used to refer broadly to public health problems in which characteristics of the natural, physical, or built environment play an important role.

This broad definition of environmental health is inherent in Healthy People 2020, a set of goals and objectives issued by the U.S. Department of Health and Human Services to guide health promotion and disease

Box 2.2

Defining Environmental Health

Different organizations, disciplines, and sectors define the term "environmental health" differently. "Environmental health research" commonly refers to toxicology, which is the study of how chemical contaminants affect the body. However, the National Institute of Environmental Health Sciences (NIEHS) has a broader definition; its mission is "to discover how the environment affects people in order to promote healthier lives" (NIEHS 2012a, 1). In other settings, "environmental health" or "healthy environments" may refer to the health of ecosystems or the nonhuman environment. The field of "One Health" focuses on the relationships between healthy ecosystems and human health (CDC 2018c). Local planners and community stakeholders often use the term "environmental health" to refer to characteristics of the built environment, like walkability, transportation safety, or even exposure to secondhand smoke. The term "environmental public health" is sometimes used to emphasize community-level concerns about local problems. Local health departments may define "environmental health" in terms of the services they provide, such as sanitation inspections, lead poisoning prevention, food safety, and vector-borne disease. The World Health Organization's 2016 report, *Preventing Disease through Healthy Environments* takes a broad view of "environmental risks to health" as including "all the physical, chemical, and biological factors external to a person, and all related behaviors, but excluding those natural environments that cannot reasonably be modified" (Prüss-Ustün et al. 2016, x). Given these diverse interpretations, it is important to be clear what is meant by "environmental health" in a particular situation, especially as it relates to the role of public health agencies.

prevention efforts. The environmental health section within these guidelines addresses six themes: outdoor air quality, surface and ground water quality, toxic substances and hazardous wastes, homes and communities, infrastructure and surveillance, and global environmental health (Office of Disease Prevention and Health Promotion 2018a). Many of the levers for managing such environmental health determinants lie outside the authority, responsibility, or capacity of local health departments. Thus, although public health agencies play an important role, environmental management is largely the responsibility of multiple agencies. Awareness of these relationships is key to understanding the kinds of partnerships required to address local environmental health problems.

Environmental Management: From Local to Federal

As described thus far, the U.S. environmental management system largely developed in response to concerns about human health and well-being. Problems with air and water quality in urban areas spurred the earliest public health efforts. Regulation of industrial chemicals, hazardous waste cleanup programs, and occupational health protections all aim to manage human exposures to environmental toxicants. The objective of most natural resource, public lands, and wildlife decisions is to manage human use and distribution of the resulting economic benefits (e.g., jobs for natural resource dependent communities; mining, grazing, and forestry uses; and the recreational use of public lands). Nonetheless, issues related to natural resources management, such as smoke from wildfires, water contamination from mine tailings, and opportunities for physical exercise, have significant implications for human health.

Most federal laws that guide environmental protection today were passed in the 1970s in response to growing public awareness of the ecologic, economic, and human health costs of environmental degradation. Environmental problems became more visible in the 1950s and 1960s, with thousands of deaths attributed to poor air quality events, the loss of biodiversity resulting from the widespread use of DDT and other pesticides, "dead" lakes, and rivers literally catching on fire (Andrews 2006). Growing concern about the environment prompted the first Earth Day in 1970. Public pressure led to a wave of federal responses including the National Environmental Policy Act of 1969, the Clean Air Act Amendments of 1970, and the Clean Water Act of 1972) (Salzman and Thompson 2014). Additional policies addressing pesticides, drinking water protection, and hazardous waste management, disposal, and cleanup followed shortly thereafter. Created in 1970, the U.S. Environmental Protection Agency (EPA) was given responsibility to implement many of these laws (Williams 1993; U.S. EPA 2018c; Andrews 2006).

A comprehensive overview of the U.S. environmental policy system is beyond the scope of this book. However, as a foundation for appreciating the significance of local environmental health initiatives, it is important to understand the general structure of the federal environmental management system. The common theme of "silos"—the separation of management of different sectors and aspects of environmental quality—and the division of roles and responsibilities between different levels of government often present barriers to addressing community environmental health concerns. The remainder of this chapter provides a foundation for understanding these and other challenges inherent in the U.S. environmental management system. First, the historical evolution of surface water quality protection in the United States is summarized to demonstrate some of the common features of the U.S. environmental management system. Second, a short summary of the National Environmental Policy Act (NEPA) highlights its function as the main federal tool for integrating environmental regulation of major developments, as well as its limitations. Third, the federal approach to promoting environmental justice—based on President Clinton's Executive Order 12898 of 1994—is briefly discussed.

The fourth section traces the evolution of tools for shaping private land use decisions that have significant implications for community health. Decisions about private land use are primarily under local control but are shaped by national policies, programs, and funding. Gaps in existing environmental management systems can contribute to environmental health disparities or make it difficult to address them. Because of these limitations of the existing policy system, local environmental health initiatives often require working outside established environmental management or public health institutions.

The U.S. Environmental Management System: The Example of Surface Water Quality

The U.S. environmental management system is stratified by a complex web of relationships between federal, state, and local government entities. A brief look at the evolution, structure, and characteristics of U.S. surface water quality management follows. This overview demonstrates how this system can leave gaps in protection of environmental public health at the local level.

When people began congregating in cities, discharge of human sewage and industrial waste into rivers and lakes contributed to spread of disease (Melosi 1980, 2001). Surface water bodies such as lakes and rivers were used both for water supply and waste disposal. If upstream industries contaminated a river, downstream cities might not be able to use it as a source of drinking water. This presented obvious limitations to individual communities' ability to protect water quality (Andrews 2006). Because of these problems, some of the earliest state environmental laws addressed water quality, primarily by restricting discharge of sewage or industrial wastes (Kneese and Schultze 1975; Patrick et al. 1992).

By the 1930s, most states had water quality control regulations, but they were generally voluntary or weakly enforced. States that strongly regulated pollution risked losing industry and economic development to areas with less costly requirements (Melosi 1980). This created a strong incentive for states to implement minimally restrictive standards. State-level agencies often lacked the technical resources to develop, enforce, and monitor standards. Additionally, rivers and lakes often cross state boundaries and state-based systems failed to protect these interstate waterways.

The first significant federal effort to create a national system for water quality protection was the 1965 Water Quality Act (Andrews 2006). This law placed primary responsibility for implementation on the states. Lacking a strong system for federal enforcement, technical support, and oversight, the law had limited effect (Salzman and Thompson 2014). When the Cuyahoga River caught on fire in June 1969, it became the symbol of a failed system to protect water quality (Rotman 2017; Stradling and Stradling 2008; Salzman and Thompson 2014). Media coverage of this event galvanized public and political pressure to improve water quality protection. Soon after, with the formation of the EPA in 1970, Congress set about developing a more robust system to protect surface water quality.

The modern system of surface water quality protection is based on the Clean Water Act of 1972 (Andrews 2006; Milazzo 2006).[2] As with most federal environmental laws, the system established by the Clean Water Act (CWA) set national standards, monitoring systems, and enforcement protocols and delegated implementation to state environmental agencies. The CWA set the lofty goal that all surface waters should be "fishable and swimmable" by 1983 (Andrews 2006). The CWA had two major approaches to protect water quality. First, it regulated discharges from new and existing point sources into waterways. Each point source (e.g., industry, wastewater treatment plant) was required to obtain a permit specifying what it was allowed to discharge (Salzman and Thompson 2014). Second, the CWA set standards for surface water quality based on designations for the desired use of different water bodies (e.g., fishing, swimming, agriculture). These standards were informed by public health and ecological research. The CWA also included a massive federal investment in wastewater treatment plant improvements (Andrews 2006).

Despite the significant improvements in surface water quality achieved under the Clean Water Act, many waterbodies still do not meet water quality standards. A 2013 assessment by the EPA found that over half of streams and rivers were in "poor condition," and a significant portion of lakes, ponds, estuaries, and bays were categorized as "impaired" (Salzman and Thompson 2014; U.S. EPA 2013b). These continued problems reflect several gaps in the existing water quality protection system.

First, although the CWA's initial focus on point sources like industries and wastewater treatment plants resulted in significant improvements, pollution from "non-point" sources (e.g., runoff from residential developments, streets, and agriculture) was not effectively controlled. The cumulative effects of non-point pollution within watersheds continued to degrade water quality. Over time, the CWA was amended to better address non-point sources, but they remained problematic (Salzman and Thompson 2014; Viessman 1990).

Second, although surface water quality has implications for public health, public health agencies do not have a direct role in surface water quality protection. For example, local health departments are typically responsible for closing beaches to water-based recreation when bacteria levels get too high. However, they are not typically responsible for setting the standards and making permit decisions that control discharges to surface waters—this falls to state environmental agencies.

Third, water quality agencies do not directly control all sources of pollution. How land is used significantly affects the amount and type of pollution that runs off into waterbodies. Since land use is largely determined by local government and private owners, these sources are difficult for federal or state agencies to control. As well, deposition of nutrients from the air can contribute to water pollution, but water quality agencies do not have direct authority to control air emissions (Salzman and Thompson 2014).

Finally, although state agencies solicit public input in designating "use" classifications of waterbodies, classifications may not reflect actual use. For example, people may fish, swim, or boat in waters that are not designated for these uses. Low-income, non-English-speaking, and recent immigrant populations are at greatest risk because of traditional practices, reliance on subsistence fishing, or lack of knowledge about hazards. Because water quality is monitored by measuring concentrations of certain pollutants rather than actual human health impacts, it is difficult to know how effectively the system of water quality protection actually protects public health

(Iannantuono and Eyles 2000). As Salzman and Thompson note (2014, 188), "Rather than studying the effects of pollution on water quality and human and aquatic health, EPA officials have more often focused their attention on engineering questions."

This brief overview of the U.S. water quality management system shows the complex roles of different levels of government and interactions between health and environmental stakeholders. Several key themes inherent in our framework for water quality protection pertain to other environmental management arenas as well. Many environmental quality issues are managed under similar systems of standards set by federal regulation with clearly specified implementing roles for state and local agencies (one exception is land use). Although these systems aim to protect public health, health stakeholders have limited input. Additionally, there are few tools for addressing the cumulative impacts of pollution from multiple media, sectors, or activities. The legacy of this system has left gaps in protecting environmental quality at the local level.

The National Environmental Policy Act of 1969

The separate silos of environmental management pose problems for protecting communities' health. The National Environmental Policy Act (NEPA) of 1969 is the federal government's main strategy to promote comprehensive consideration of impacts of all federal actions, including permits, policies, and projects funded by non-environmental agencies (Carruth and Goldstein 2014; Andrews 2006; U.S. EPA 2018f). NEPA's primary tool is the environmental impact statement (EIS) process, in which the agency proposing the action must analyze its potential environmental effects. Although NEPA itself is a short law, its implementation is complex (Eccleston 2008; Andrews 1976; Clark and Canter 1997). There are several key features and limitations of NEPA as they pertain to local environmental health issues.

First, it is important to understand the limits of NEPA's scope. NEPA applies only to major federal actions. These actions include projects conducted by federal agencies (e.g., building roads, dams, or bridges), private actions that require certain federal permits, and projects funded by federal agencies (Carruth and Goldstein 2014; Andrews 2006). The first step of the NEPA process is to determine whether the action is likely to have "significant" environmental impacts. The initial environmental assessment is usually conducted by the agency or industry proposing the action and provides an opportunity for public comment. If the originating agency or EPA reviews the Environmental Assessment and finds there is no significant impact, no further action is required. Otherwise, the agency proposing the action must produce a full EIS (Clark and Canter 1997).

Thus, NEPA is a process rather than a source of enforceable regulations like the Clean Water Act. There are clear procedural standards for conducting an EIS, including evaluating multiple alternatives to the proposed action, consideration of a wide range of environmental impacts, and opportunities for public input. Although NEPA reviews nominally include human health, the health parameters evaluated are often restricted to toxic exposures (Bhatia and Wernham 2008; Steinemann 2000). It is also important to recognize that while the lead agency is required to respond to all comments received, it is not required to select the least environmentally damaging alternative. Litigation is a common part of NEPA actions: if stakeholders are not satisfied with the EIS, they can sue on the basis that the proper process was not followed or that scientific information was ignored, but not based on the outcome of the decision (Carruth and Goldstein 2014; Clark and Canter 1997).

Effective participation in the review and comment process of NEPA requires significant technical, financial, and organizational capacity. Local stakeholders are typically less able than industry and larger organizations to critique highly technical documents, provide substantive analyses, and draft detailed comments within the time frames allowed. Legal action is expensive and time-consuming. Thus, although NEPA provides for public comment, local communities with limited resources may not be able to participate effectively.

Although NEPA applies only to federal actions, many states have a similar process that applies to state actions (Council on Environmental Quality 2018). These laws differ from state to state, but similar to NEPA, most of them provide opportunities for public comment as part of a nonbinding review process (Bhatia and Wernham 2008). These processes provide an important opportunity for stakeholders to get information about proposed actions, submit new information, and consider alternatives (Andrews 2006). However, NEPA is a limited tool—it applies to a subset of public decisions, addresses a narrow set of impacts, can be daunting to community groups, and does not require implementation of the least-damaging alternative. NEPA is a reactive process: an EIS is conducted on a specific proposed action. Public comments must respond to the proposal and alternatives put forward by the initiating agency, rather than suggesting new possibilities. NEPA is not a framework for comprehensively considering how future development trends may affect environmental health and equity. Although it offers an important tool for communities concerned about local environmental health problems, NEPA alone cannot address longstanding environmental health inequities in a comprehensive, sustainable, cumulative way.

Governmental Approaches to Environmental Justice

The environmental justice movement arose in response to the disproportionate burden of environmental hazards on low-income neighborhoods and communities of color. These disparities persisted despite the implementation of federal and state environmental laws enacted in the 1970s and 1980s. To address these concerns, in 1994 President Clinton signed Executive Order 12898 ("Federal Actions to Address Environmental Justice in Minority Populations and Low-Income Populations"), which requires federal agencies to consider the equity impacts of their actions (Presidential Documents 1994; U.S. EPA 2016e). This executive order instructed agencies to build environmental justice into their work and to "identify and address the disproportionately high and adverse human health or environmental effects of their actions on minority and low-income populations" (U.S. EPA 2016e). While not legally binding, this executive order is supported through several mechanisms, including an Office of Environmental Justice within the EPA's Office of Enforcement and Compliance Assurance (OECA), an Environmental Justice Intergovernmental Working Group (EJ IWG) with representatives from eleven agencies, and a National Environmental Justice Advisory Council composed of nongovernmental and community stakeholders (U.S. EPA 2016a). These groups have developed resources, provided advice, and encouraged agencies to integrate communities' environmental justice concerns in their policies, programs, and funding (U.S. EPA 2016e). For example, the Environmental Justice Intergovernmental Working Group developed guidelines for consideration of environmental justice in NEPA reviews (U.S. EPA 2017b; Federal Interagency Working Group on Environmental Justice and NEPA Committee 2016). The Office of Environmental Justice operates several grant programs to support local environmental justice efforts (U.S. EPA 2017c, 2018b). Public participation and direct involvement by affected communities is a key aspect of these efforts (Federal Interagency Working Group on Environmental Justice and NEPA Committee 2016).

Several states mirror the approach of Executive Order 12898. California has adopted a goal of "fair treatment of people of all races, cultures, and incomes with respect to the development, adoption, implementation, and enforcement of environmental laws, regulations, and policies" (State of California Department of Justice 2017a). California's online "CalEnviro-Screen" is an open-access mapping tool that identifies communities disproportionally burdened by multiple sources of pollution and socioeconomic factors, like unemployment and poverty, that have been found to increase sensitivity of populations to pollution exposure (Office of Environmental Health and Hazard Assessment 2018). Communities identified as disadvantaged are designated to receive a significant portion of funds generated by the state's cap and trade program (State of California Department of Justice 2017a; Richard 2017). SB 535 (2012) directs that 25 percent of the proceeds from the cap and trade program provide benefit to disadvantaged communities, as identified by CalEnviroScreen. In 2012, Attorney General Kamala Harris issued guidance on advancing environmental justice within existing legal frameworks, particularly the California Environmental Quality Act (CEQA), the state's analog to NEPA (Harris 2012).

Several other states also promote environmental justice through small grant programs, mapping, and other resources (New York State Department of Environmental Conservation 2018; Massachusetts Department of Environmental Conservation 2018). Some of these efforts provide technical and financial resources to local groups to address environmental justice concerns. They may also encourage governmental actions such as prioritizing improvement projects for federal funding that are located in disproportionately burdened communities. However, few localities have adopted systematic efforts to promote environmental justice throughout their decisions, funding, and operations. As described in chapter 3, the movement to comprehensively promote health equity in all policies aims to provide such a framework.

Urban Land Use and Public Health

Many environmental justice issues arise because of the concentration of hazardous land uses and lack of health-supportive resources near low-income neighborhoods and communities of color. These common geographical patterns in cities reflect historical, political, and economic forces (Maantay 2002). Addressing these issues in the future depends on aligning community and local, state, and federal government efforts to influence future land use decisions. Although land use is managed at the local level, it is shaped over time by larger political, social, and economic forces that together determine the distribution of environmental hazards and resources within neighborhoods. Because community geographies are relevant to all three case studies in this book, a brief overview of how land use patterns are shaped over time is called for.

As previously mentioned, federal and state agencies aim to manage environmental impacts of developments by setting health-based standards. However, these federal systems do not directly determine what land gets developed, when, and where. Many powers to regulate land use rest within local jurisdictions, although this balance varies from state to state (Dannenberg, Frumkin, and Jackson 2011).[3] Local land use tools influence the private and public sector decisions that shape urban development over time.

Rapid industrialization and uncontrolled growth of cities in the nineteenth century resulted in overcrowded and dangerous conditions. Systems to control land use were developed in part to address public health concerns arising from industries located adjacent to residences. Before government began to regulate urban land use, the only recourse was for affected private property owners to sue for trespass or nuisance based on pollution, odors, or noise that impaired their ability to enjoy their property (Carruth and Goldstein 2014). This approach was inefficient and insufficient to create a healthy separation of incompatible land uses. The worsening health problems in cities gave rise to the idea of land use planning—setting out the desired layout of a city before problems arose, regulating existing uses, and regulating future development to fit that plan (Corburn 2009). The first land use plans in the United States were adopted in the early twentieth century and were modeled on German and British systems (Corburn 2009; Dannenberg, Frumkin, and Jackson 2011). Over time, cities across the United States developed land use plans and agencies to implement them that operated in isolation from public health institutions. In many cities, these planning tools were used to exclude low-income people and communities of color (Babcock 1966; Wilson, Hutson, and Mujahid 2008). A comprehensive description of how municipal planning for land use, transportation, housing, and economic development interfaced with public health goals over time is beyond the scope of this chapter; however, a robust literature has grown up around the theme of reconnecting these fields (Dannenberg, Frumkin, and Jackson 2011; Corburn 2009; Kochtitzky et al. 2006).

Shaping the Future City: Local Management of Land Use

Today, most U.S. cities have planning departments that develop and implement a range of plans, policies, and codes to manage existing and future development. The right of local governments to regulate private behavior in order to protect public welfare allows them to regulate land use, but within certain limitations. Government cannot regulate land in such a way as to restrict all profitable use; this would be considered a violation of the "Takings Clause" of the Fifth Amendment to the U.S. Constitution. However, the power of eminent domain allows governments to take ownership of private property after paying fair market value if there is a compelling public need. While governments can control how public land is used, most urban land is privately owned. The government cannot mandate what is built on private land; it can only incentivize and regulate development (Dannenberg, Frumkin, and Jackson 2011).

Land use regulation is based on "comprehensive plans" (sometimes called "master" or "general" plans) that express a city's vision for the future of their community (Dannenberg, Frumkin, and Jackson 2011). Local governments typically implement comprehensive plans through more detailed land use plans, zoning ordinances, and building codes. Chapter 5 provides additional detail on these tools and approaches.

Although most cities have land use plans and codes, their actual control over land use varies. Cities that are struggling economically often lack resources or political will to regulate new development. Small cities may also have limited staff, financial, or technical capacity to review development plans, inspect new or existing buildings, and enforce codes and may not have updated their comprehensive plans for decades (Bunnell 2002). Others have well-resourced planning departments with the capacity to effectively inform, update, monitor, and implement a comprehensive set of planning tools.

In addition to these legal approaches to shaping private development, cities use a range of financial mechanisms to encourage development consistent with their comprehensive plans. Publicly financed infrastructure can support desired private development. For example, when a city improves roads, water systems, or sidewalks in an area, it becomes more attractive to private investors. Similarly, public facilities like parks, libraries, and schools can attract new private residential developments.

Local governments' capacity to promote changes in the built environment is key to solving many local environmental health problems, particularly because local stakeholders tend to have more influence with local governments than with state or federal agencies. Nonetheless, changes in land use patterns are typically very slow, especially in economically depressed urban areas. As a practical matter, city planning, zoning, and finance can shape future development over time, but it is usually a gradual evolution from existing geographic patterns.

Historical social, economic, and political forces at every level of government created the inequities observed today in the built environment of many cities. In an effort to counter these existing inequities, a number of municipalities have embedded environmental justice goals into their comprehensive plans. For example, as of 2018, all local governments in California are required to have an "environmental justice element" in their general plans if the local jurisdiction has a disadvantaged community identified within its boundaries (State of California 2016).[4] Local government alone cannot reverse existing racial segregation, concentrated poverty, and generations of disinvestments in certain neighborhoods without state or federal support. Nonetheless, the role of local government in shaping land use is key to addressing many local environmental justice problems. Although local land use tools are not usually considered part of the environmental management system, local policies strongly influence which communities are disproportionately impacted by environmental burdens.

Summary

The histories of environmental and public health are intimately intertwined: Both arose from concerns about human health and well-being in urban environments. However, as the systems to address these concerns developed, connections between the agencies that manage them were not maintained. As Jason Corburn noted, "As new agencies were established and separate disciplinary 'silos' emerged for urban issues, professional specialization increased and collaborative work between the fields decreased, further separating public health from urban planning" (Corburn 2009, 39).

Although environmental health is within the purview of the practice of public health, most health departments are directly responsible for only a small subset of environmental health determinants. The United States has a complex system for environmental management with interactions between federal, state, and local government entities separated by sector. As a result, local governments have limited ability to directly control environmental quality within their jurisdictions.

The concept of preemption is crucial to appreciating the limits that can be placed on local governments and their capacity to advance appropriate, innovative, health-protective strategies within their jurisdictions. Preemption is a legal doctrine whereby a higher level of government may limit, or even eliminate, the power of a lower level of government to regulate a certain issue. This is an essential foundation of federal environmental protection laws which provide consistent regulation of pollution and goals for environmental quality nationwide (Andrews 2006). As a consequence of preemption, however, there may be limits to local innovation, flexibility, and ability to respond to community priorities. Recently, preemption has been used by state legislatures to constrain localities' ability to adopt policies that are more protective of health or the environment, effectively setting a "ceiling" on public health protection (Change Lab Solutions 2013). For example, in 2018 California and Washington passed bills blocking localities from enacting taxes on sugary beverages (Sanger-Katz 2018). Conversely, states may have laws explicitly allowing localities to pass stricter regulations, or may be silent on the issue (ChangeLab Solutions 2013). Local initiatives need to clearly understand how existing federal and state environmental protection systems may constrain local discretion to respond to their particular environmental health concerns.

To be effective, local environmental health initiatives must be aware of the federal, state, and municipal environmental policy frameworks that impact the problems facing their communities. They also need to determine whether the problem at hand results from inadequate standards, insufficient enforcement of existing standards, or cumulative impacts of activities in multiple sectors. Sometimes significant scientific uncertainties, limited environmental monitoring, and data gaps make it difficult to characterize exposures at the community level.

A starting point for many local initiatives is recognizing that while environmental regulations aim to protect human health, standards may be based on old science, balanced with economic considerations, or monitored on such a large geographic scale that local "hot spots" are missed. As a result, local populations may experience environmental health problems even when relevant federal regulations are being met. In order to pursue effective systems changes, local environmental health initiatives must understand the history, institutional structure, and limitations of the existing federal and state environmental health policies affecting their issue of concern. It is particularly important to appreciate the abilities and limitations of local governments, including regulation of land use, infrastructure, development, and housing. Initiatives targeting local systems are often better suited than are state or federal efforts to coordinate among various sectors, shape cumulative patterns of development in the urban environment, and respond to stakeholders' concerns. Thus, local environmental health initiatives have the potential to form bridges spanning the gaps between public health and environmental management.

3 Building Bridges: Systems Approaches to Local Environmental Health Problems

Chapter 2 outlined the separate evolution of the U.S. systems for protecting public health and managing the environment. Although one of the main goals of environmental management is to protect human health, there are significant gaps in the current system's ability to identify, prevent, or address health hazards resulting from cumulative environmental exposures at local scales. At the same time, the public health community has become more aware of how social, economic, and environmental health determinants contribute to the health problems facing our society and particularly to the health disparities facing low-income urban areas and communities of color.

The widely recognized paradox of the U.S. health care system is that it spends more per person than any other country, and yet its health status is worse than many countries that spend far less on health care (Brink 2017; Fox 2016). The diseases that dominate health costs and drive health inequities are chronic conditions like obesity, diabetes, and heart disease. These same diseases are influenced by factors including people's education, income, and environment. Such social determinants of health may affect health directly through increasing people's exposure to environmental hazards, crime, and poor nutrition or indirectly by shaping individual behaviors and people's access to preventive services and care. Social determinants of health, in turn, are shaped by policies, systems, environments, and institutions outside the purview of the health care system.

Recognition of the importance of social determinants of health has encouraged public health professionals to work toward changing policies that shape social, economic, and environmental conditions. This "Health in All Policies" (HiAP) approach encompasses a range of environmental policy arenas, including housing, air quality, neighborhood design, and exposure to toxic chemicals. However, public health agencies have limited opportunities to impact the social determinants of health that lie outside the scope of health agencies. Local environmental health collaborations provide such opportunities.

Local environmental health initiatives have diverse structures, processes, and strategies and their most significant outcomes are often indirect, multilevel, multisector, and long-term. Because of this, it is difficult to assess their contributions to systems change. Similar challenges faced scholars studying the collaborative ecosystem management institutions that emerged to fill the gaps in federal environmental policies in the 1990s. Over time, however, social scientists developed frameworks to characterize, evaluate, and disseminate these efforts. This chapter presents a conceptual framework developed to assess collaborative ecosystem management efforts and adapts it to the context of local environmental health initiatives. This framework guides analysis of the case studies presented in subsequent chapters.

Signs of Failure: Public Health, Health Care Costs, and Health Inequities

Rising health care costs and growing disparities in health status (see box 3.1) within the United States suggest that our health system is ineffective, inefficient, and inequitable. These indications of failure have driven government leaders, health care systems, and public health professionals to look for new ways to address the causes of disease, poor health, and the high costs of health care.

A recent Commonwealth Fund analysis found that the United States spends more on health care per person than any of the other thirteen high-income countries studied—over $9,000 per person annually (Squires and Anderson 2015). Health care costs accounted for 17.1 percent of the U.S. gross domestic product in 2013; the runner-up, France, spent 11.1 percent. Nonetheless, the United States had the lowest life expectancy in this group (78.8 years). This trend is reflected in other measures of population health, including infant mortality, in which the United States ranks just below Poland, Hungary, and Slovakia (MacDorman et al. 2014). Health care costs are projected to exceed 20 percent of gross domestic product by 2025 (Keehan et al. 2017). In response to these problems, in 2007 the Institute

Box 3.1

What Are Health Inequities?

> According to Paula Braveman et al. (2017, 2), "Health equity means that everyone has a fair and just opportunity to be as healthy as possible. This requires removing obstacles to health such as poverty, discrimination, and their consequences, including powerlessness and lack of access to good jobs with fair pay, quality education and housing, safe environments, and health care. Health equity is the ethical and human rights principle that motivates us to eliminate health disparities; health disparities—worse health in excluded or marginalized groups—are … how we measure progress toward health equity."
>
> Health disparities are often linked with social or economic disadvantage, historical discrimination, or exclusion. Health inequities may be thought of as a special kind of health disparity that are "systematic, avoidable, and unjust." For example, "health inequities include the increased rates of asthma hospitalization in children living near freeways or the lower life expectancies for African Americans living in low-income neighborhoods" (Rudolph et al. 2013, 9).
>
> Since people may disagree about what is "believed to reflect injustice" (health inequity) versus merely "morally suspect" (health disparity), there are variations in use of these terms. As the environmental justice movement has shown, many differences in exposure to environmental harms are the cumulative result of unfair, racist, or discriminatory policies, practices, or decisions. Therefore, environmental health disparities are usually considered to be inequities.

for Health Care Improvement proposed a "Triple Aim" framework, the goals of which are to "improve the patient experience, reduce per capita costs and improve the health of populations" (Berwick, Nolan, and Whittington 2008).

The primary causes of mortality and morbidity in the United States, according to the Centers for Disease Control and Prevention (CDC), are chronic diseases such as heart disease, cancer, respiratory disease, and stroke that result in high health care costs, reduced productivity, and susceptibility to other health problems over many years (CDC 2017f; Johnson et al. 2014). Obesity contributes to many of the leading causes of preventable death, including heart disease, stroke, diabetes, and some cancers (CDC 2017e). These diseases are strongly linked to behaviors, environment, and access to preventive care.

Health Inequities in the United States

Significant health disparities exist within the United States by race, income, and geography. The gap in life expectancy for blacks is 3.6 years shorter than for whites and 14.6 years shorter for those with the lowest 1 percent of income than those with the highest 1 percent of income (Chetty et al. 2016; Kochanek, Arias, and Anderson 2015). In fact, life expectancy has been decreasing among the poor (DeSalvo et al. 2016; National Academies of Sciences 2015). Many cities have documented dramatic differences in health status between people living in adjacent communities (May et al. 2013). For example, in 2013, life expectancy for babies born in one neighborhood in New Orleans was twenty-five years lower than for those born just a few miles away (Robert Wood Johnson Foundation 2015). Such disparities are frequently correlated with an increased burden of chronic disease among communities of color and people with lower socioeconomic status (Gillespie, Wigington, and Hong 2013; Osborn, de Groot, and Wagner 2013; Healthy People 2013; CDC 2017a; Ogden et al. 2010; National Cancer Institute 2008; Meyer et al. 2013). For example, the national infant mortality rate in 2010 was 5.18 per 1,000 live births among non-Hispanic whites but more than double that rate (11.14) among non-Hispanic blacks (CDC 2014c). Geographically, infant mortality is highest in the southeastern states and among low-income mothers (CDC 2018e; Chen, Oster, and Williams 2016; Mathews, MacDorman, and Thoma 2015). Disparities in health between more and less advantaged populations is a growing concern within the U.S., especially because economic inequality is increasing (Rudolph et al. 2013). Race is associated with health above and beyond socioeconomic differences (Williams 2012). In response to these disturbing trends, U.S. public health efforts have focused on promoting health equity, as reflected in Healthy People 2020, the government's statement of national goals for health promotion and disease prevention (see box 3.2) (CDC 2014b).

A Historical Perspective on Health Equity

The observation that poorer people have poorer health dates back to the origins of the field of public health, when the health problems in London's slums were attributed to unsafe living and working conditions (Dannenberg, Frumkin, and Jackson 2011). In 1842, Edwin Chadwick's *Report on the Sanitary Conditions of the Labouring Population in Great Britain* documented

Box 3.2
Healthy People 2020

Healthy People 2020 Vision: A society in which all people live long, healthy lives.

Overarching Goals:

- Attain high-quality, longer lives free of preventable disease, disability, injury, and premature death;
- Achieve health equity, eliminate disparities, and improve the health of all groups;
- Create social and physical environments that promote good health for all; and
- Promote quality of life, healthy development, and healthy behaviors across all life stages (Office of Disease Prevention and Health Promotion 2018b).

---

that the "gentry and professional" classes lived longer than lower classes. Chadwick attributed this to differences in the social and environmental characteristics of their neighborhoods (Chadwick 1842). Sanitary surveys in Massachusetts and New York came to similar conclusions (Corburn 2009). Maps of poverty and health trends conducted by settlement houses in several cities in the late nineteenth century documented a strong association between poverty and poor health. Even after sanitary reforms and declines in infectious disease in more modern times, George Rosen (2015, 319) wrote that "the appalling inequalities in health conditions that exist throughout the world today are directly and intimately connected with the fundamental problem of wealth and poverty." In 1980, the Black Report showed that income was the strongest predictor of health among British workers, a finding that was affirmed by the Whitehall studies that correlated the incidence of disease with grade of work within the British civil service (Gray 1982; Marmot et al. 1991; Marmot, Shipley, and Rose 1984). Studies continue to find connections between income and health to this day (White and Edgar 2010). The persistence of these trends despite widespread improvements in health care suggests a multifaceted relationship between wealth and health.

Efforts to address health disparities have had varied rationales, approaches, and goals. Concern for the health of the poor had a clear component of self-interest when epidemics of contagious disease festered in low-income neighborhoods and could readily spread to adjacent areas. As Rosen wrote,

"Without being his brother's keeper, anyone who valued his life felt it eminently desirable not to have virulent diseases and the conditions that foster them too close at hand" (Rosen 2015, 184). Beyond this utilitarian concern, many initiatives to address health disparities are based on a normative goal to promote the well-being of all citizens. The argument that societies have an ethical obligation to help the poor has long justified public health efforts. This argument is countered by the socially conservative view that government should not limit individual choice or "incentivize" unproductive behaviors through public health programs (Schneider 2016). An economic rationale for prevention is that it saves taxpayers money if excessive health care costs are avoided by preventive efforts. This logic is particularly persuasive in countries with government-funded health services. However, even in the United States, which lacks a single-payer health system, the costs of treating people who cannot afford to pay is passed on to wealthier citizens through tax revenues used to support Medicare, Medicaid, and charity care at hospitals. Another long-standing perspective on reducing health disparities is enlightened self-interest. Some American sanitarians of the nineteenth century argued for investment in prevention because sick workers could not be productive. Emerging research shows that modern societies with greater inequality have worse health status for all citizens, which suggests that reducing health disparities may improve society's overall well-being (Wilkinson and Pickett 2009). These different ways of framing the problem of health disparities lead to different views of appropriate public health policies to reduce disparities and address the social determinants that contribute to them.

Social Determinants and Health Equity

In the past decade, global public health professionals have focused on the role of social determinants of health (WHO 2018).[1] A 2008 report emphasized that social and physical environmental determinants may have equal or greater impacts on health than genetics, behavior, and health services combined (Commission on Social Determinants of Health and World Health Organization 2008). Although estimates vary, there is consensus that medical care explains only a small increment of health status compared to behaviors, social factors, and environmental conditions (McGovern, Miller, and Hughes-Cromwick 2014). This stands in contrast to the small percentage

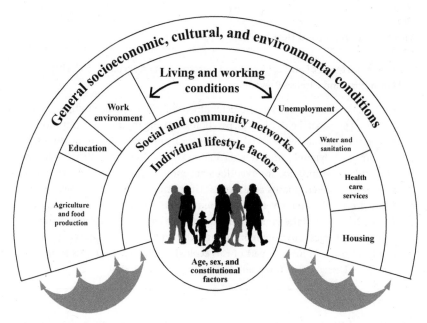

Figure 3.1
The broad determinants of health
Source: G. Dahlgren and M. Whitehead. 1991. *Policies and Strategies to Promote Social Equity in Health* (Stockholm, Sweden: Institute for Futures Studies).

of the U.S. health care budget that is spent on prevention programs aimed at social determinants of health (McGinnis, Williams-Russo, and Knickman 2002). In fact, some have suggested that the low social services expenditures contribute to the United States' high health care costs compared with countries that invest more in prevention (Squires and Anderson 2015; Avendano and Kawachi 2014; DeSalvo et al. 2017).

Health professionals recognize that social factors outside the sphere of public health contribute to the chronic conditions and diseases that drive U.S. health care costs (Marmot and Bell 2009). According to the socioecological model of health, these determinants interact in complex ways to cause or exacerbate disease (WHO 2009; Institute of Medicine 2002; Dahlgren and Whitehead 1991). Figure 3.1, sometimes called the "policy rainbow," emphasizes the multilevel impacts of society, environment, community, and family on the health of individuals (Dahlgren and Whitehead 1991; Rudolph et al. 2013). The Centers for Disease Control and Prevention

Box 3.3
Health Determinants in Healthy People 2020

The Importance of an Ecological and Determinants Approach to Health Promotion and Disease Prevention

Health and health behaviors are determined by influences at multiple levels, including personal (i.e., biological, psychological), organizational/institutional, environmental (i.e., both social and physical), and policy levels. Because significant and dynamic inter-relationships exist among these different levels of health determinants, interventions are most likely to be effective when they address determinants at all levels. Historically, many health fields have focused on individual-level health determinants and interventions. Healthy People 2020 should therefore expand its focus to emphasize health-enhancing social and physical environments. Integrating prevention into the continuum of education is an integral part of this ecological and determinants approach (Office of Disease Prevention and Health Promotion 2018b).

---

highlighted the importance of social and physical environmental determinants of health as part of the Healthy People 2020 goals (See box 3.3, *Health Determinants in Healthy People 2020*).

Thomas Frieden (2010) proposed a "Health Impact Pyramid" as a framework for understanding the multiple roles of public health and the power of systems-change approaches to improving social health determinants (see figure 3.2). The pyramid has five "levels of public health action." The base of the pyramid represents actions addressing socioeconomic factors such as poverty and racism. The next level is changes in environments that make it easier for people to make healthy choices. As Frieden (2010, 591) noted, "The defining characteristic of this tier of intervention is that individuals would have to expend significant effort not to benefit from them." At the top of the pyramid are clinical care and health education efforts. Actions at the bottom levels of the pyramid have the largest potential for sustained positive impacts. Public health professionals have limited ability to address the fundamental factors at the base of the pyramid (e.g., poverty). However, there are opportunities to impact the next level of the pyramid to make healthy choices the "default choice" through systems change.

There are multidirectional relationships between these social determinants of health. Most significantly, there is a two-way relationship between poverty and health. Being unhealthy can contribute to poverty, since health

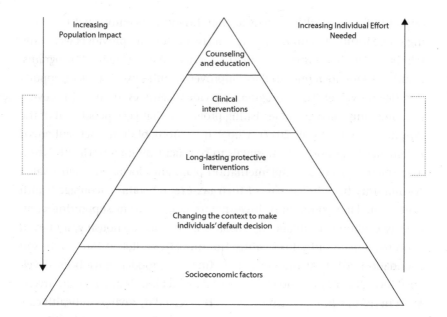

Figure 3.2

Health Impact Pyramid

Source: Thomas R. Friedan. 2010. "A Framework for Public Health Action: The Health Impact Pyramid." *American Journal of Public Health* 100 (4): 509–595.

problems can interfere with education, make it harder to work, limit one's ability to travel to needed services, and require expensive medication. As well, being poor can increase health problems through multiple pathways, including limited access to health education, preventive services, and care; insufficient resources to pay for quality food and housing; being exposed to more air, water, or soil pollution; likelihood of having a hazardous job; and chronic stress from economic hardship and exposure to violence. These complex interactions make it difficult to prove that any particular economic, social, and environmental factor causes a health condition or to predict the impact of changing social determinants on any individual's health. Nonetheless, it is clear that multiple health determinants connected with poverty contribute to health inequities.

Despite the potential for systems-level interventions to improve social health determinants, address health disparities, and reduce health care costs, there have been few incentives for health professionals and institutions to engage in such work. Recently, health care reform has introduced opportunities for health systems to align financial incentives with improving social health determinants. Previously, health care providers were only reimbursed for treating patients (fee for service). With value-based programs, health systems are reimbursed for improved health of their patient population (fee for value). These programs provide incentives to invest in prevention programs, such as home visiting programs, that keep people out of the hospital (DeSalvo et al. 2017). Under the Affordable Care Act, enhanced requirements for nonprofit hospitals to conduct Community Health Needs Assessments, create an implementation plan, and document their related "community benefits" as part of their tax-exempt status encourage health systems making community investments ranging from supporting community coalitions to financing education, low-income housing, and even parks (National Center for Healthy Housing 2018a; Robert Wood Johnson Foundation 2012). At the same time, financing models have been developed including pay for success and social impact bonds in which an investment in nonmedical prevention projects is repaid by savings in health care costs (Galloway 2014). These financial incentives may encourage health care organizations to support systems changes that affect social determinants, including environmental quality.

These developments in policies and institutional frameworks have led to calls for an expanded role for public health in addressing social determinants. DeSalvo and others (2016) describe this new role as "Public Health 3.0." They refer to the history of public health prior to the 1988 Institute of Medicine report as Public Health 1.0, and that report's call for a reinvigorated public health infrastructure is termed Public Health 2.0 (DeSalvo et al. 2016, 621). Public Health 3.0 refers to a new era of enhanced and broadened public health practice that goes beyond traditional public department functions and programs. This vision calls for public health professionals to be strategic leaders in building community capacity, cross-sector collaboration, and "environmental, policy, and system-level actions that directly affect the social determinants of health" (DeSalvo et al. 2016, 622).

Environmental Determinants of Health

Within this focus on social determinants of health, health professionals increasingly recognize the key role of the physical environment (figure 3.3). The World Health Organization estimates that 23 percent of deaths in the world are caused by "modifiable" environmental factors (Prüss-Ustün et al. 2016). Both environmental risks and resources can interact with social factors, stress, poverty, and racism to cumulatively affect health (Kjellstrom et al. 2007; Payne-Sturges et al. 2015; Northridge, Sclar, and Biswas 2003). Changes in the built environment—particularly access to healthy food and opportunities for physical activity—can help people live healthier lives (Northridge, Sclar, and Biswas 2003; Dannenberg, Frumkin, and Jackson 2011; Kochtitzky et al. 2006). Inclusion of environment in the Healthy People 2020 goals encouraged public health professionals' renewed focus on the built environment (Corburn 2009; CDC 2015b; Brennan Ramirez, Baker, and Metzler 2008; Northridge, Sclar, and Biswas 2003).

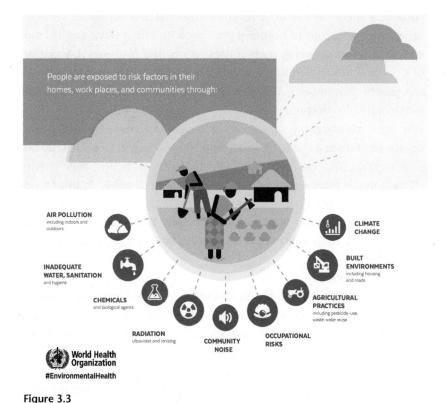

Figure 3.3
How the environment impacts our health
Source: http://www.who.int/quantifying_ehimpacts/publications/PHE-prevention-diseases-infographic-EN.pdf?ua=1.

Environmental factors may be more actionable than some of the more fundamental social determinants of health such as economic status. Environmental improvements may be objectively measured, making it easier to document progress. Physical changes in the environment are durable and can continue to impact people positively over time, even as other socioeconomic conditions change. Environmental factors influence many other determinants including poverty, education, and social capacity. For example, creating bike paths in low-income neighborhoods may help residents more easily reach food stores, jobs, and schools while reducing their transportation costs so they have more money for food, housing, and health care. Thus, improvements in the physical environment often have ripple effects on other social determinants of health.

Recognizing these connections, many public health professionals have enhanced their involvement in environmental health, either through expanding their scope of work or partnering with others (Kent and Thompson 2012). To encourage such collaboration, the National Association of County and City Health Officials (NACCHO), in its Resolution 99–13 (adopted on November 7, 1999), called for better integration between environmental protection and public health (see box 3.4, NACCHO 1999). However, the decreasing staff capacity in local and state environmental health departments poses a challenge to accomplishing this goal (NACCHO 2017).

Addressing the environmental determinants of health may require changes in the roles, resources, tools, and training of public health professionals. The next section introduces approaches that aim to support efforts by public health professionals and others to integrate health into decisions that shape social determinants of health, including environmental conditions.

Health in All Policies

Improving environmental health determinants often requires changing policies and systems in non-health sectors. The idea of Health in All Polices (HiAP) is that human health should be considered in all policies that shape social determinants of health. This sounds like common sense. In fact, community members are often surprised to discover that many public decision processes do not directly consider health outcomes. Those that do often address a only narrow set of health concerns. Increased concern about the contributions of social determinants to health disparities has focused attention on how to better incorporate health considerations into non-health

Box 3.4

The Integration of Environmental Health and Public Health Practice

---

WHEREAS, the Institute of Medicine's 1988 Future of Public Health Report states that "The removal of environmental health authority from public health has led to fragmented responsibility, lack of coordination, and inadequate attention to the public health dimensions of environmental health issues;" and

WHEREAS, environment and health are intimately related, and environmental health is a public health activity, yet the two fields are often isolated and overly distinct in their current missions; and

WHEREAS, local public health agencies bring a unique, population-based approach to environmental health issues and an emphasis on prevention and system-wide approaches to health;

THEREFORE, BE IT RESOLVED that the National Association of County and City Health Officials (NACCHO) advocates for resources, policies, programs, and legislation that promote the integration of environmental health and public health practice; and

BE IT FURTHER RESOLVED that NACCHO endorses the development and/or enhancement of coordinated training for the environmental health workforce in public health sciences such as epidemiology, social and behavioral sciences, physiology and biology, and for the public health workforce in environmental sciences such as ecology and urban planning (NACCHO 1999).

---

decisions. Health in All Policies, "health impact assessment," and "policy, systems, and environmental" change work are all concepts that relate to improving health equity through action in multiple sectors (Browne and Rutherfurd 2017).

International public health organizations were among the first to use the phrase Health in All Policies (WHO 2015). The idea dates back at least four decades to the 1978 Alma-Ata Declaration on Primary Health Care (WHO 1978).[2] The theme was developed through a series of global meetings and articulated in the "Helsinki Statement on Health in All Policies" in 2013: "Health inequities between and within countries are politically, socially and economically unacceptable, as well as unfair and avoidable. Policies made in all sectors can have a profound effect on population health and health equity" (WHO 2014).

Within the United States, HiAP has been promoted by public health organizations such as the National Association of County and City Health

Officials (NACCHO), the Association of State and Territorial Health Officials (ASTHO), the National Academies of Medicine (NAM), and the American Public Health Association (APHA) through webinars, publications, training programs, and conferences. The Affordable Care Act incorporated the concept through its National Prevention Council (Shearer 2010). The first report of the National Prevention Council (2011, 7) envisioned "a prevention-oriented society where all sectors recognize the value of health for individuals, families, and society and work together to achieve better health for Americans" and named "healthy and safe community environments" as one of four "strategic directions."

The Centers for Disease Control and Prevention has promoted HiAP by providing technical resources and community grants (CDC 2015a). At the state level, California has been a leader in implementing this idea through a statewide HiAP Task Force established in 2010 (State of California Department of Justice 2017b). To encourage other states to pursue this approach, the APHA and the Public Health Institute published "Health in All Policies: A Guide for Local and State Governments," which drew on California's experiences related to environmental determinants of health (Rudolph et al. 2013). Several localities have committed to integrating HiAP into their decisions, programs, and practices. For example, Multnomah County, Oregon, established a Health Equity Initiative in 2007 that aimed to address "the root causes of socioeconomic and racial injustices that lead to health disparities" through local policy change (Multnomah County 2018).

A closely related concept to HiAP is "policies, systems, and environments" (PSE). The terms PSE and HiAP are sometimes used interchangeably (ChangeLab Solutions 2018b; Public Health Institute 2018). HiAP emphasizes the need to infuse health into non-health policies, whereas PSE highlights the importance of multilevel systems change by private, public, and nonprofit stakeholders in addition to changes in the policy sector. These approaches are sometimes referred to as "upstream" health promotion to distinguish them from public health's traditional focus on individual education and behavior change (Ehlinger 2015; Butterfield 2017; Rudolph et al. 2013; Williams et al. 2008). In this book, the terms HiAP, PSE, upstream health, and "integrating health into non-health policies" are used depending on context to refer to systems-change approaches.

Many public health stakeholders developed experience in PSE work through tobacco control efforts (American Cancer Society 2015; Trochim

2006). Decades of public education campaigns about the dangers of smoking failed to reduce smoking rates. Significant reductions in smoking rates did not occur until higher taxes on cigarettes, restrictions on advertising, banning cigarette sales to minors, and smoke-free environment policies were implemented (Task Force on Community Preventive Services 2000). The success of this effort encouraged public health professionals to address other complex health issues with comprehensive, community-based, multilevel systems-change approaches (Sallis et al. 2006; Schneider 2016). More recently, PSE has been promoted as a framework for active living and healthy-eating initiatives seeking to make the "healthy choice the easy choice" (Honeycutt et al. 2015; Levi 2012; Oakar 2017).

Advocates of HiAP and PSE encourage their integration into private-sector and nonprofit decision-making as well as public policy. For example, the nonprofit Active Living by Design promotes wellness through its human resources, workplace, and institutional food procurement choices. Several health care organizations have made similar efforts throughout their operations by reducing chemicals use, providing healthier food options in cafeterias, supporting active transportation by employees and patients, and hosting farmers' markets (Ashe et al. 2016; HERO 2018). The Robert Wood Johnson Foundation has advanced these ideas through its Culture of Health campaign (Plough 2015).

The concepts of HiAP and PSE emphasize inclusive decision processes and the need to build community capacity. For example, the Minnesota Health Department developed a "triple aim for health equity" that sets forth HiAP as a means to promote health equity and emphasizes the importance of community engagement in these efforts (Ehlinger 2015). These efforts are described further in chapter 5.

Despite these initiatives, integrating health into non-health sectors remains a challenge. As noted previously, one barrier is that non-health agencies, policies, and practices seldom *require* consideration of health. Therefore, integration of health is voluntary. A second challenge is that "considering human health" is a very broad goal with multiple possible (and potentially conflicting) interpretations. Third, even when there is consensus about health equity goals, integrating health into non-health decisions may require data, assessment strategies, expertise, and expense beyond the institution's existing resources. In other words, simply setting health equity as a goal does not clarify which health outcomes to assess, how to balance impacts on disadvantaged communities versus the whole population, or what to do when there are gaps in information.

One framework for integrating health in non-health policies is called Health Impact Assessment (Harris-Roxas et al. 2012; Bhatia et al. 2011). A Health Impact Assessment (HIA) is a voluntary, collaborative process to analyze the health outcomes of proposed decisions. Government agencies, foundations, and nongovernmental public health organizations have promoted HIA through grants, training programs, and policy statements. HIAs begin by building consensus around what are the most critical health equity implications of a decision, thus creating a shared definition of what impacts should be assessed. By involving decision makers and other stakeholders, the process aims to recommend solutions that are feasible within the context at hand. By providing a structure for cross-sector collaboration, HIAs can help integrate multiple types of information to clarify the health equity impacts of a decision (Pew Charitable Trusts 2018a, 2018b).

HIAs have been conducted in a wide range of sectors, including education, criminal justice, transportation, education, and land use (Pew Charitable Trusts 2018a). The land use planning sector, in particular, has promoted the practice of HIA (American Planning Association 2016). Several federal agencies have funded HIA efforts and provided technical support (CDC 2018d, 2015a). Private foundations have also played a role in developing HIA capacity across the country, notably through the Health Impact Project of the Robert Wood Johnson Foundation and Pew Charitable Trusts, as well as several regional health foundations (Pew Charitable Trusts 2018a). HIA courses are offered in many planning and public health programs, and a professional society supports development of the practice (Society of Practitioners of Health Impact Assessment 2018). Together, these efforts have informed hundreds of decisions across the country and raised awareness of the health equity impacts of non-health decisions (Bourcier et al. 2014; Pew Charitable Trusts 2018a).

Nonetheless, HIA has several limitations. First, it is reactive—HIAs are conducted to inform pending decisions, not to create new initiatives. Furthermore, decision-making processes seldom allow time for a full HIA. However, "prospective" HIAs have been conducted when decisions can be anticipated, as in the expansion of wind power developments in Oregon (Oregon Health Authority 2013). As voluntary processes, HIAs are limited by available funding and staff resources. Most HIAs in the United States have been grant-supported, although there are efforts to institutionalize HIA in some jurisdictions. Agencies in the land use sector have developed toolkits to streamline health assessment, including San Francisco's Healthy Development Measurement Tool and the Mid-Michigan Mapping and Impact Assessment Toolkit (Farhang et al. 2008; Wernham and Teutsch 2015; Mid-Michigan Regional HIA Program 2018). Lower-cost "desktop HIAs" that rely on existing tools, data, and analyses have also become more common (Dannenberg et al. 2008; Pew Charitable Trusts 2018b). Some have advocated for integrating HIA into the National Environmental Policy Act (NEPA) Environmental Impact Statement process; others caution against such a formalized process (Bhatia and Wernham 2008).

The practice of HiAP, PSE, and HIA have increased public health professionals' opportunities to engage in systems change to impact social determinants of health. These approaches provide models for integrating data across sectors, encouraging collaboration between institutions, and promoting multilevel solutions. Many of the local environmental health initiatives discussed in this book were informed by these concepts and related experience.

Collaborative Ecosystem Management

Public health professionals' growing interest in systems change is similar to environmental and natural resource managers' development of ecosystem management several decades ago. By the 1990s, environmental managers had recognized that existing institutions often failed to protect ecosystems. U.S. environmental policies had evolved to manage each resource individually, with different goals, separate agencies, and specific technical expertise, usually along politically determined boundaries (e.g., cities, states, park boundaries, water districts) with limited opportunities for input from resource users and the public. These gaps contributed to slow progress in addressing environmental problems and resolving natural resource use conflicts. In response, new institutions were developed to manage ecosystems more holistically, proactively, and collaboratively. This section describes the evolution of these efforts (referred to as "ecosystem" or "collaborative environmental" management efforts), similarities and differences to local environmental health initiatives, and how conceptual frameworks for ecosystem management may inform environmental public health protection.[3]

Ecosystem management focuses on the complex interactions between physical, human, and biological components of the environment and the geographic scale at which these forces interact (John 1994; Koontz 2004). Managing resources separately makes it difficult to account for cumulative impacts and interactions across different resources and political units (John 1994). Place-based ecosystem management collaborations were developed to manage systems more comprehensively. Ecosystem management's key features include enhanced public participation (particularly by those dependent on a natural resource), decisions based on multidisciplinary science, and collaboration between multiple institutions that affect the ecosystem (Koontz 2004; Wondolleck and Yaffee 2000; Yaffee 1996).

The surface water quality management example given in chapter 2 demonstrates some of the problems of single resource management. The Clean Water Act's focus on point sources like industries and wastewater treatment plants only addressed a small portion of surface water pollution sources, which include runoff from residential development, farms, industries, and extraction of natural resources. There was no comprehensive system to avoid overpollution by point and non-point sources throughout the watershed. Decisions by individual landowners that had a significant impact on water quality—for example, how much fertilizer to apply, where, and when—were beyond the scope of the Clean Water Act (CWA). The CWA did not create institutions within which water quality managers, private developers, municipal wastewater plants, farmers, agriculture agencies, local land use planners, and community groups could coordinate their activities to protect water quality.

Given these gaps, it is not surprising that some of the earliest collaborative environmental management efforts developed to manage watersheds. Watershed management organizations span a range from community-based coalitions to public-private partnerships to government-sponsored participatory planning groups (Koontz 2004; Sabatier et al. 2005). Many watershed protection organizations are community-led (Steelman 2010; Koontz 2004). Some work closely with private industry to gain voluntary compliance with their goals. Others are organized and funded by government agencies. For example, in 1987, the Great Lakes Water Quality Agreement established a model for collaborative ecosystem management of forty-three Areas of Concern (AOC). Each AOC received financial support to develop a Remedial Action Plan that involved multiple agencies and stakeholders, public participation, scientific assessment, and public education (U.S. EPA 2018l; Vallentyne and Beeton 1988; MacKenzie 1996). Over time, the idea of collaborative watershed management was integrated into the federal system of water quality management—for example, through the Stormwater Management Phase II rule, which provides for education, watershed planning, and public participation to reduce non-point sources of pollution (U.S. EPA 2005).

Collaborative institutions for environmental management evolved in other sectors, including forest, fisheries, and wildlife management. Many of these collaborations were led by government agencies, such as U.S. Forest Service (USFS) efforts to increase collaboration in forest planning and management in the 1990s (Wondolleck and Yaffee 2000; Lee 1993). Today, collaboration is an established part of USFS practice, including a "collaboration cadre" of staff that supports these efforts (U.S. Forest Service 2018). By 1994, eighteen federal agencies had adopted ecosystem management approaches that incorporated collaboration (Koontz 2004; Morrissey, Zinn, and Corn 1994; MacKenzie 1996).

Environmental policy scholars studied these varied collaborative institutions from a wide range of perspectives, asking questions like: What are criteria for success of ecosystem management? What contributes to their success? How successful are they compared to existing environmental institutions? Several common themes emerged from this research (Sabatier et al. 2005; Koontz 2004; Wondolleck and Yaffee 2000; Koontz and Thomas 2006; Yaffee 1996). First, ecosystem management requires multidisciplinary information, including the knowledge of communities that use natural resources. The knowledge of diverse technical specialists, user groups, and managers is also important. Second, public participation is critical throughout the process. Third, the effort must facilitate collaboration among multiple institutions involved in managing different aspects of the system. Finally, the ability to adapt to changes in the ecosystem, political landscape, or partners' resources is key (Lee 1993; John 1994).

Studies of ecosystem management efforts revealed that their impacts are often indirect, long-term, or even invisible (Koontz 2004; Korfmacher 1998). Therefore, in order to assess ecosystem management efforts, it is important to evaluate their processes and indirect effects as well as their short-term outcomes and likely future trends. Sometimes the process of collaboration establishes new relationships that then lead to positive changes in other parts of the system. Because of these complexities, most studies of collaborative environmental management have focused on understanding both the collaborative process and the outcomes initiated by these efforts. This generally requires in-depth, multimethod case studies that can capture the varied goals, perspectives, and experiences of the participants (Yin 1984).

Before applying lessons learned from ecosystem management to local environmental health initiatives, it is important to consider some critical differences between the two fields. The goal of collaborative environmental management is to maintain a healthy ecosystem while sustaining desired human uses, whereas the goal of local environmental health initiatives is usually to promote health equity without disrupting the local economy. Both goals require choices about values, priorities, and distribution of costs and benefits about which stakeholders may disagree. The scale of a local environmental health initiative is usually defined by political boundaries, whereas many collaborative environmental efforts aim to manage entire watersheds or ecosystems that cross jurisdictions. Many ecosystem management efforts are established by government agencies with significant control over the sector being managed, as is the case with public lands (e.g., national parks or forests). Although most of the local environmental health initiatives explored in this book involved government agency staff, none was led primarily by government. As a result, ecosystem management partners often have the power to implement at least some of the changes the effort recommends, whereas local environmental health collaborators may need to advocate for decision makers external to the partnership to change their behaviors, practices, or policies.

The Local Environmental Health Initiative Framework

One framework for analyzing ecosystem management efforts was set forth by Tomas Koontz and others in *Collaborative Environmental Management* (Koontz et al. 2004). This framework emphasizes how collaborative environmental management initiatives frame the issue of concern, leverage diverse resources, structure their efforts, and produce diverse kinds of impacts (Koontz 2006). It is adapted here to reflect the nature of local environmental health efforts, including the roles of diverse collaborators and multiple kinds of outcomes (figure 3.4). This Local Environmental Health Initiative Framework provides a structure for examining four aspects of collaborative initiatives: (1) problem definition, (2) resources for collaboration, (3) structure and decision processes, and (4) impacts of the efforts. Each of these elements is briefly described below.

Problem definition and issue framing refer to how stakeholders characterize the scope, scale, and nature of the issue of concern. This process often shapes the initiative's approach. For example, framing a polluted lake as a problem of industrial discharges suggests a very different strategy than portraying the problem as a failure of all watershed actors including farmers, cities, residents, and businesses to manage their wastewater responsibly. In the case of local environmental health initiatives, framing may emphasize fairness, equity, and vulnerable populations. Defining an actionable geographic scale may be challenging when the environmental determinant is managed on a regional basis but negative health impacts of concern are concentrated among a local population. Problem definition also involves focusing on a limited scope of targets, which determines the interests and expertise the initiative needs to engage. Thus, how an issue is defined and framed affects which stakeholders are involved, the scope of solutions considered, and the types of knowledge that are invoked.

Research on collaborative efforts emphasizes that their accomplishments depend largely on the resources they are able to garner. Diverse types of resources in addition to funding can support an initiative's progress. The Local Environmental Health Initiative Framework characterizes resources for collaboration as *human, knowledge,* and *financial.*

Human resources are the people who contribute time, attention, or skills to the overall effort. Human resources may be paid or volunteer staff and their skills, including technical expertise, leadership abilities, past experiences, credibility, social connections, and professional networks. One key human resource is staff time to convene meetings, communicate with group members, and carry out coalition tasks. Staff time may be donated by member organizations or paid for by the group's financial resources.

Knowledge resources include the information available to the initiative, as well as the ability to generate, translate, and use knowledge (Ascher, Steelman, and Healy 2010). Generating knowledge encompasses collecting new data, synthesizing the experiences of others, or analyzing existing information in new ways. The ability to interpret and communicate information to diverse stakeholders is also a "knowledge resource" and is essential to promoting the use of information in decision processes. In addition to scientific information and quantitative data, knowledge resources may include community members' knowledge about the issue, qualitative information about community health, cultural practices, public preferences, opinions, or beliefs and recollections of past social, economic, political, and ecologic conditions. Knowledge resources may be contributed by partners or purchased with the group's financial resources (e.g., paid consultants, contracts). Collaborations often enhance their credibility by engaging technical experts, respected local leaders, or national groups with knowledge of the issue at hand.

Financial resources may come from discretionary funding of partner groups, donations, contracts, or grants. Lack of funding is a common barrier to collaboration, particularly when it limits the initiative's ability to maintain its convening functions. The source of funds, constraints on types of expenditures, and control over allocation also has a significant impact on the effort's progress. Donation of services that would normally cost money, such as airtime for public service announcements, may also be considered a financial resource.

Human, knowledge, and financial resources are clearly interrelated. The ability to identify funders, write proposals, and implement projects depends on the human and knowledge resources of the group. Grant funding (*financial resources*) can support the time of personnel (*human resources*) who can access data (*knowledge resources*) that contribute to the overall effort. Taken together, these resources support opportunities for partners to interact with each other, provide access to multidisciplinary expertise, and allow staff to coordinate meetings, communicate the group's messages, and carry out programmatic activities. Distinguishing different types of resources helps clarify who controls them, limiting factors, and how they evolve over time.

The third factor in the framework is the group's structure and decision-making processes. Collaborative efforts may or may not have formal goals, decision processes, committee structures, membership rules, and leadership roles. Some collaborative initiatives are incorporated as independent nonprofit organizations. Others operate under the auspices of a convening organization. In such cases, the discussion of group structure and decision processes focuses on how the key stakeholders interact, who the leaders are, how the collaboration functions, and whether it changes over time. Even when there is a formal institution overseeing the collaboration, mapping

out the *functional* structure and decision processes helps clarify collaborative processes and how they affect outcomes and impacts.

The final component of the framework is "impacts of collaboration." For
the purposes of analyzing local environmental health efforts, it is helpful
to distinguish impacts in terms of outputs, social outcomes, and impacts
on policies, systems, and environments. *Outputs* include activities, programs, analyses, educational materials, events, and other short-term, direct
products of the collaborative effort. *Social outcomes* are the ways in which
the effort changed individuals and their relationships with others, such
as development of participants' capacity, credibility, networks, and experiences that enable them to contribute to future change. Social outcomes
may also include factors like reducing conflict, improving coordination, or
changing how participating group members make decisions. *Impacts on policies, systems, and environments* include the decisions, practices, programs, or
processes to which these efforts contributed. It is seldom possible to directly
attribute a change in health equity to a collaborative effort in the near term.
However, it may be feasible to identify how the local environmental health
initiative contributed to changes in environmental conditions, policies, or
decision processes that are expected to result in health improvement over

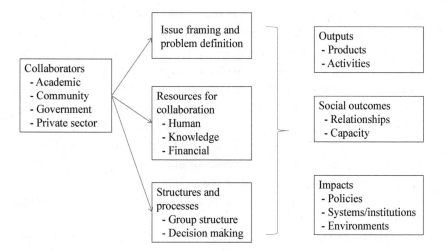

Figure 3.4
The Local Environmental Health Initiative Framework
Source: Adapted from Koontz et al. (2004) *Collaborative Environmental Management:
What Roles for Government?*

time. Or, the collaborative effort may encourage partner or external organizations to produce new materials, programs, or practices. Such indirect
impacts are important contributions of local environmental health initiatives but can be challenging to identify, attribute, and evaluate.

Assessing Local Environmental Health Initiatives

The Local Environmental Health Initiative Framework provides a structure
for describing, analyzing, and comparing local environmental health initiatives. Unlike programs or projects with defined goals and measurable outcomes, by definition these initiatives had a more "developmental" approach,
in which goals, objectives, and metrics of success evolved over time as a
function of the collaborative process (Patton 2010). They generated new
understanding of an existing problem, refined their objectives accordingly,
created new solutions, and promoted multiple strategies to address the
problem.

Table 3.1 sets forth questions that explore how the collaborative initiative redefined the problem, marshaled resources, and organized its internal
processes as well as its accomplishments in terms of outputs (what it did),
social outcomes (how it affected participants), and impacts on policies, systems, and environments. These questions guided the case study analyses.

One of the most fundamental challenges in evaluating the impacts of
local environmental health initiatives and defining appropriate measures
of success is that any changes observed must be considered in the context
of the "counterfactual" (NIEHS 2013): What would likely have happened
in this situation had the initiative not existed? One avenue for addressing
this question is through comparison to other communities that lack such
collaborative initiatives. Another is to consider the conditions and trends
prior to the initiative's work. The questions in table 3.1 guide assessment of
the initiative's problem definition, resources marshaled, internal processes,
and impacts in terms of moving from the status quo toward promoting
health equity.

Characterizing the initiative's problem definition, resources, and structures
focuses on how the initiative changed how the problem was addressed in the
community. Questions about problem definition focus on how the initiative reframed the issue with respect to environmental health equity, mobilized new constellations of stakeholders, and identified the problem's scope

Table 3.1

Applying the Local Environmental Health Initiative Framework

Local Environmental Health Initiative Function	Questions for Analysis
Issue framing and problem definition	Did the problem definition and framing inform the strategy to engage appropriate resources, stakeholders, and approaches to create systems change?
	Were the scope and scale of the problem defined in an actionable way?
	How did the initiative frame the issue with respect to environmental health equity?
Resources for collaboration	How did the initiative's resources contribute to the credibility, effectiveness, and impact of the effort?
	Did the initiative bring new human, financial, and knowledge resources to bear on developing solutions to the problem?
	Did it integrate multiple sources of knowledge to develop and promote science-based solutions?
Structure and decision-making process	Did the initiative's structure for collaboration allow it to function effectively over a long enough time to affect systems?
	Who were the primary conveners? What were the various stakeholders' roles in the collaborative structure and decision-making process?
	How did the process engage affected community members or groups?
Impacts of collaboration:	What evidence is there that the initiative made progress toward addressing the identified problem?
Outputs	What activities, programs, and materials did it produce to expand awareness, build support, or promote solutions that enhance health equity?
Social outcomes	Did it develop participants' capacity (skills, relationships, resources) to address the problem beyond the scope of the collaboration?
Impacts on policies, systems, and environments (PSE)	How did the initiative affect decision-making processes, policies, or practices?
	Is there any evidence the initiative impacted environmental determinants or health outcomes?
	Did the initiative have impacts beyond its central scope and scale?

in an actionable way. The framework emphasizes on examining whether the initiative mobilized new and diverse kinds of resources to address the problem, and also its ability to integrate them to develop credible, well-informed solutions. In addition to clarifying the structure and decision-making processes of the effort, the framework acknowledges that these may be informal, decentralized, and evolving. It particularly highlights how these structures enhanced community engagement in problem-solving.

The framework guides assessment of the initiatives' impacts in terms of outputs, development of participants' capacity and relationships, and changes in policy processes and outcomes. It is relatively straightforward to document the "outputs" of collaborative initiatives (e.g., meetings held, educational materials produced, reports issued, trainings conducted), but the success of these products depends on how they changed policies, systems, or environments. These impacts are frequently indirect and long term. Sometimes the impacts of systems-change efforts are simply categorized into short-, medium-, and long-term outcomes, in which case outputs are normally considered short-term outcomes (NIEHS 2013). The Local Environmental Health Initiative Framework distinguishes outputs from social and systems impacts to focus attention on the role of the collaborative initiative in affecting the behaviors of member and external organizations (indirect effects) versus those activities directly accomplished by the convened group.

Research on collaborative efforts suggests that social outcomes are important to implementing, supporting, and sustaining the goals of the core initiative. Therefore, the framework examines the impacts on individual participants and their relationships with others (i.e., do they bring new approaches into their organization's work, partner on projects outside of the collaboration, or engage other individuals within their organization?). Participation in a collaborative effort may enhance an individual's or an organization's credibility, skills, and experience in ways that increase their ability to be effective in future policy initiatives. It may give them access to new technical or financial resources. Relationships among participants may create networks for collaborative action that outlast the original initiative.

The complexities of evaluating collaborative efforts' impacts on policies, systems, and environments are well recognized, including the long timescale of impacts, importance of indirect effects, and the multiple factors influencing complex policy systems (Korfmacher et al. 2016; NIEHS 2013;

Patton 2010). Documenting trends in health and environmental outcomes can provide important context to understanding the long-term impact of these initiatives. It may be more feasible to identify changes in the physical environment that occurred as a result of the initiative's efforts than to link these changes to reductions in health disparities, particularly in the short term. However, population and environmental health outcomes depend on multiple factors (e.g., policies in many sectors, economic forces, cultural shifts) over long periods of time. Intermediate indicators may include shifts in funding streams, programs, or statements by political leaders.

Assessing an initiative's impact on policy and systems change is also challenging. While a collaborative effort may contribute to a policy change, it can seldom claim full credit. Local policy systems are also influenced by external forces—for example, a change in a federal law may make a local policy campaign moot. Systems change can take a long time. Therefore, failure to observe improvements in environmental public health within the lifespan of a collaborative effort may not mean that the initiative was a failure. Finally, as Garry Brewer and Peter DeLeon (1983, 322) note, criteria for a successful policy outcome depends on "who one is, where one sits, and what one intends." Thus, different stakeholders may have different views about the appropriateness, effectiveness, or impacts of the effort.

Because of these complexities, local environmental health initiatives are most appropriately studied through exploratory, in-depth case studies (Yin 1984). In-depth case studies can document ongoing processes, internal dynamics, "invisible successes," and potential for future systems change (Korfmacher 1998). The Local Environmental Health Initiative Framework guides exploration of the initiative's impacts on its partners' skills, relationships, and capacity as well as how it influenced changes in decision processes, policy outcomes, and systems that affect the environment.

Summary

Existing systems for environmental and public health management often fail to protect the most vulnerable populations in society from environmental health risks. These inequitable environmental conditions can create or compound health disparities. Diverse local environmental health initiatives have arisen to develop innovative ways to address these problems. However, little is known about what leads to initiation of such efforts, what promising strategies or critical barriers will emerge, or how to promote their success. These collaborative efforts are diverse, complex, and therefore difficult to evaluate.

The Local Environmental Health Initiative Framework is used to guide analysis of the three case studies and understanding their impacts. Chapters 4 through 6 present in-depth explorations of how three collaborative local environmental health initiatives unfolded in New York, Minnesota, and Southern California. These local initiatives worked at multiple levels to improve environmental health. Each chose different strategies to pursue its goals, tapped different resources, developed the capacity of its participants, and played different roles (direct or indirect) in changing policies, systems, and environments.

4 The Coalition to Prevent Lead Poisoning: Promoting Primary Prevention in Rochester, New York

Case Summary

In 2002, rates of childhood lead poisoning in certain high-risk neighborhoods in Rochester, New York, were more than ten times the national average. In the context of failing schools, child poverty, and high crime rates, local advocates coalesced around the idea that addressing lead in older housing could make a difference in children's lives—and the community's well-being. The resulting Coalition to Prevent Lead Poisoning (CPLP) focused its efforts on promoting systems changes to prevent lead exposure. CPLP worked to develop awareness of the problem, support for policy change, and a framework for a cost-efficient local lead law. Although many older cities have similar lead problems, Rochester is one of the few that has successfully passed and implemented a housing law to prevent lead poisoning. The lead law includes provisions for reporting and data sharing, which CPLP leveraged to monitor implementation and adaptation over time. In addition to the law, CPLP fostered collaboration between community, government, and academic partners to sustain, support, and adapt Rochester's lead poisoning prevention efforts over time. A decade on, lead poisoning rates in Rochester have decreased more than twice as steeply as those in the rest of upstate New York. This case demonstrates how bringing together diverse stakeholders and reframing the problem of lead poisoning from a "health issue" to a "housing issue" were key to developing a new, locally appropriate solution to a longstanding problem.

Introduction

Home is where most of us spend the majority of our time. Although the air, dust, water, and materials inside homes are not typically considered within the realm of environmental management, home-based exposures can have significant impacts on health (Saegert et al. 2003). However, lead hazards in housing built before 1978, when lead was banned from residential paint in the United States, remain a major environmental health threat. Despite solid medical understanding of the dangers of lead toxicity, proven techniques to address home-based lead hazards, and decades of federal and state prevention programs, many children are still at risk of lead poisoning. Lead remains a particular problem in cities with older housing in poor condition. This case examines a collaborative effort in Rochester, New York, to prevent lead poisoning in neighborhoods with high rates of lead hazards in housing.

The story of how humans spread lead throughout the environment goes back thousands of years (Lewis 1985). Lead is a soft metal that melts at relatively low temperatures. It was one of the first metals humans processed and used, resulting in exposures as a result of mining, processing, and making lead into a wide variety of products (Chisolm 2001a; Lewis 1985). Lead colic was attributed to children putting lead toys in their mouths as early as 1848. At the same time, however, lead chromate ("chrome yellow") was used as a yellow dye for bread and candies (Rosner, Markowitz, and Lanphear 2005; Weis 2012). Lead use expanded in the industrial era, vastly increasing the amount of lead distributed into the environment.

Starting in the 1920s, lead was added to gasoline as an "anti-knock" agent to improve the performance of engines (Rosner and Markowitz 1985). Although public health professionals raised concerns about the use of lead in gasoline, industrial interests successfully prevented federal regulation until the 1970s. Lead was also used in water pipes, plumbing fixtures, and solder; although use of lead in pipes declined by the 1930s, it was not banned until 1986 (U.S. EPA 2018k; Rabin 2008).[1] Most significantly for modern children's health, lead was increasingly used in house paint in the late nineteenth century. J. Lockhart Gibson, an Australian physician, was first to document children poisoned from lead in household paint in 1904 (Rosner, Markowitz, and Lanphear 2005; Gibson et al. 1892; Gibson 1904). However, corporate interests downplayed the evidence of harm and continued to produce lead paint. Companies actively marketed lead paints to families, citing the bright colors, durability, and "easy to clean" finish imparted by high lead content (Markowitz and Rosner 2000, 40). As a result of these industrial, commercial, and consumer uses, lead was distributed throughout homes, yards, and neighborhoods. Lead does not disappear over time and remains a threat unless it is removed or permanently covered. As a result, lead in paint, dust, and soil is still a significant source of exposure for children in the United States (Lanphear et al. 1998; Levin et al. 2008).

Environmental Health Policy and Lead Poisoning

Understanding of lead's wide-ranging health impacts has grown over time (Chisolm 2001a; Needleman 2009). By the middle of the twentieth century, neurological effects and even death were documented in cases of workers who were exposed to high levels of lead through mining, smelting, and other industries in the United States (Rosner and Markowitz 1985; Markowitz and Rosner 2013). Meanwhile, the number of cases of children exposed to lead in housing mounted as lead-painted surfaces began to deteriorate, particularly in lower-income neighborhoods (Jacobs 1995). The symptoms exhibited by these children added to the evidence that lead affects health and development. Despite the accumulated medical understanding of the causes and consequences of lead exposure, even today there is no effective treatment that can reverse lead's permanent damage to children's growing brains, bones, and organs. Therefore, lead poisoning is known as a disease that can be prevented but not cured (Cole and Winsler 2010; Ryan et al. 1999).

As a result of this growing understanding of lead's harms, public health professionals and community advocates pushed for policies to remove lead from children's environments (Chisolm 2001b). In the 1960s, cities including Baltimore, Boston, Chicago, and New York developed lead-screening programs, with public health nurses visiting the homes of children with elevated blood lead levels to provide hygiene education. Even at that time, many health professionals recognized that education alone was insufficient and that a solution could "only be mounted through an attack on slum housing" (Colgrove 2011, 48). In 1969, Dr. Rene Dubos of the Rockefeller Institute was quoted as saying, "The problem is so well defined, so neatly packaged with both causes and cures known, that if we don't eliminate this social crime, our society deserves all the disasters that have been forecast for it" (Oberle 1969, 992).

Lead was banned from paint in most of Europe in the 1920s (Chisolm 2001a; Pueschel and Fadden 1975; International Labour Organization 2018). However, in the United States, lead industries resisted efforts to regulate lead for decades. Just as the tobacco industry undermined medical research and efforts to restrict smoking, the lead industries argued against evidence of lead's harm (Markowitz and Rosner 2000; Rosner and Markowitz 1985). Childhood lead poisoning was blamed on "slum dwelling and relatively ignorant parents" who allowed their children to eat paint chips and failed to clean properly (Markowitz and Rosner 2000, 43). Meanwhile, lead in gasoline and paint continued to spread lead throughout the country.

Pressure from physicians and public health professionals prompted several states and municipalities to restrict the use of lead paint (Pueschel and Fadden 1975; Freudenberg and Golub 1987). In 1960, both New York City and the state of Massachusetts banned lead paint from being used inside homes (Pueschel and Fadden 1975). Eventually, the federal government followed suit, banning lead in residential paint in 1978 and initiating the phase-out of lead in gasoline in 1976. Lead poisoning rates in the United States dropped dramatically after the federal policies to remove lead from paint and gasoline were implemented. The percentage of children ages 1–5 with blood lead levels greater than 10 micrograms per deciliter (µg/dL) dropped from 88 percent in 1980 to 0.8 percent in 2010 (CDC 2013). However, restricting lead from new paint did not eliminate risks from existing leaded paint in older homes. Even when covered over by new lead-free paint, old lead paint can still get into household dust from deterioration, friction (doors and windows opening and closing), or impact (walking on floors). Lead can also be tracked or blown into homes from bare soil in the yard or neighborhood (Mielke et al. 1999).

In addition to banning lead in paint and gasoline, the federal government took other steps to reduce the hazards posed by leaded paint in older housing. As part of the 1992 Housing and Community Development Act, the Lead-Based Paint Disclosure Rule (Section 1018 of Title X) required sellers and landlords of housing built before 1978 to provide information about known lead hazards (Korfmacher 2014). Also, as part of this law, the U.S. Department of Housing and Urban Development (HUD) developed lead-safety requirements for federally assisted housing and grant programs to reduce lead hazards in private housing (HUD 2018a). These grant programs initially emphasized removal or permanent "abatement" of lead hazards. Subsequent housing research showed that hazards could be largely controlled through removal of lead on friction surfaces (e.g., windows, floors, and doors) using lead-safe work practices, but also that without careful work and cleanup, disturbing lead paint could increase hazards (Dixon et al. 2012; Ryan et al. 1999; Amitai et al. 1987). HUD also set forth standards for "interim controls," lower-cost methods for controlling lead hazards without removing all lead paint (HUD 2012). Whereas the HUD rules applied primarily to federally-assisted housing, in 2010, the U.S. Environmental Protection Agency (EPA) implemented regulations for safe renovation, repair, and painting practices (the "RRP rule") that also applied to most privately owned pre-1978 housing (U.S. EPA 2014c).

Many states have adopted additional policies to reduce childhood lead poisoning. Medicaid requires health care providers to screen all young children for exposure to lead and to test at-risk children's blood; many state health departments have similar requirements. Since low levels of lead seldom cause immediately visible symptoms, blood tests are the only way to detect exposure. When children are identified with elevated blood lead levels (EBLLs), health departments work to identify and require removal of the lead hazards from the children's environments. This "secondary prevention" approach aims to prevent further exposure in children who have already been identified as exposed (CDC 2004b; Ettinger et al. 2019). Unfortunately, secondary prevention does not protect children from the permanent injuries caused by lead poisoning. Because there is no effective medical treatment for most children with lead poisoning, public health professionals emphasize "primary prevention" (box 4.1)—that is, identifying and removing hazards before children are poisoned (Brown and Meehan 2004; Lanphear, Hornung, and Ho 2005).

Housing-based sources (paint, dust, and soil) are responsible for the majority of EBLL cases. However, other contributors such as imported folk medicines, consumer products, water contaminated by passing through lead pipes or solder, industrial emissions, and "take-home" lead from hobbies or occupations may be significant for some populations (Levin et al. 2008; Franko et al. 2009; Newman et al. 2015; Spanier et al. 2013). Such nonpaint sources may contribute to over 30 percent of EBLL cases in the United States (Levin et al. 2008).

Box 4.1
A Renewed Call for Primary Prevention

In 2012, the Centers for Disease Control and Prevention's Advisory Committee on Childhood Lead Poisoning Prevention issued a seminal report on low-
level lead exposure that included this "Renewed Call for Primary Prevention"
(ACCLPP 2012, 15):

The [aforementioned] arguments as well as those that follow all underscore
the critical importance of primary prevention. Using a strategy of identifying
lead poisoning or elevated BLLs relies on detection in the child, relegating
the child to the function of a sensing device for poor/contaminated housing,
contaminated water, and/or tainted consumer products. Thus, the child can
be considered the proverbial "canary in the coal mine." The current strategy,
which relies on identifying extant elevated BLLs, while still warranted to some
extent, does not prevent the damage already incurred. Moreover, while agents
such as chelators can be used to treat overt lead poisoning and possibly reduce
the case fatality rate, these agents have been demonstrated not to improve IQ
or behavioral consequences of lead exposure. Therefore, primary prevention
is the most important and significant strategy.

Because housing-based lead hazards remain the dominant source of exposure for most children, several states, including Maryland, Massachusetts,
and Vermont, as well as a handful of municipalities have adopted laws that
aim to identify and fix lead hazards in housing before children become poisoned (Brown et al. 2001; Mares 2003; Breysse et al. 2007; National Center
for Healthy Housing 2018b).

New York City has been a notable leader in lead poisoning prevention (Freudenberg and Golub 1987; Pueschel and Fadden 1975). In 1960,
New York City required the city's health department to inspect the homes
of children with elevated blood lead levels and order abatement of lead
paint (Freudenberg and Golub 1987; Chachere 2018). New York City Citizens to End Lead Poisoning was formed in 1968 by scientists, health care
providers, and community organizers to advocate for stronger municipal
health department action on lead (Colgrove 2011; Freudenberg 2004). This
group worked directly with affected communities and groups such as the
Black Panthers and Young Lords, which made lead "part of their platform
against racial injustice" (Colgrove 2011, 50). It was succeeded in 1983 by
the New York City Coalition to End Lead Poisoning (NYCCELP), which

continued to push for programs to address lead poisoning, which it viewed as a "symptom of sick housing" (Colgrove 2011; Freudenberg and Golub 1987; NYCCELP 2016). It supported the passage of Local Law 1 in 1982, which required landlords to annually inspect and remediate lead hazards in most child-occupied units; legal actions and advocacy by groups including NYCCELP prompted further updates to this law over the next thirty years, culminating in adoption of a new, stronger lead law coincidentally also named Local Law 1 of 2004 (Chachere 2018).

More recently, a number of innovative state and local policies have been enacted to promote housing-based primary prevention with mixed results (Korfmacher and Hanley 2013; Brown et al. 2001; Brown 2002; Korfmacher 2014; Pew Charitable Trusts 2017). However, accessing, testing, and repairing pre-1978 housing—even just rental units—is expensive and logistically challenging. Therefore, housing-based primary prevention laws are rare and unevenly enforced (Korfmacher and Hanley 2013).

Despite these many policy interventions, lead poisoning remains a significant environmental health threat, particularly for low-income children who live in older housing (Landrigan et al. 2002; Gould 2009; Pew Charitable Trusts 2017). Because lead is a neurotoxicant that affects the developing brain, lead-poisoned children may experience behavioral and learning problems (Brown and Meehan 2004; Lanphear et al. 2000; Canfield et al. 2003; Lanphear et al. 2005; Jurewicz, Polanska, and Hanke 2013; Winneke 2011). Later in life, they are at greater risk for health problems including hypertension, osteoporosis, and cognitive deficits (Cole and Winsler 2010; Campbell and Auinger 2007; Navas-Acien et al. 2007; Beier et al. 2013). Although population blood lead levels have declined, new medical research showing a wide range of learning, behavioral, and health effects from very low lead exposures has sustained public health concerns about lead (Lanphear et al. 2005; Brown and Meehan 2004). In 2012, the National Toxicology Program concluded that children can experience decreased academic achievement, lowered IQ, and increased incidence of attention behavioral problems below blood lead levels of 10 micrograms per deciliter (μg/dL) (National Toxicology Program 2012). Accordingly, the Centers for Disease Control and Prevention (CDC) set a new "reference value" of 5 μg/dL, while emphasizing that there is no known lower threshold for lead's negative effects on children (CDC 2012). CDC estimated that more than half a million children in the United States had blood lead levels above the new reference value (CDC 2013).

Geographic analyses demonstrate that the children of lower-income families of color living in older housing exposed to lead are disproportionately exposed to lead (Levin et al. 2008; Lanphear et al. 1998). Many cities have delineated specific neighborhoods that produce the majority of cases of lead poisoning, emphasizing the connection between lead and older housing in poor repair (Sargent et al. 1997; Boyce and Hood 2002; Haley and Talbot 2004; Meyer et al. 2005; Reyes et al. 2006; Korfmacher and Kuholski 2007; Hanley 2007). These localized concentrations of lead poisoning persist despite significant population-wide reductions of lead poisoning, prompting some to call lead a "public health success but an environmental justice failure."

In summary, most cities and states do not proactively regulate lead hazards in pre-1978 private rental housing. In addition, low-income owner-occupants often lack resources to maintain lead-safe homes. As a result, by 2000, federal government-assisted housing had fewer lead paint hazards compared to privately owned low-income housing (Jacobs et al. 2002; Ahrens et al. 2016). As recent cases in New York City and elsewhere show, public housing can still pose risks because of funding cuts, deteriorated conditions, and lax enforcement of federal law (Weiser and Goodman 2018; Parker 2018). However, lead hazards in privately owned pre-1978 housing—both rental units and owner-occupied properties—are largely unregulated and remain a major source of children's exposure to lead and resulting elevated blood lead levels.

Childhood Lead Poisoning in Rochester, NY

Rochester was typical of many cities with high rates of lead poisoning at the turn of the millenium. Most of its housing was built before 1978, with 87 percent built before 1950. The oldest homes generally had the highest risk of lead hazards because paint produced before 1950 had higher amounts of lead, many were repainted with lead multiple times, and their painted surfaces may have deteriorated over time (Boyce and Hood 2002; HUD 2011; Jacobs et al. 2002). Rochester also had a depressed housing market—the median sale price of a single-family home was under $50,000. In 2000, around 220,000 people lived in Rochester, down from over 330,000 in 1950.

Citywide, 60 percent of families rented their homes. In some neighborhoods, there were fewer than 10 percent owner-occupants. Because of the low housing values, many low-income owner-occupants lacked the capital to maintain their homes and ensure they were free of lead paint hazards.

In addition to Rochester having high lead-risk housing, many families lacked resources to avoid or respond to lead exposure. Child poverty rates climbed from 38 percent to 52 percent from 2000 to 2014, the second highest rate in the country for cities with populations over 200,000 (ACT Rochester 2015; Sharp 2014). High school graduation rates remained just over 40 percent during this period, and in 2012 the Schott Foundation for Public Education found that only 9 percent of black male students graduated from high school—the lowest rate in the country (Hofer 2012). Child poverty and educational attainment were therefore key community concerns.

Because of strong implementation in Monroe County of the state law requiring blood lead testing of all one- and two-year-olds, there was good data on lead poisoning trends. According to a 2002 report, the citywide childhood lead poisoning rate in 2000 was 23.6 percent (Boyce and Hood 2002). In twelve "extreme risk" census tracts, over 35 percent of screened children were identified as having elevated blood lead levels—over twenty times the national rate (figure 4.1) (Meyer et al. 2003). Black and Hispanic children were most likely to live in high-lead-risk neighborhoods (Boyce and Hood 2002).[2]

Many older cities, particularly in the Northeast and Midwest, have similar housing risks, demographics, and lead poisoning rates. Rochester is one of the few to have adopted a comprehensive housing-based lead ordinance. This case explores the collaborative effort that developed, promoted, and implemented the law, the resources that supported the effort, and the potential for dissemination to other cities.

Case Overview: The Rochester Coalition to Prevent Lead Poisoning

In 1999, Rochester Elementary School 17 Principal Ralph Spezio heard nurses in his school talking about the high rate of lead poisoning among special education students. He began researching lead's impacts on children's ability to learn and connected this information to his students' struggles to succeed in school. Working with the local health department, he

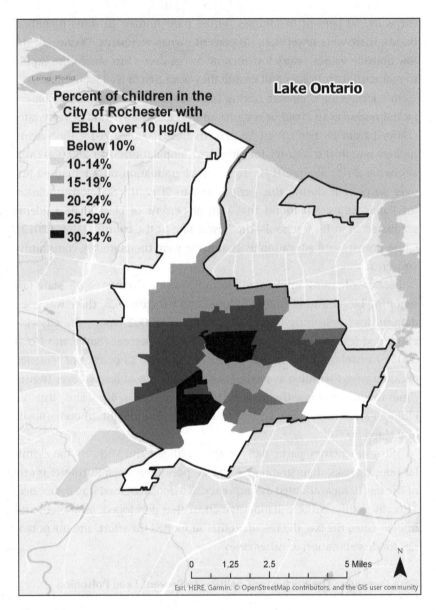

Figure 4.1
Rates of tested children found to have elevated blood lead levels in Rochester, New York, in 2000
Data source: Sarah Boyce and Kim Hood. 2002. *Lead Poisoning among Young Children in Monroe County, NY: A Needs Assessment, Projection Model, and Next Steps* (Rochester, NY: Center for Governmental Research). (Map credit: Karl Korfmacher)

discovered that 41 percent of the children entering his school had a history of elevated blood lead levels (EBLLs) (McDade 2018; Spezio 2017; Tevlock 2014; Spezio 2011; McGarvey 2010).

With the findings of this analysis in hand, he organized a meeting of nearly 100 community stakeholders at School 17 in 2000. Although concern about the issue was high, the City of Rochester's housing commissioner cautioned that abating lead in all of Rochester's housing would take all of the city's federal grant money for fifty years and could bankrupt the city. Nonetheless, the meeting inspired educators, community leaders, doctors, nurses, and researchers to organize a coalition to address the problem. Their collaboration has spanned nearly twenty years (table 4.1) and included the development and implementation of Rochester's lead law in 2006. This overview provides context for the discussion of the CPLP's collaborative activities, which are explored in greater detail in the sections that follow.

Initially called the Rochester Lead Free Coalition, the group soon changed its name to the Coalition to Prevent Lead Poisoning (CPLP) to better reflect its focus on cost-effective primary prevention, rather than full lead removal. One of CPLP's first steps was to gather more information about childhood

Table 4.1
Rochester Coalition to Prevent Lead Poisoning timeline

1998	First HUD Lead Hazard Control grant awarded to Monroe County.
1999	Principal Ralph Spezio finds 41% of incoming students have a history of elevated blood lead levels.
2000	Rochester Lead Free Coalition is formed.
2001	Coalition changes name to Coalition to Prevent Lead Poisoning (CPLP).
2004	Community Lead Summit held.
2005	Rochester lead law passes.
2006	Implementation of Rochester's lead law begins on July 1.
2007	Rochester City School District adopts school lead policy.
2009	CPLP and partners receive U.S. EPA Environmental Justice Award.
2014	County health department paper finds the decline in EBLL is 2.4 times faster than in other upstate counties (Kennedy, 2014).
2016	Lead law's tenth anniversary celebration; Over 140,000 city lead inspections completed.
2017	CPLP transitions administrative home to Causewave Community Partners.

lead poisoning in Rochester. In 2002 the Monroe County Department of Public Health commissioned a study that found the prevalence of lead poisoning in the highest-risk neighborhoods was nearly 24 percent, compared with a statewide rate of 5.8 percent and a national rate of 2.2 percent (Boyce and Hood 2002; Meyer et al. 2003).

Initial membership of CPLP included educators, public interest lawyers, primary care providers, academics, neighborhood group leaders, and the local health department. They met monthly in space provided by the Rochester Primary Care Network (RPCN), an organization that serves the region's federally qualified health centers. The group reached out to additional stakeholders, including housing professionals, community action agencies, the United Way, the local public television/radio affiliate, and civic and religious leaders.

By 2003, members were organized into seven working committees (Finance, Government Relations, Housing, Membership, Outreach, Science, and Screening/Professional Education) that carried out the bulk of CPLP activities. At CPLP's peak of engagement in 2004, each committee had between five and ten regularly attending members and most of them met on a monthly basis, as did the Board (with ten to twenty regular attendees). Active participation attenuated after passage of the Rochester lead law in 2005. By 2013, CPLP had reorganized into two monthly committee meetings (Screening/Professional Education and Government Relations) plus quarterly executive committee meetings and an annual membership meeting. These committees developed programs, conducted analyses, researched other communities' experiences, and drafted policy positions. The committees made recommendations to the Board, which finalized the organizations' decisions.

Committee members included both volunteers and professionals whose time was contributed by their employers. Table 4.2 provides a brief overview of members of CPLP and their roles. Professional educators, health care providers, community groups, and public interest lawyers were active participants. Local government agencies—particularly housing and inspections staff from the City of Rochester and the Monroe County Department of Public Health—were represented on committees but did not serve in leadership positions.

The University of Rochester engaged with CPLP in several ways (HUD 2018c). Many of the health care providers who worked with CPLP were

Table 4.2

Coalition to Prevent Lead Poisoning membership*

Organization Name or Type	Description of Role in CPLP
City of Rochester	Housing department and inspections staff served on committees; funded some CPLP educational efforts.
Community groups	Neighborhood and community groups, community action agency, child advocacy organizations, environmental and social justice groups sent staff and volunteers to committee meetings and events.
Educators	Principal Ralph Spezio initiated CPLP; Head Start staff served on committees; Rochester City School District environmental services staff sat on committees, developed Lead Safe Schools Policy.
Health care providers	5–10 individuals served on committees and in leadership roles over time; summarized medical literature; shared patient stories.
Lead professionals	Several private lead risk assessors served on housing committees; provided lead assessments for Get the Lead Out (GLO) project.
Monroe County Department of Public Health	Director commissioned 2002 Needs Assessment; appointed staff to sit on committees; funded several CPLP educational efforts.
Public interest lawyers	Staff attorneys from Empire Justice Center served on committees, drafted legislation, analyzed case law.
United Way	Staff served on committees; provided partial funding for Lead Summit and for CPLP staff.
University of Rochester	Health care professionals and Environmental Health Sciences Center outreach staff (COEC) served on multiple committees; arranged for talks by researchers; supported Lead Summit.

*CPLP had over 100 active committee members and 700 members on its mailing list. This chart does not encompass all the key stakeholders, but rather provides an overview of the types of organizations and members involved over time.

based at the University of Rochester Medical Center. The university's Environmental Health Sciences Center (EHSC) included nationally known experts on lead. The National Institute of Environmental Health Sciences supported the EHSC's Community Outreach and Engagement Core (COEC), whose goal was to translate research to meet community needs. Because of the importance of childhood lead poisoning to the Rochester community, the COEC staff focused much of their time on this issue. This amounted to commitment of around a half-time staff person during CPLP's most active period.

The CPLP bylaws required that at least 30 percent of Board members must represent "affected communities," meaning low-income and predominantly African American and Latino neighborhoods with the highest rates of lead poisoning. One co-chair position was also designated to be an affected community representative. Community seats were often filled by paid staff members of neighborhood or community groups that served high-lead-risk neighborhoods (i.e., community health center staff); others were volunteers. Around 2005, a "leadership development" group was formed to help recruit, train, and sustain community representation in these positions.

CPLP committees included only a small number of parents of lead-poisoned children. CPLP co-chair Mel Callan said, "I wish we had more direct participation from the affected families, but there is always that tension between not wanting to exploit their situation and being able to get the message out based on their stories" (Callan 2018). To protect the privacy and respect the time constraints of families affected by lead poisoning, CPLP aimed to understand their needs through individual interactions and involvement of community representatives rather than direct parent engagement in committees. Several parents of lead poisoned children also contributed their stories to CPLP communications materials or press events.

The CPLP Board made decisions by consensus, with a provision for a supermajority vote (75 percent) if consensus could not be achieved. In response to concerns that CPLP's open membership and meetings could attract individuals whose interests might undermine the organization's objectives, the Board developed Guiding Principles to which participants committed as a condition of membership (box 4.2, CPLP 2006).

The CPLP leadership debated obtaining 501(c) status several times but decided to instead use the services of a host organization as "fiscal agent."

Box 4.2

Guiding Principles of the Coalition to Prevent Lead Poisoning

Primary Prevention—The only way to truly protect children and their families from environmental health hazards is to identify hazards and take corrective and preventive action before harm occurs.

Right to Know—Community members have the right to know about environmental hazards in their homes, neighborhoods, and communities.

Community Organizing—Communicating directly, exchanging ideas regularly, and developing projects jointly with local communities is our organizing strategy. We understand that for solutions to be sustainable, those directly affected must be full partners in the project design and implementation.

Community Empowerment—Community residents are effective agents of change when they are provided with information and resources. Information about primary prevention is the most effective means to maintain a long-term lead safe community. Resources to test housing stock and abate lead hazards are required to establish lead safe environments for our children and families.

Environmental Justice—All people, regardless of income or color, deserve to live in housing that is decent, affordable, and safe from environmental hazards and to live, work, learn, and play in healthy communities.

Responsibility—Our responsibility is to communicate the best health hazard information and to educate the residents about steps they can take to reduce health risks.

Accountability—The central purpose of this effort is to hold property owners, governmental agencies, health care providers, insurers, and the legal system accountable for protecting the health and safety of our children and families.

Outcome-Oriented—The Coalition will consistently be outcome-oriented. Hence, its goals, objectives and actions will be directed toward achieving measurable outcomes within a specified period of time.

Collaboration—Coalition members will work together as a team to make this community's environment lead-safe. Because we recognize and value the differing perspectives of our Members, we seek to achieve a consensus on all Coalition decisions and use a formal consensus-building model to that end.

Science-Based—All initiatives, reports, and proposals publicly issued by the Coalition shall be based on the best scientific evidence available.

Respect—Individuals and organizations that share common values and work on kindred issues deserve mutual respect, honesty, trust, and candor, even when they may differ on tactics or short-term objectives (CPLP 2006).

Initially, this was the Rochester Primary Care Network (now known as Regional Primary Care Network), which also provided meeting space. When CPLP was able to hire full time staff in 2003, it rented office space in and moved most of its meetings to the United Way's building. Several years later, its administrative home transitioned to the Finger Lakes Health Systems Agency (now known as Common Ground Health), a not-for-profit regional health planning agency. In 2017, Causewave Communications, long-time partner in CPLP's communications campaign, became CPLP's fiscal agent.[3]

Initial funding for a part-time communications director came from a small community grant from the Eastman Kodak Company. This staff person worked with the Board to obtain additional funding from local foundations, the United Way, and government agencies. Most grants were identified and written by CPLP staff with support of Board members. Board members also worked with state elected officials to obtain partial funding from the state legislature to support operations of CPLP for several years. CPLP's budget consisted primarily of staff salaries, a communications campaign, and overhead costs. CPLP funding also paid for office space and administrative services through its host organizations.[4]

Levels of staffing for CPLP fluctuated over time, peaking around 2007, when staff included a full-time executive director, a communications director, and a part-time outreach specialist. Reflecting the reduction in the CPLP's membership, the formal bylaws were set aside in 2013 and replaced with a less-formal system of information-sharing, coordination, and planning by the working committees. In 2014, CPLP had just one part-time staff member focused on outreach and supporting the two active committees (Government Relations and Screening/Professional Education). By 2016, CPLP had no paid staff, but its two working committees and executive committee continued to meet, and Coalition activities were undertaken by committee members on a voluntary basis.

CPLP initially faced several significant challenges to motivating action on lead. First, many community leaders believed that the lead problem had already been solved by the federal bans on lead in paint and gasoline decades earlier. Second, childhood lead poisoning fell under the purview of the local health department. Indeed, the Monroe County Department of Public Health (MCDPH) was a leader in implementing New York State's secondary prevention system for children identified with elevated blood lead levels. MCDPH served the entire county, but the majority of lead-poisoned children lived in the city of Rochester. However, housing inspections, permits, and planning were controlled by city government. Although the county health department shared information on lead violations with the city, the city housing inspections office had no role other than to help enforce these violations reactively. Third, many key leaders, including housing professionals in city government, believed that lead remediation was prohibitively expensive and that any systematic effort to address lead in Rochester would destroy the housing market. HUD's lead abatement protocols required expensive abatement of lead, which seemed infeasible in a city with such low housing values (U.S. Census 2000; HUD 2018a).[5] Since housing professionals were most familiar with HUD's approach to lead, they accordingly used cost estimates based on HUD's abatement protocols, which projected prohibitively high costs to make the city lead-safe. Fourth, the elected leadership of county government was Republican while the mayor and City Council were Democrats. This posed an additional challenge to coordinated action. Finally, those most affected by lead—low-income families of color—were not politically powerful voices in the community.

To address these challenges, CPLP articulated a clear goal: to end childhood lead poisoning in Rochester by 2010 (Korfmacher 2008). CPLP recognized the need to reframe the issue as one of children's health and well-being with a housing solution. Its messaging called lead poisoning "an invisible and silent monster" sapping children's intellectual potential and "a disease kids catch from their houses" (Korfmacher 2010; Drmacich 2011). To overcome fears that housing-based primary prevention was prohibitively expensive, CPLP first aimed to make it "morally, economically, and politically unacceptable" for lead poisoning to continue, then to design and implement cost-effective solutions (Hetherington and Brantingham 2004).

CPLP members worked together over the next five years to increase public awareness of the problem, build support among community leaders, and pass a local lead law. Adopted in 2005, the Rochester lead law has been widely hailed as a national model. It mandated lead inspections of rental housing as part of the city's existing Certificate of Occupancy program. Between 2006 and 2018, lead inspections were conducted in over 166,000 rental units (City of Rochester 2018). The Monroe County health department provided data on areas where children identified with elevated blood lead levels lived and funded part of the city's inspection costs. The Rochester

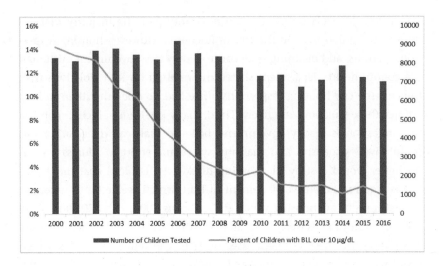

Figure 4.2
Number of tested children and percentage of tested children with elevated blood lead levels in Rochester, New York, 2000–2016 (includes tested children living in zip codes approximating the Rochester municipal boundary)
Data source: Monroe County Department of Public Health, 2018. Blood Lead Screening Data, 2003–2016,
https://www2.monroecounty.gov/files/health/Lead/2016%20FINAL%20Screening%20Totals.pdf.

Housing Authority (RHA), housing grant programs, and social service agencies also coordinated their programs in support of this policy. Soon after passage of the lead law, the Rochester City School District passed its own policy to identify and address lead hazards in school buildings (Rochester City School District 2007). CPLP helped coordinate this comprehensive system of awareness, hazard identification, remediation, and implementation.

CPLP continued to educate the public, support ongoing lead prevention programs, and monitor implementation after passage of the law. By 2012, the City of Rochester had seen more than an 85 percent decline in children with elevated blood lead levels (figure 4.2); this decline was nearly two and a half times faster than in the rest of the state (Kennedy et al. 2014). This rapid decline in lead poisoning suggests that the community was able to create an effective local system for lead poisoning prevention. Its approach integrated a comprehensive communications strategy to promote lead prevention messages to a range of key stakeholders, a system for translating science to address stakeholders' concerns and questions, and a strategy to support the design, passage, and implementation of a local lead law. An overview of each of these functions is provided next, followed by an analysis of the resources and approaches that successfully supported this work.

Collaborative Activities of the Coalition to Prevent Lead Poisoning

From the outset, CPLP promoted multipronged action to protect children from lead in their homes. First, it needed to define and communicate the problem effectively to the community at large, but particularly to community leaders who could voice persuasive support. Second, CPLP bolstered its credibility by bringing the best science to bear on addressing stakeholders' questions and concerns. CPLP members mined the published literature, experience in other communities, and local and national expertise to develop science-based solutions. Third, the group developed an organizing strategy to build support for local systems change.

Communicating the Problem to the Community

CPLP recognized that before promoting a specific systems change, it needed to address the community's lack of awareness of the extent, distribution, impacts, and tractability of childhood lead poisoning. Many CPLP members with experience in community organizing understood that politicians would only act if the public expressed strong concern. They developed a communications strategy tailored to raise key stakeholders' understanding of the problem, how it affected different community interests, and how various groups could contribute. CPLP devoted much of its staff time, committee attention, and funding to carrying out these communication efforts.

CPLP's communications reconceptualized childhood lead poisoning as a child health problem with a feasible housing solution. There were three main components of this message (Korfmacher 2008):

- Lead is costly to our entire community.
- We are all responsible for ending lead poisoning.
- Ending childhood lead poisoning in Rochester by 2010 is an attainable goal.

CPLP also balanced highlighting the environmental justice implications of childhood lead poisoning with the reality that all children living in pre-1978 housing were at risk. CPLP produced maps that showed clusters of elevated blood lead levels (EBLLs) in older towns and shared stories of lead-poisoned children in rural, pre-1978 housing. However, CPLP emphasized the concentration of EBLL in the lowest-income neighborhoods around the center city that also had high rates of crime, low educational attainment, and low incomes. CPLP shared New York State Department of Health data showing that high percentages of black and Latino children lived in high lead risk zip codes. These same children were most likely to struggle in school, engage with the juvenile justice system, and be enrolled in Medicaid. Tabulating the data by race, income, and ethnicity helped mobilize community groups in these neighborhoods and captured the attention of educators, religious leaders, health care providers, and advocates for low-income children. At the same time, CPLP sought the support of the broader community by noting that all pre-1978 housing, including older housing in suburban and rural areas, could pose a lead risk. CPLP was clear, however, that its advocacy would focus primarily on protecting children at highest risk. This tied into the second message of shared responsibility. CPLP emphasized that while property owners are responsible for maintaining rental units in a safe condition, our entire society held historical responsibility for lead paint's legacy. To make their case, CPLP worked to design affordable solutions for property owners and helped secure funding for hazard control grants. The third point—that primary prevention was attainable—was based on experiences in other communities. CPLP emphasized to Rochester's leadership that lead poisoning prevention could be an important community "win" in a city that had suffered many recent setbacks (CGR 2015).

CPLP's vision was summarized in the catchphrase: "Find the hazards, fix the hazards, and fund the fix" (Hetherington and Brantingham 2004). This vision statement was used in many CPLP materials and was elucidated in a 2004 guest essay in the *Democrat and Chronicle* by Board Chair Bryan Hetherington and Executive Director Patricia Brantingham (Hetherington and Brantingham 2004): "We will find lead hazards before they poison children. We will fix the hazards using proven, cost-effective control measures. And we will fund the work through a combination of public and private financing that acknowledges that we as a society allowed this toxin to be used in homes and so we as a society must share in the cost of making homes lead-safe." Rather than focusing immediately on specific strategies for accomplishing these objectives, CPLP first set about communicating these general principles as a basis for a community-wide discussion about solutions appropriate for Rochester. This strategy refrained from pointing fingers at government, landlords, or paint companies, common tactics for organizing in other communities. Instead, they framed the issue as a community problem that everyone had responsibility to solve.

"Lead 101" CPLP encouraged health, housing, and community organizations to think about lead poisoning in a new way. CPLP developed publications, a website, and training materials that expressed its reformulation of the lead problem as an issue of community well-being with a solution based on improving housing quality. CPLP developed a "Lead 101" Power-Point presentation that included an overview of the effects of lead on children's health, behavior, and educational outcomes; the sources of lead in homes; maps of Rochester showing areas with high rates of EBLL children; the proposed solution of housing-based primary prevention; and ways to get involved with CPLP. This presentation was adapted for a wide range of stakeholders. In one instance, a pediatrician shared the presentation with city inspectors, adding personal stories of the problems his patients faced as a result of lead poisoning. This helped the inspectors appreciate that their efforts to pursue strong enforcement of housing violations would protect children's health. Similarly, Principal Ralph Spezio's presentations to groups of educators, community leaders, and children's advocates linked the issue to their core interests, emphasizing that lead prevention efforts could improve educational outcomes.

CPLP leaders also used the Lead 101 materials to explain their approach to the United Way of Greater Rochester. In 2004, the United Way was exploring how it could use its community credibility and role as convener to positively affect local conditions. It established a policy committee charged with selecting a local challenge that could be impacted by the addition of the United Way's advocacy voice. According to United Way Policy Committee staff member Kathy Lewis, "Childhood lead poisoning was not even a blip on United Way's radar screen, but the nascent Coalition to Prevent Lead Poisoning approached us with an impressive and cogent proposal that asked only for United Way's influence to help change specific local policies. This proposal rose to the top of the group, and United Way agreed to make ending childhood lead poisoning its top advocacy issue" (Lewis

2018). United Way also subsequently provided several years of core funding for CPLP (Prevention Institute 2010).

Whenever CPLP gave the Lead 101 presentation, audience members were encouraged to join CPLP and to do what they could to support its work by encouraging blood lead testing, providing funding, and sharing the message with others. A key message to these stakeholders was that the existing system of secondary prevention was "using kids as canaries in the coal mine" to identify lead hazards. This message gave a moral imperative to CPLP's approach of primary prevention through proactively addressing housing hazards.

Public Communications Campaign   The goal of CPLP's communications campaign was to raise awareness among the general public—especially the parents of young children—and to reinforce the targeted outreach to community leaders. CPLP applied and was chosen in 2004 by Causewave Community Partners as a "Community Impact Campaign" (Causewave Community Partners 2018). This gave the group access to pro bono public relations and graphic design support from Roberts Communications, a private marketing and communications firm. A team of Causewave and Roberts Communications staff members contributed their time and talents to CPLP over a decade to develop messages and images to support their efforts. They created a slogan, "Let's make lead history," and a design template that was used throughout CPLP's communication materials. In subsequent years, Causewave and Roberts helped CPLP refine its messages about blood lead testing and the dangers of lead poisoning that were used in brochures, billboards, and public service announcements. As part of this arrangement, CPLP received free advertising from local television, radio, and print media outlets valued at around $250,000 per year. These efforts were supplemented with regular press releases, events, and editorials by CPLP members to keep the lead issue alive in the local media. In addition, staff regularly posted CPLP activities, scientific summaries, recent research, and news articles from Rochester and elsewhere on the CPLP website. CPLP also developed several issue-specific communications materials. For example, a task force was established to research, summarize, and communicate the workforce development needs and employment opportunities lead hazard reduction work could provide for low-income residents. The task force published a short booklet on workforce development for lead hazard reduction. Finally, CPLP published a newsletter to provide resources to community members and organizations trying to learn more about the issue. This newsletter was delivered electronically to CPLP's membership list, which by 2016 included over 700 organizations and individuals.

Community Lead Summit By 2004, CPLP members decided that a local lead law held the most promise for addressing the problem. They also understood that passage of such a law would require strong community pressure. With support from staff at the United Way, CPLP leaders organized a Community Lead Summit in June 2004. The two-day event included an hour-long live show on the local public television station, featuring local and national experts on lead followed by a public call-in session with phone lines staffed by CPLP members. The Community Lead Summit attracted nearly 500 people, far exceeding the organizers' initial goal of 150 attendees (Hetherington and Brantingham 2004; Prevention Institute 2010). Several nationally known keynote speakers, including Mary Jean Brown, then director of the Centers for Disease Control and Prevention Lead Branch, and Don Ryan, executive director of the National Alliance for Healthy Homes, voiced their support for the local efforts.

At the end of the Lead Summit, participants were invited to take the podium in a "commitment session" to state how they personally would help end childhood lead poisoning by 2010. Speakers included parents who pledged to test their children. Religious leaders promised to speak about lead to their congregations and "to declare lead poisoning morally unacceptable" (Lewis 2018). Several key commitments had been carefully mapped out by CPLP in advance of the Lead Summit. Most significantly, Rochester Mayor William Johnson, a Democrat, stated that he would pass a comprehensive lead law before leaving office in December 2005. Republican County Executive Maggie Brooks then pledged to mirror the city's approach in the county's Quality Housing Inspections (QHI) program so that if the county was paying direct rent for residents receiving public housing assistance, those units would be inspected (Prevention Institute 2010; Korfmacher 2010; Korfmacher and Hanley 2013). As Coalition leaders noted in an editorial, "The Community Lead Summit demonstrated conclusively that Rochester and Monroe County have both the knowledge and the will to eliminate what the county health director has called the greatest environmental threat to our young children. In an extraordinary display of unity, Democrats stood with Republicans, labor stood with business, teachers stood with school administrators and boards. All agreed that while much may still divide us, on this issue the community speaks with a single voice: We can and we must end childhood lead poisoning by 2010" (Hetherington and Brantingham 2004). These commitments made in a highly visible public forum paved the way to develop the city's lead law, which was unanimously adopted by the Rochester City Council on December 20, 2005.

Ongoing Support, Coordination, and Community Communications   One of three "Resolutions" passed by the Rochester City Council as part of the lead law package was a commitment to continue community education (City of Rochester 2018). This resolution recognized that part of keeping children lead-safe depended on the actions of their parents—getting their homes tested, testing children at ages one and two, providing proper nutrition, using lead-safe cleaning practices, and calling the city or county for help if they suspected a lead hazard in the home. CPLP recognized that implementation and enforcement of the law would require ongoing political and financial support; therefore, keeping lead in the public's eye was essential. Maintaining public attention posed a challenge after the lead law went into effect and funders perceived that the lead mission had been accomplished. As a result, CPLP's resources declined, as did its communications capacity. Nonetheless, the organization continued to prioritize communications strategies through its partnership with Roberts Communications. For example, in 2011, CPLP received funding from the City and the local health foundation to update, translate, print, and distribute lead brochures in seven languages to community partners. Each year, CPLP partnered with the county health department to create a press release announcing the previous year's lead testing rates and number of children with elevated blood lead levels. These ongoing efforts to communicate about lead were critical to maintaining public, political, and government support for primary prevention efforts.

Translating Information to Meet Stakeholders' Needs

Throughout its work, CPLP emphasized that its positions were based on the best available science. The process of seeking, translating, and, when necessary, generating information was integrated into CPLP communications strategies. CPLP assembled information to include in its presentations, website, and other outreach materials. It also used feedback from engaging with stakeholders about additional key questions that needed to be answered in order to move forward. These processes drove the agenda for summarizing science, synthesizing community knowledge, and analyzing existing data.

Costs of *Not* Preventing Lead Poisoning   Early on, CPLP members heard in their conversations with stakeholders that the most significant barrier to action on lead was concern about costs. CPLP leaders therefore decided that data on the costs of *not* preventing lead poisoning might help to counterbalance these fears. CPLP's messages emphasized lead's effects on the immediate and long-term physical health of children, the need for special education services, and the increased risk of juvenile delinquency. In 2002, the CPLP Board Chair Bryan Hetherington asked the staff of the University of Rochester (UR) Community Outreach and Engagement Core (COEC) to search for cost estimates of lead poisoning. Most of the existing estimates of the costs of lead poisoning were extrapolated from projections of lead's impact on IQ and reduced future earning potential (Landrigan et al. 2002; Prevention Institute 2010). Local leaders were not persuaded by predictions of lost future earning potential since this did not affect their annual budgets. Instead, the COEC staff searched for short-term costs related to medical treatment, special education services, and the juvenile justice system and applied these estimates to local EBLL data. The resulting analysis projected the annual costs of lead in Monroe County to be nearly $500,000 for medical treatment and $1,000,000 for special education, with additional unquantified juvenile justice costs (Korfmacher 2010; Stefanak, Diorio, and Frisch 2005). CPLP later included these calculations in its Lead 101 presentation to show that avoided costs of ending lead poisoning would be enough to make over 400 units lead-safe each year.

Communicating the State of the Science   Opponents of a strong housing-based lead law argued that it was unnecessary, excessively costly, and would be ineffective in preventing lead poisoning. Instead, they suggested that if parents cleaned their homes, fed children better diets, and washed their hands more frequently lead poisoning would be reduced. These arguments were repeatedly raised by landlords and some city council members. CPLP countered that focusing on nutrition and housekeeping implied that parents were to blame for their children's lead poisoning. Because the nutrition and cleaning issues were complex, controversial, and had the potential to undermine its housing-based policy strategy, CPLP leaders asked several physicians and researchers on its science committee to summarize the relevant scientific literature. Their short, plain-language summaries were posted on the CPLP website and delivered in hard copy to all city council members. Because they were written by health care providers and cited peer-reviewed research, these summaries were credible counters to some of the criticisms of the housing-based policy approach. This effort supported the CPLP's argument that while education about good nutrition and housekeeping complemented a housing-based prevention law, educational strategies alone would not prevent lead poisoning.

CPLP members effectively leveraged additional resources from their organizations. Several University of Rochester researchers were nationally known for their work on topics including the contributions of lead in dust to children's blood lead levels, lead's role in osteoporosis, and the effects of low levels of lead on neurodevelopment. CPLP regularly invited University of Rochester researchers to present their latest findings about the human health effects of lead to its members and other key stakeholders. Although these detailed research findings did not directly influence the community's policy choices, such presentations enhanced the community's knowledge about lead, boosted CPLP's credibility, and helped keep lead "in the news."

Finally, CPLP secured technical support from national groups such as the Alliance for Healthy Homes and the National Center for Healthy Housing. These groups shared experiences from other cities, gave feedback on emerging proposals, and conducted new analyses of unpublished data to address Rochester's specific information needs. CPLP members also maintained connections with federal agency staff, including the Centers for Disease Control and Prevention Lead Branch and the HUD Office of Healthy Homes. Committee members maintained these connections by attending national lead and healthy homes meetings, participating in online networks, and communicating with national groups about ongoing local projects, emerging questions, and policy proposals.

Get the Lead Out (GLO)   Dr. Richard Kennedy, then a family physician at the Orchard Street Community Health Center at School 17, worked directly with Principal Ralph Spezio and joined CPLP early on. As he learned more about the causes of lead poisoning, he grew frustrated by his inability to prevent lead poisoning among his young patients. As he said, "When you learn that 41 percent of your patients are lead poisoned, what is a community doctor to do?" Kennedy responded by securing a small grant to test the homes of children in his practice for lead hazards. Partnering with the University of Rochester COEC, medical students, a VISTA volunteer, a lead risk assessor, and the neighborhood group JOSANA (the Jay and Orchard Street Area Neighborhood Association), he initiated the "Get the Lead Out" (GLO) project (O'Fallon 2004). GLO found lead hazards in 98 percent of the homes it tested and estimated an average cost of lead hazard repairs using interim controls at $3,300 (Korfmacher 2010). These homes were mostly private rental properties. GLO educated families to help them avoid lead hazards, notified the property owner of the hazards, referred them to existing funding sources, coordinated with the local code enforcement office, and, when necessary, helped the families locate safer housing. Despite this support system, GLO found that fewer than a third of the properties it assessed were made lead-safe as a result of its information and education efforts. This finding supported the CPLP's claim that education and knowledge alone were not sufficient to protect children.

GLO demonstrated the need for an improved housing quality policy system. The rental properties assessed by GLO were subject to the city's existing Certificate of Occupancy inspection system, which prohibited deteriorated paint. Nonetheless, GLO found deteriorated paint in nearly all of these properties. It concluded that the system of rental housing inspection and enforcement was not effectively protecting children.

In addition, GLO documented the stories of families facing lead hazards in their homes. For example, GLO staff told the city council about testing the house of a one-year-old child with blood lead levels just above the public health level of concern, which at the time was 10 µg/dL. GLO's risk assessor reported the lead hazards to the landlord and referred him to a local housing grant program and free lead-safe work practices training, but no action was taken. Meanwhile, the child's blood lead level continued to rise to over 20 µg/dL, at which point state law required the health department to assess lead hazards in the home and require repairs. Subsequent investigation by GLO showed that city inspectors had previously cited fifty-nine code violations in the house, but that deteriorated paint on windows—the most significant lead risk to the child—had not been cited. This child was poisoned despite the best efforts of her parents, her doctor, and GLO staff to

use existing systems to protect her. This case further demonstrated that neither the existing housing code inspection system nor education to promote
voluntary action were effective. Perhaps most important, GLO showed that
without a change in policy, the community was powerless to prevent continued poisoning of its most vulnerable members. GLO convinced CPLP
that simply informing residents, landlords, and government agencies about
lead hazards was not enough: a policy change was needed.

Identifying Cost-Efficient Lead Hazard Control Solutions   The 2002 Center for Governmental Research needs assessment report estimated the total
cost to make Rochester lead-safe was between $605 million and $5.6 billion.
These figures were based on per-unit costs of $7,556 to make a unit lead-
safe and up to $70,000 for complete rehabilitation, respectively (Boyce and
Hood 2002). These figures reinforced fears that pursuing lead safety would
bankrupt the city. The higher cost estimates reflected full lead abatement,
which involves removing all lead hazards according to standards set by
the Environmental Protection Agency (U.S. EPA 2000). Other, more recent
housing-based lead laws, such as the Massachusetts law, had required partial abatement; however, even this approach was deemed to be too costly
for Rochester because of its low property values and weak rental housing
market (State of Massachusetts 2016; Brown 2002; Mares 2003).

To inform an alternative, less costly approach, CPLP summarized emerging research on housing interventions to reduce lead hazards. These summaries showed that lower-cost interim controls could effectively control
lead hazards if combined with proper maintenance and monitoring (Dixon
et al. 2005). CPLP also reviewed local experience with lower cost lead
hazard controls. Local data came from a housing rehabilitation program
funded by a 2002 HUD Lead Hazard Control grant to the Monroe County
Department of Public Health. Health department staff reported that the
average cost to make a unit lead-safe under this program was $3,253 per
unit for interim controls ($5,598 for interim controls with window replace-
ment) (Korfmacher 2010). The GLO project had estimated similar repair
costs. These figures were well below the lowest cost estimated in the Center
for Government Research needs assessment report (Boyce and Hood 2002).
Thus, emerging national data on efficacy of interim controls combined with
local data on costs of interim controls supported CPLP's arguments for
this cost-effective strategy. This approach reduced the anticipated costs of

making the city's highest risk housing lead-safe, addressing a key barrier to policy change.

Informing the Inspection Approach While the cost of lead hazard controls was the biggest concern of landlords, city officials were also concerned about the costs, logistics, and liabilities involved in testing houses for lead. One option was to contract out inspections to private EPA-certified risk assessors, who would conduct a thorough assessment of each house at a cost of around $400 per unit. City officials argued that this was too expensive for the city to subsidize and landlords insisted that they could not afford to pay for private risk assessments. Instead, both city staff and landlord groups initially maintained that visual inspections for deteriorated paint would be sufficient.

CPLP argued that visual inspections could not detect invisible lead in dust. The Rochester Lead in Dust Study had previously shown lead in dust to be correlated with children's blood lead levels (Boyce and Hood 2002; Lanphear et al. 1995). CPLP asked the University of Rochester COEC staff to help identify an inspection protocol that would be more cost-effective. The COEC staff worked with the National Center for Healthy Housing (NCHH) to summarize recent research and found that a significant percentage of homes with no observable lead hazards had hazardous levels of lead in dust (Breysse et al. 2007; Jacobs et al. 2002). Based on these findings, CPLP proposed that the city use the EPA's lead clearance protocol for testing after lead hazard control work is completed. In "clearance testing," a certified Lead Dust Sampling Technician does a visual inspection and takes at least eight dust wipe samples, which are sent to a certified laboratory for analysis (U.S. EPA 2009c). The average cost of a clearance test was around $150, much less than the cost of a full lead-risk assessment (Korfmacher 2010).

CPLP staff and members coordinated with stakeholders and decision makers throughout the policy process to assemble data, research, and community knowledge to address their concerns, answer questions, and inform a cost-effective approach to prevent childhood lead poisoning. One city council member complained to the CPLP co-chair that it was impossible to find experts who were *not* part of CPLP when they wanted an "independent expert" to critique CPLP's positions (Hetherington 2016). Another noted that, because of the complexity of the lead issue and the scientific credibility of and breadth of expertise accessed by CPLP, this was the first time he had seen the city council rely more on an outside group than on city staff to inform policy development (Korfmacher 2008, 2010). Thus, collaborating with local researchers, health care professionals, community members, government agencies, and national organizations to generate, use, and translate information was a critical part of CPLP's efforts to promote systems change.

Supporting Policy Change

CPLP interacted extensively with city council members, staff, and key stakeholders to provide the knowledge needed to design and pass a cost-effective lead law. CPLP's research and analysis capacity was accessed regularly during development of the Rochester lead law. After the law was passed, CPLP continued to coordinate with multiple stakeholders to support implementation, evaluation, and adaptation of the law and related efforts. Thus, CPLP's collaborative efforts supported systems change through multiple phases of the policy process (Korfmacher et al. 2016).

Developing the Rochester Lead Law   Mayor William Johnson's commitment at the 2004 Community Lead Summit to pass a comprehensive lead law before leaving office launched a policy process that produced three separate legislative proposals, an environmental impact statement, and dozens of public meetings over 18 months. On December 20, 2005, the Rochester City Council unanimously passed the state's first local lead poisoning prevention ordinance outside New York City. The new local law went into effect in July 2006 (City of Rochester 2005). This law has been heralded as a national model, embodying the most recent medical and housing research on lead poisoning prevention in an economically feasible approach (Prevention Institute 2010; Pew Charitable Trusts 2017).

Importantly, CPLP's policy approach was also informed by community representatives on its committees and input from residents through GLO. For example, renters' fears of retaliatory eviction reinforced CPLP's position that the law must not rely on tenant complaints. Their concerns about housing discrimination against families convinced CPLP that the law must target all high-risk housing, not just child-occupied housing. This decision was reinforced by community and social service agency members' reports about how frequently low-income families moved and how many children may be exposed to lead from spending time in multiple older facilities, including in-home informal day care centers and friends' or grandparents' homes. The observation that children frequently play on porches because of concerns about crime in high-risk neighborhoods led CPLP to insist on a porch dust standard in the final proposal.

Rather than promoting a single specific policy proposal, CPLP developed five "principles for an effective lead law" (Korfmacher 2008):

1. Targeted Roll-Out: Protect the kids who are at the greatest risk first.
2. Required Inspection and Lead Hazard Control: Inspect buildings, not bodies, to find hazards before kids are poisoned.
3. Lead-Safe Work Practices: Do the work safely—don't make the problem worse!
4. Disclosure: Warn people about lead poisoning risks when they buy or rent, and when work is being done.
5. Tenant Protection: Don't let the tenants be punished for asking for safe housing!

CPLP gathered information from the health department, Get the Lead Out, and the city to project the impacts of various proposals. It also relied on information from other cities, national healthy housing groups, and housing research to comment on how effectively each of the successive policy proposals met these five principles.

An additional underlying criterion was to develop a policy that would not significantly disrupt the Rochester economy, housing market, or availability of low-income rental housing. As a result of this commitment, CPLP's objectives for the lead law focused on maintaining lead-safe housing, not removing all lead.

One proposal, drafted by a public interest attorney who served on the CPLP housing committee and submitted by City Councilman Tim Mains, who was also a Rochester elementary school principal, would have required landlords to pay for risk assessments. Another proposal developed by a coalition of landlords relied on publicly funded inspection of child-occupied homes (both rental and owner-occupied units). City staff developed a third proposal that added lead to the city's existing inspections process.

The final lead law was based on the third model. As adopted, it added lead to the "Certificate of Occupancy" inspections already being carried out by the city in all rental housing. Under the city's longstanding Certificate of Occupancy program, inspections must be carried out every three years in buildings with three or more rental units, and every six years for one- and two-unit rental buildings (Korfmacher and Holt 2018; City of Rochester 2018). Although the statewide Property Maintenance Code that guided these inspections already prohibited deteriorated paint, as GLO had discovered, minor deterioration of paint was sometimes overlooked by city inspectors and there was no presumption that deteriorated paint posed a lead hazard.

Based on the information it had collected, CPLP argued for including dust wipes as part of the new lead law (Korfmacher 2010). City staff countered that this would be cost-prohibitive. As a compromise, they agreed to use Monroe County Department of Public Health data on the location of homes of children with elevated blood lead levels to designate "high risk" areas within the city. Under this compromise, only houses in the high-risk area that passed a visual inspection for deteriorated paint inside the house would also receive dust wipes. While this approach may appear counter-intuitive (i.e., requiring additional testing in the *absence* of deteriorated paint), it was based on research showing that dust hazards exist in a significant proportion of homes with intact paint (Jacobs et al. 2002; HUD 2011). This scenario is particularly likely when painters disturb old paint and leave lead dust behind. If interior deteriorated paint was observed or a dust wipe test failed, the city would issue a compliance notice requiring the owner to address the hazard and obtain a lead clearance by a certified lead inspector or risk assessor. This system added a degree of protection in high-risk areas. The dust wipe lab test also provided built-in quality control for inspectors' visual assessment of paint condition.

The Rochester law included two triggers for inspection in addition to the periodic Certificate of Occupancy inspections. The first mechanism allowed occupants, community groups, or doctors to request inspections on a "complaint" basis. Second, as promised by Monroe County Executive Maggie Brooks at the 2004 Community Lead Summit, the county added lead inspections to its Quality Housing Inspections (QHI) program for county-subsidized housing (Korfmacher 2010). The QHI program had been established years earlier to protect the county from fraudulent damage claims. In order to receive direct payment of rent from the county, a property owner could request a QHI to document the condition of the apartment before and after the Department of Human Services client's tenure.

As of 2005, the city was conducting around 2,000 of these inspections under contract from the county each year. CPLP argued that these were by definition high-lead-risk units that merited more frequent inspection (CGR 2015). According to CPLP co-chair Bryan Hetherington, "We reached out to county executives and said that tax dollars were being used for housing that was poisoning kids," which persuaded the county to add lead to the QHI program (Hetherington 2016). These two additional mechanisms, complaint and QHI, ensured more frequent inspections of high-risk units (Korfmacher and Hanley 2013).

It is important to note that the Rochester lead law did not set forth standards for *how* to repair lead hazards. Thus, property owners cited for lead hazards could simply repaint and clean without removing paint from friction and impact surfaces as required by HUD's guidelines for "interim controls" (HUD 2012). CPLP acknowledged that these temporary control measures could fail within a few years. Proponents hoped property owners would be incentivized by the periodic reinspections to invest in more permanent controls and to maintain units free of lead hazards.

After incorporation of the dust wipe protocol, targeting of highest-risk neighborhoods, and the ability for tenants to request extra inspections on demand, CPLP leadership decided the city's proposal met its five principles for a sufficiently protective law. Accordingly, CPLP encouraged its members to show their support by attending the city council meeting on December 20, 2005, at which a vote on the law was expected. Over fifty supporters filled the council chambers holding signs on paint sticks reading, "Let's Make Lead History." Numerous rental property owners also attended to voice their opposition to the proposed ordinance. Going into the meeting, three of the nine council members were expected to oppose the proposal. Just before the vote, one city council member, elementary school principal Tim Mains, gave an impassioned speech about how important the law was to children in his school. This emotional appeal appeared to sway several additional members of council. Another city council member, Wade Norwood, later said that "there was a tidal wave of facts" and "a moral, scientific, and community imperative that the ordinance pass" (Dissell and Zeltner 2015a). The law passed unanimously, along with three accompanying resolutions:

1. Resolution 2005–23, requiring the city to report annually on the progress of inspections over time and establishing a process to update the

"high risk area" based on county health department data on where 90 percent of children with elevated blood lead levels reside.

2. Resolution 2005–24, encouraging funding and implementation of education campaigns and establishing a community-based advisory committee to monitor initial implementation.

3. Resolution 2005–25, establishing a voluntary program for owner-occupants to receive free lead inspections and establishing a registry of lead-safe properties.

The date for implementation was set as July 1, 2006, to give the city inspectors and property owners time to prepare for the new lead inspections.

After the lead law was passed, the city presented it to the Codes Council of the New York State Department of State for review to make sure it was not preempted by the statewide Uniform Fire Prevention and Building Code. The Codes Council determined that because lead paint was not explicitly addressed in the state code, the Rochester code was therefore neither more nor less restrictive and it was allowed to stand (Kirkmire 2018).

Implementing Systems Change   CPLP recognized that passing an inspections law alone would not address lead hazards. It actively supported the city's implementation efforts, maintained public education and communications, and pursued other local systems changes to complement the law.

The city of Rochester's Division of Inspections was responsible for training inspectors, developing protocols, and educating property owners about compliance with the new law. The CPLP role included public communication about the lead law to help tenants, community groups, and property owners know what to expect and how to comply. In addition, CPLP advocated that the county health department contribute funds from its lead Primary Prevention Program to help subsidize the added costs of inspections by the city. The county agreed to give the city over $200,000 per year to defray dust wipe costs.

CPLP also promoted other local primary prevention efforts. CPLP worked closely with the Rochester City School District to develop a lead-safety inspection and maintenance program for school buildings, which was adopted in 2007 (Rochester City School District 2007). CPLP's government relations subcommittee provided a forum for the Rochester Housing Authority and the city to coordinate—for example, by harmonizing their inspection protocols—which saved money by reducing duplicate inspections. CPLP wrote letters of support for the city's and the county's lead hazard control grant proposals to HUD; between 2002 and 2016, HUD provided over $30 million in grants to make low-income owner- and investor-owned properties in Rochester lead-safe. CPLP continued to advocate that outlying towns in Monroe County adopt lead laws, albeit with limited success. For example, in 2014 the adjacent Town of Irondequoit started requiring contractors to show proof of EPA Renovation, Repair, and Painting (RRP) certification as part of certain building permits (Town of Irondequoit 2018). CPLP's promotion of primary prevention helped ensure effective implementation, community support, and coordination among local government agencies after the lead law passed.

Notably, CPLP's successful collaborative approach caught the attention of other initiatives to change social determinants of health in Rochester. For example, the Finger Lakes Health Systems Agency modeled its Healthy Kids anti-obesity initiative on the lead coalition. CPLP also informed the Rochester Safe and Efficient Homes Initiative, a cooperative effort to integrate healthy housing into other grant-funded housing repair work. CPLP members have given numerous presentations on coalition-building to other communities within and outside New York.

Adaptation The CPLP Government Relations committee continued to meet monthly after passage of the law. One regular function of this committee was to review inspection data and consult on potential changes to the law. The first proposed change came in January 2006, when a group of landlords petitioned newly elected Mayor Robert Duffy to block implementation. They noted that although the Rochester law generally followed the EPA's clearance protocols, there was no precedent for Rochester's porch dust lead standard. CPLP responded that parents had reported that children frequently play on porches to avoid dangers in the neighborhood, so there were concerns both about lead exposure on porches and dust tracked into homes. Nonetheless, the landlord group was successful in getting this provision removed. CPLP later worked with the National Center for Healthy Housing and the City of Rochester's HUD grant program on a study that informed efforts to establish a national porch dust lead standard (Wilson et al. 2015). In 2017, HUD modified its clearance protocols to include a porch dust lead standard (HUD 2017). Thus, Rochester's local effort played a role in changing federal policy.

In 2010, Monroe County eliminated its Quality Housing Inspections (QHI) program because of budgetary concerns unrelated to lead. CPLP noted that this left a crucial gap in testing of high-risk homes. To fill that gap, CPLP worked with the City of Rochester and the Monroe County Department of Public Health and the Monroe County Department of Human Services (DHS) on a pilot to reinspect homes with earlier violations and found hazards in the majority of these children's homes. As a result, in January 2014, the city amended its lead law to provide more frequent inspections in units where lead hazards were previously found. The county DHS made lack of a valid Certificate of Occupancy a "health and safety" violation, triggering rent withholding in units with unaddressed hazards. This change greatly increased compliance with the city's inspection program.

The lead law also gave the city authority to audit and, if necessary, sanction third-party clearance testing firms found to have poor quality control. The lead law required property owners to obtain a clearance from a private firm after lead hazards were identified and repaired. Over time, a number of the private clearance firms were found to be falsifying dust wipe tests. In response, the City of Rochester suspended several clearance providers from doing dust wipe tests for a year.

In 2008, the U.S. EPA issued its Renovation, Repair, and Painting rule (RRP), which included training requirements, standards, and enforcement mechanisms for renovations that disturb paint in pre-1978 homes and child-occupied facilities (U.S. EPA 2014c). With support from CPLP, the city introduced and passed an amendment to the Rochester law to make the requirement for lead-safe work practices consistent with the new federal standards. The city also leveraged the RRP by requiring that all contractors receiving city permits for renovation of pre-1978 homes—both rented and owner-occupied—show proof of RRP certification. This approach allowed the city to reinforce the federal rule, augmenting the U.S. EPA's limited capacity to enforce at the local level. CPLP's ongoing involvement helped identify such needs for adaptation, develop appropriate responses, and promote community understanding of changes to local policies.

CPLP recognized that evaluation was key because (1) Rochester's lead law was a unique new model that might need adaptation; (2) documentation of progress could sustain support for implementation; and (3) it was an opportunity to learn lessons to share with other communities. CPLP was involved in several efforts to evaluate the progress of the lead law.

Evaluation was embedded in the law itself, which required the city to pub-licly report annual data on the number of inspections conducted, passing rates for visual, dust, and exterior inspections, and clearance rates. This data showed that inspections were keeping pace with the city's goal of inspect-ing all high-risk rental units before 2010. Passing rates for both visual and dust wipe inspections were over 90 percent, much higher than had been anticipated. This indicated that property owners understood and were able to successfully address the law's requirements prior to inspection. Passing rates continued to increase over time, suggesting that landlords were learn-ing to successfully maintain lead-safe units. Another built-in evaluation mechanism was a requirement to review requests for emergency housing received by the county related to lead. This provision was included as a safeguard to make sure the lead law was not inadvertently causing housing disruptions for low-income families. The review found that lead was cited as a cause in only a handful of the hundreds of emergency housing cases each year (Korfmacher, Ayoob, and Morley 2012).

In collaboration with CPLP, the Center for Governmental Research (CGR) received funding in 2007 from the Greater Rochester Health Foundation to conduct an evaluation of the first four years of the lead law (Boyce, Ruffer, and Ayoob 2008; Korfmacher, Ayoob, and Morley 2012). CGR analyzed the county's EBLL data alongside the city's inspections data, conducted a land-lord survey, and convened focus groups to explore the law's impacts. This study found that implementation had proceeded as planned with nearly all target units inspected in the first four years, higher than expected inspec-tion passing rates, and no major disruptions of the Rochester housing mar-ket (Korfmacher, Ayoob, and Morley 2012). The Monroe County health director published a paper in 2014 showing a decline in EBLL cases from 13.4 percent to 1.1 percent of children tested in Monroe County between 1997 and 2011, 2.4 times faster than in upstate New York as a whole, and noting that "the experience of Monroe County demonstrates the role of local health department capacity and community-based efforts in reducing sources of environmental lead exposure for children beyond national and statewide policies" (Kennedy et al. 2014, 263).

Promoting Primary Prevention beyond Rochester   In addition to support-ing lead poisoning prevention in Rochester, CPLP promoted policy changes at state and national levels. CPLP contributed to efforts to revise state lead policies and increase state resources for primary prevention. CPLP members were active in the New York State Coalition to End Lead Poisoning, a loose statewide affiliation of stakeholders that supported a comprehensive primary prevention bill. With CPLP's support, this bill was introduced by Rochester-area elected officials. It passed in 2008 but was vetoed by Governor David Patterson because of concerns about its economic impact following that year's stock market crash. Nonetheless, this legislation paved the way for expansion of the state's Primary Prevention Program, which eventually provided funding to health departments in fifteen high-risk counties to conduct additional lead prevention activities (New York State Department of Health 2019).

Despite this failure to achieve statewide primary prevention legislation, CPLP continued to advocate for changes in state policy to fill needs identified through its local work. For example, at the urging of its Screening and Professional Education committee, CPLP successfully advocated for a state policy change to allow school nurses to access students' lead levels in their health records. They were also successful in changing the language on blood test reports statewide to call attention to the dangers of lead levels below 10 µg/dL.

CPLP contributed to national lead poisoning prevention efforts by disseminating the story of the Rochester lead law through presentations, publications, news media, and outreach. In 2009, CPLP received an Environmental Justice Achievement Award in recognition of its efforts (U.S. EPA 2009a).

Through this publicity, staff at a local health department in Michigan heard about the Rochester lead law and encouraged the City of Benton Harbor to adopt a similar law. Benton Harbor is an older city with high-risk housing and elevated rates of lead poisoning, so the Rochester approach seemed an appropriate analogue. Health department staff invited representatives from Rochester to brief Benton Harbor city staff about the law, which was passed without significant discussion or opposition. However, Benton Harbor had only two housing inspectors and no proactive code enforcement. In addition, soon after the law was passed, the city government was taken over by the state of Michigan because of financial troubles. As a result, no lead inspections were conducted. Thus, while Benton Harbor had a nearly identical lead law to Rochester's "on the books," it had little if any impact on childhood lead poisoning prevention.

National interest in lead poisoning prevention spiked after the Flint water crisis was publicized in 2015 (Bellinger 2016; Butler, Scammell, and Benson 2016). Soon after, national advocates organized a "Find It, Fix It, Fund It" campaign—coincidentally adopting one of CPLP's early slogans—to push for national policy changes and resources to address childhood lead poisoning (National Center for Healthy Housing 2017). Several projects were undertaken to identify promising local models, and Rochester was frequently cited as an example (Pew Charitable Trusts 2017; National League of Cities 2017).

In the wake of this renewed interest in lead poisoning prevention, many cities contacted Rochester for advice on developing their own local housing-based lead laws (Dissell and Zeltner 2015a, 2015b, 2019; Lindstrom 2017; Tevlock 2014). In responding, CPLP members and city staff explained that the lead law was developed to work in the context of Rochester's community resources, its housing market, and, most important, its preexisting system of proactive code enforcement. Instead of recommending "replication" of the Rochester code, they advised building a community coalition to determine the best approach for each city and developing broad-based support for its implementation (Korfmacher and Hanley 2013). CPLP also highlighted the fact that the Rochester lead law was actually a rather modest, low-cost intervention appropriate to local context: because Rochester already had proactive code enforcement, adding lead to the inspection cost relatively little. In contrast, most smaller cities lack a proactive rental housing inspection system (Korfmacher and Holt 2018; ChangeLab Solutions 2014). CPLP members pointed to Benton Harbor as a cautionary tale of adopting a policy without first developing a strong local consensus about what works for each unique community, municipal governance system, financial resources, and housing market.

Summary　CPLP's role in the policy process evolved over time. By first developing community support for ending childhood lead poisoning, CPLP generated support for the "what"—a comprehensive local lead law—that was able to minimize conflict about the "how"—which specific policy measures should be adopted. With the policy in place, the organization stayed involved in monitoring progress, coordinating implementation, and adapting the law.

Applying the Local Environmental Health Initiative Framework to CPLP

Rochester is similar to many cities with high rates of childhood lead poisoning. However, CPLP's collaborative process and the resulting local lead law are fairly unique. CPLP brought together a wide range of stakeholders, marshaled diverse evidence, and participated in a policy process to pass a housing-based lead law and supportive systems changes. Using the framework set forth in chapter 3, table 4.3 characterizes how CPLP supported local policy change.

Issue Framing and Problem Definition

CPLP realized early in its formation that since solutions lie in the housing sector, framing lead primarily as a medical issue was a significant barrier to lead poisoning prevention. Therefore, its communications, information, and policy efforts reframed the issue as a "disease kids catch from their houses." By focusing on geographic concentrations of children with lead poisoning in low-income neighborhoods and among communities of color, CPLP also highlighted lead as an issue of environmental justice. CPLP's messages connected with community concerns about the health, education, and economic future of Rochester's children. Additionally, CPLP broadened the definition of the "health" impacts of lead to include impacts of childhood lead poisoning on the whole community, including failing schools, increased criminal incidents, long-term health costs, and reduced earning potential by affected children.

Resources for Collaboration

Rochester is a relatively small city with a high poverty rate. It has a large number of active community, health, and advocacy organizations, but the resources of these groups shrank during the period CPLP was most active, as did the budgets of the city housing and county health departments. The University of Rochester has a medical school and an Environmental Health Sciences Center with a commitment to outreach. By leveraging these and other community assets, CPLP was able to sustain collaborative efforts to educate stakeholders, build support, and pass a local lead law that became a national model.

Human Resources The CPLP's committee members provided human resources that were the primary strength of the collaboration. The seven working committees engaged over a hundred people at the height of

Table 4.3
CPLP and the Local Environmental Health Initiative Framework

Collaborative Function	Analysis of CPLP
Issue framing and problem definition	Redefined childhood lead poisoning as threat to children's well-being caused largely by hazards in low-income pre-1978 rental housing.
	Highlighted concentration of hazards in low-income urban communities of color, as well as pockets of cases throughout county.
	Framing called for engagement of housing, children's advocates, educators, health professionals, and community leaders.
Resources for collaboration	Wide range of skills accessed through members' professional and volunteer roles, lending credibility, skills, and visibility to the effort.
	Modest funding raised to support core functions of coalition (activities and staff).
Structure and decision-making process	Sustained core committees and structure for over 18 years.
	Hosted and fiscally administered by series of community organizations.
	Structure and decision processes changed over time. In early years, detailed bylaws ensured a strong decision role for affected communities. Structures became more informal as CPLP transitioned to a coordinating role.
	Board included 30% affected community members; others included through outreach events and community group partners.
	Decisions made by consensus.
Impacts of collaboration:	
Outputs	Presentations, articles, media interviews, press releases, PSA's and written educational materials.
	Analyses, research summaries, and policy proposals.
	Community Lead Summit and other events.
Social outcomes	CPLP members collaborated on other issues and contributed to subsequent community coalitions in Rochester (healthy homes, obesity, etc.).
Impacts on policies, systems, and environments (PSE)	Built community support for policy change (city lead law, school lead policy, county government practices).
	Prevalence of lead hazards in inspected housing declined.
	Rate of lead poisoning declined more rapidly than in other cities.
	Helped bring $30 million in housing grants to city.
	Informed lead policy efforts in other communities.

activities, with several hundred additional people signed up as members. The CPLP was able to leverage human resources because individuals believed that the issue was important and the collaborative process was promising. As former CPLP co-chair Bryan Hetherington said, "We are not going to end poverty in my lifetime, but this one we can win!" (Hetherington 2016). This sense of optimism grew with the credibility, size, and activity of the organization. The CPLP staff and leadership also excelled at defining roles and tasks for members that gave them a sense of concrete contribution to the effort's success (Korfmacher 2010).

CPLP staff provided direct community outreach and public communications support. Staffing was limited by funding, so CPLP relied on the working committees to accomplish CPLP's objectives and goals.

Knowledge Resources   CPLP's broad-based membership provided technical expertise, community knowledge, and access to data. Knowledge resources were provided through the expertise of working committee members, technical information members obtained through their organizations, and connections with national nonprofits and government agencies involved in lead poisoning prevention. CPLP's science-based approach, clear structure, and strategic process made it safe, straightforward, and rewarding for local experts—including health care providers, lawyers, and researchers—to provide input, thus boosting the group's credibility. Sometimes experts hesitate to get involved in advocacy groups for fear their technical contributions will be disregarded or manipulated for political gain, thus damaging their credibility. CPLP's demonstrated commitment to science and medical expertise assuaged these concerns. CPLP's efforts to maintain representation by affected community members provided knowledge about low-income families' preferences, priorities, and perceptions about lead. As former city councilman Wade Norwood noted when asked about CPLP's access to expertise, "Understanding can't become wisdom without context. ... So, the experts need to be embedded in the community to help them gain this understanding" (Norwood 2007). CPLP was a place where this productive exchange could happen.

Financial Resources   Funding for CPLP came from a variety of sources, including government agencies, the charitable giving of private companies, and foundations. Some of CPLP's funding was used to support production and dissemination of communications materials. Other funds were project-based, and staff was directed by grant deliverables such as conducting a certain number of training and outreach events. For most of its existence, CPLP was able to maintain core support for dedicated staff time to lead the organization, support committee work, and seek additional funding. A number of funders, particularly United Way, were attracted to CPLP's efforts to promote lasting community benefits through systems change.

Group Structure and Decision-Making Processes   CPLP's structure and decision-making processes changed over time from a robust group of seven committees and a decision-making board to a more informal coordinating organization led by a small executive committee. CPLP's approach to consensus-building both internally and externally made it an effective policy advocate despite its limited financial resources. Even when CPLP set aside its original bylaws, the organization maintained clear processes for obtaining consensus and approval for actions taken on behalf of the organization.

Although CPLP had strong involvement by government staff, none held a decision-making role. This reflected both government and community members' recognition that CPLP would advocate for policy change that would affect their agencies. As former school principal Spezio recalled, the county health director visited a CPLP meeting and "as he was leaving, he said, 'it's very difficult for me to change this from the inside. Bureaucracies need external pushes. Keep pushing me.' ... That was courageous of him!" (Spezio 2017). This balance between collaboration and advocacy was an ongoing dynamic in CPLP's approach.

CPLP never had independent status as a not-for-profit organization; instead, it operated under the auspices of a series of host agencies. Nonetheless, the CPLP Board maintained primary responsibility for fund-raising, staff decisions, strategy, and activities. During each transition to a new fiscal agent, the CPLP Board members considered carefully whether the host agency would try to control the initiative's activities and received clear assurances of their independence. Despite these changes, CPLP was able to sustain a functional decision process and committee structure over nearly twenty years.

Collaborative Outputs and Outcomes

CPLP's activities contributed to systems changes in the Rochester community and beyond. The CPLP's primary outputs were its information materials, presentations, and communications. Its applied analyses, research summaries, and policy proposals also informed the policy process. Another "output" of the organization was the multiple opportunities it created to engage stakeholders, ranging from committee meetings to the Community Lead Summit.

The most visible outcome of these efforts was the passage of the Rochester lead law. The accompanying commitment by Monroe County to inspect homes of families receiving public housing assistance through the Quality Housing Inspections program was also important. The increased community awareness of the lead problem, incorporation of lead prevention into multiple organizations' activities, and the ongoing collaboration between city and county governments around housing, health, and children's well-being were less tangible but important outcomes.

To what extent CPLP's efforts contributed to the decline in lead poisoning rates in the City of Rochester cannot be definitively determined. Lead poisoning rates have been consistently decreasing throughout the country, even in cities without lead laws. Other factors, including changes in the housing market, demolition of high-risk housing, community education, and ongoing public health programs have contributed to this trend. Furthermore, lead is a multimedia toxicant that may be present in soil, dust, water, or consumer products, so changes in housing alone are unlikely to fully explain trends in population blood lead levels. However, inspection data, program evaluations, and reports by key informants suggest that CPLP's efforts significantly helped Rochester reduce childhood lead poisoning more rapidly than other similar cities. Finally, CPLP actively disseminated lessons learned from its experiences and advised other localities on how to address lead, contributing to national lead poisoning prevention efforts.

Conclusions

Despite CPLP's significant progress, it is important to remember that the local law that is the lynchpin of Rochester's housing-based system does not require full removal of lead and therefore relies on regular inspections and constant community vigilance. If the ongoing inspections and educational efforts were to cease, lead hazards could increase. The economic pressures on property owners, decreasing budgets of local governments, and continued declines in the number of lead-poisoned children could reduce the sense of social urgency around childhood lead poisoning over time. There may be future pressures to weaken these local lead programs. To the extent that CPLP's educational efforts, the city's integration of lead into ongoing inspections, and the county's commitment to help fund these inspections continue, these accomplishments may be considered sustainable. Since they do not rely on removing all lead from buildings, however, in a physical sense these reductions in environmental health risk are not permanent. Nonetheless, the continuity of Rochester's lead inspection program despite the city's fiscal hardships suggests that it is a durable change in practice.

As innovative and unique as the Rochester experience may appear, the story of CPLP has been played out in similar fashion multiple times, notably in New York City, decades before passage of Rochester's law (Freudenberg and Golub 1987; Pueschel and Fadden 1975). Efforts elsewhere resulted in very different systems to address lead (Korfmacher and Hanley 2013). Thus, the particulars of lead laws are not necessarily transferable from place to place. At the same time, experiences like that of Benton Harbor where local lead policy efforts have been passed but not effectively implemented suggest that developing community support for the policy may be as important as the specific approach adopted (Laker, Ruderman, and Purcell 2016).

Looking back at CPLP's history, former county health director Dr. Andrew Doniger said, "It was such a wonderful sequence of events that it's hard to be critical in any way" (Doniger 2017). What made this successful process possible in Rochester? A combination of community context, leadership, and resources all contributed. The question of what might promote similar conditions in other communities is further explored in chapter 8.

5 Healthy Duluth: Toward Equity in the Built Environment

Case Summary

In 2008, local health department staff in Duluth, Minnesota, viewed *Unnatural Causes,* a video series about the contribution of social determinants to health disparities. These ideas resonated with their observations about health problems in low-income neighborhoods in their city. Since then, community groups, public health professionals, and city staff have engaged in a range of efforts to promote health equity by improving the built environment. These organizations integrated health considerations into their plans, activities, analyses, grant proposals, policies, and projects, focusing on increasing opportunities for physical activity and food access. Many communities have engaged in one-time projects or grant-funded programs to improve environmental health determinants, but Duluth's efforts stand out with respect to breadth of scope, collaboration, and sustainability. This work culminated in Mayor Emily Larson's 2016 announcement that health and fairness would be adopted as key goals of the city's new Comprehensive Plan. This chapter traces how these innovative initiatives evolved in what might seem an unlikely place: a small, postindustrial city ringed by Superfund sites that thirty years ago had one of the highest unemployment rates in the nation. This case offers insights about how state and national efforts to promote health-supportive environments can be institutionalized at the local level. The Healthy Duluth partners overcame barriers to collaboration between community and government stakeholders, promoted engagement to target the needs of disadvantaged communities, and leveraged diverse resources to sustain this work over time.

Introduction

Every day, we make decisions that affect our health. Should I walk, take a bus, or drive to work? Should I pick up fast food or buy vegetables for a salad? Should I stay inside and watch television or go outside for a walk with my friends? These health-affecting decisions are shaped in part by the accessibility, convenience, safety, and cost of the options available where we live, work, and play. However, public health has not historically been a primary goal of policies that shape neighborhood environments. Some people have better access to healthy food and physical activity opportunities in their neighborhoods than do others. Within many cities, lower-income neighborhoods have fewer health-supporting resources than do wealthier areas. These neighborhoods also tend to have higher rates of obesity, diabetes, heart disease, and other chronic health problems. Communities, government agencies, and researchers have worked to understand these connections and explore whether changing the built environment can improve health.

In Duluth, Minnesota, citizens, foundations, and agencies concerned about health inequities in their community have undertaken a range of efforts to improve the built environments of low-income neighborhoods. Their initiatives evolved from a focus on encouraging healthy eating and physical activity to improving food access and equitable opportunities for active transportation. A core focus was on how the built environment—including recreational trails, sidewalks, roadways, public transportation systems, food stores, restaurants, and community gardens—supports the health of diverse residents. A brief summary of emerging national movements to promote public health through the built environment provides context for explaining Duluth's efforts.

Historically, health policies focused on health *care*—its quality, accessibility, and cost. However, public health professionals increasingly recognize that people's health depends on their social conditions, economic status, and physical environments. The saying that "your zip code is a better predictor of your health than your genetic code" has become a popular refrain of public health advocates (Roeder 2014). Neighborhood characteristics such as walkability, safety, and the presence of grocery stores and other health-supportive services can significantly affect people's long-term health. However, the decisions that shape built environments do not explicitly take health into account. Because these decisions are often local, communities across the country are working to bring health into the decision processes of local governments, health systems, schools, philanthropic funders, and private developers.

Geographic differences in health outcomes are often associated with neighborhoods with concentrated poverty and higher proportions of racial and ethnic minorities (Murray et al. 2006). These neighborhoods also tend to have fewer environmental amenities and more hazards. The built environment in urban areas with a history of disinvestment, industrial pollution, and high concentrations of low-income residents is of particular concern. This section begins with an overview of how the built environment affects public health, especially as relates to obesity. This is followed by a brief history of how U.S. cities developed historically and the multiple decision processes that control future land use decisions.

Built Environment and Public Health: Food Access and Physical Activity

The built environment includes the buildings, roads, public spaces, and parks that make up our neighborhoods (Dannenberg, Frumkin, and Jackson 2011). Features of the built environment can directly affect health by exposing people to air pollution, contaminated water, or toxic waste. The built environment also indirectly affects health by shaping the opportunities, choices, and resources available to people. Public health professionals, researchers, and communities focus especially on characteristics of the built environment that shape residents' access to healthy food and physical activity. This renewed interest emerged from recognition of the startling and growing disparities in chronic health conditions like obesity, diabetes, and heart disease. The high cost of treating chronic diseases associated with obesity has focused attention on changing people's eating and exercise behaviors. Health care costs related to obesity were estimated at $147 billion in 2008 (CDC 2017a; Carlson et al. 2015; Lee et al. 2012). The limited success of behavior education efforts led public health professionals to recognize how difficult it is for low-income people to make healthy choices, especially when they live in neighborhoods with few healthy food and physical activity options. Thus, public health professionals shifted from a focus on shaping individuals' choices to changing the polices, systems, and environments that shape a community's access to healthy food and opportunities for physical activity.

The observation that the built environment impacts people's health is not new. As described in chapter 2, concerns about high rates of disease among low-income communities drove early policies to improve sanitation, food safety, housing, and air quality, but these connections weakened over time (Kochtitzky et al. 2006). More recently, this insight was the foundation of the "Healthy Communities" movement—a diverse range of public, private, and community efforts to shape communities' built environments to promote healthy eating and physical activity (Dannenberg, Frumkin, and Jackson 2011; Robert Wood Johnson Foundation 2018a).

The Healthy Communities Movement

With growing concern about the U.S. obesity epidemic in the early 2000s, government, nonprofit, and academic initiatives began trying to improve neighborhood resources. Many programs promoted food access and physical activity opportunities as "healthy living" or "healthy community" initiatives (Blackwell 2009). The Centers for Disease Control and Prevention (CDC) led early efforts to advance healthy living through community-level change. Between 2008 and 2012, the CDC's Healthy Communities program provided training, grants, and technical assistance to support community physical activity, healthy eating, and tobacco control efforts through a variety of initiatives, including grants from Pioneering Healthy Communities and Communities Putting Prevention to Work (CDC 2017b, 2017c).

Private foundations also played an important role. For example, starting around 2000, the Robert Wood Johnson Foundation (RWJF) made a significant commitment to funding active living research and pilot programs. The approach was explicitly modeled on earlier successes in tobacco control. The aim was to both build a research base and support systems-change initiatives in communities across the country (Orleans et al. 2009). The "Active Living by Design" initiative was launched in 2002 to promote environmental changes that encourage physical activity (Active Living by Design 2018). Over time, the program also grew to include healthy eating and other social determinants of health and in 2018 was renamed Healthy Places by Design (2018).

Programs such as Active Living by Design and many others initially focused on creating opportunities for recreational activities like walking and biking. However, they soon recognized that increasing physical activity as part of people's daily transportation routines was essential, especially in communities where people did not have the time, flexibility, discretionary income, or social support to engage in recreational physical activity (Community Prevention Services Task Force 2018). Public transportation was integrated in the active transportation initiatives because getting to transit stops often involves walking or biking.

One approach to creating more walkable and bikeable neighborhoods is improving the availability, safety, and design of sidewalks and trails. The concept of "complete streets" encourages active transportation by slowing motorized traffic, marking bike lanes, improving crosswalks, and enhancing transit facilities (e.g., bus stops) (Smart Growth America 2018). Crime prevention through environmental design (CPTED) principles were developed to improve lighting and other environmental features that discourage crime and increase people's feeling of safety so they are more likely to walk and bike (Crowe 2000; Mair and Mair 2003). Other initiatives like "Safe Routes to School" integrated infrastructure changes with programs such as working with schools to organize "walking school buses" for children (U.S. DOT 2012; CDC 2018a).

On the other side of the obesity equation, new initiatives promoted healthy food environments. Starting around 1990, the term "food desert" was used to describe neighborhoods lacking access to healthy foods (e.g a full-service grocery store) (Beaulac, Kristjansson, and Cummins 2009). Food deserts are most common in both low-income urban and rural neighborhoods (Grimm, Moore, and Scanlon 2013; Ver Ploeg 2010). However, in urban areas the term "food swamp" may be more accurate, since these neighborhoods frequently have many food outlets selling low-cost, unhealthy fast food (Luan, Law, and Quick 2015; Osorio, Corradini, and Williams 2013). One strategy to increase community sources of affordable healthy food focuses on developing local food production (CDC 2017d; ChangeLab Solutions 2018a; Harvard School of Public Health 2018). Community gardens and urban agriculture figure prominently in these strategies, as does increasing options for buying food by "greening" corner stores, bringing in farmers' markets, innovative financing for full-service grocery stores, and "mobile markets." A second strategy is to discourage unhealthy food sources by limiting the establishment of new fast-food and corner stores. Yet other programs work with school systems to improve the nutritional quality of school meals (Robert Wood Johnson Foundation 2018b).

No single approach is effective in combating obesity alone (Sallis et al. 2006; Grimm, Moore, and Scanlon 2013; Khan et al. 2009). Instead, as with reducing tobacco use, it appears that a multilevel combination of individual, institutional, and environmental changes is needed (Grimm, Moore, and Scanlon 2013). It is difficult to evaluate the impacts of such "complex systems comprised of diverse stakeholders engaging in multiple, inter-related activities across multiple levels" (Leeman et al. 2015). As a result, "despite the almost universal acceptance that changes in PSEs [policies, systems, and environments] will improve healthful behaviors, the hard evidence for their effectiveness is just beginning to emerge" (Honeycutt et al. 2015). Nonetheless, there is an emerging consensus that built environment strategies are an important component of integrated efforts to combat obesity.

The pursuit of built environment changes that support health requires new connections between public health, communities, the private sector, and multiple government agencies (Fulton et al. 2018). As stakeholders in Duluth realized, creating an environment where healthy eating and exercising is easier for everyone requires interaction with multiple decision-making systems at many levels. The next section explains some of the policy tools available to small, postindustrial cities like Duluth as they strive to redevelop in ways that promote health equity. It builds on the brief overview of local land use management provided in chapter 2 by highlighting the primary decision processes that affect land use, transportation resources, and food access in small cities like Duluth.

Policies, Institutions, and Actors That Shape the Local Built Environment
A comprehensive plan is a guide for a community's future (Peterson et al. 2018; American Planning Association 2015). A comprehensive plan sets forth a city's goals in a range of sectors, including land use, transportation, economic development, environment, and public facilities (Berke and Kaiser 2006; Dannenberg, Frumkin, and Jackson 2011; Cooperative Extension Service 2018). Comprehensive planning is ideally a participatory process that builds a public consensus around the future of the community. However, many cities—particularly smaller, less affluent cities—lack the staff capacity, resources, or political will to regularly update their plans, and these plans are generally nonbinding. Implementation of comprehensive plans requires sustained commitment from the city, private developers, and community organizations over time. Therefore, the planning process is important for

building the connections to support implementation, since it involves solic-
iting input from communities, businesses, and other stakeholders, collecting data from multiple sectors, and analyzing regional economic trends.

Land use plans usually feature prominently in comprehensive plans,
providing a geographical vision of what types of developments and uses
should occur, where, and how (Dannenberg, Frumkin, and Jackson 2011).
Zoning ordinances set forth what types of uses are allowed in which areas to
implement this vision (Maantay 2001, 2002). Building codes specify characteristics of developments and address matters such as fire safety, plumbing,
and electric and mechanical systems (Dannenberg, Frumkin, and Jackson
2011; Listokin and Hattis 2005). Cities also have property maintenance
codes that guide upkeep of existing buildings and facilities (International
Code Council 2015).

Once adopted, comprehensive plans may inform cities' applications for
grant funding, neighborhood land use plans, infrastructure improvements,
and development priorities. Implementing plans is complicated by the fact
that most land is privately owned, so decisions by housing, commercial,
and industrial developers determine what actually gets built. However,
cities control significant resources, including infrastructure, public facilities, parks, trails, and other public spaces. As well, cities may use tools like
reducing taxes, grants, or offering variances to encourage desired types of
private development.

Most cities have an office that plans, promotes, and oversees economic
development. Cities may partner with private or not-for-profit corporations
to build housing, commercial space, or industrial parks. Being involved in
project financing and design gives municipalities some control over when,
where, and how development happens. Cities can manage public infrastructure, including roads, water, and sewer, to influence this process. Some
cities charge private developers impact fees to help offset anticipated costs
to public infrastructure (Nelson and Moody 2003). Governments can serve
as a "land bank," buying up land as it becomes available and holding it
until a private developer comes forward (Dannenberg, Frumkin, and Jackson
2011). Thus, in addition to influencing development through planning
and zoning functions, a city may employ a wide range of tools to promote
development that fits its comprehensive plan.

Transportation planning is particularly complex. Although municipalities are responsible for planning, building, and maintaining local roads

within their borders, they must do so in accordance with federal and state design standards and in coordination with regional plans and programs. This makes sense, since local roadways connect with state and national highways, and there is a common national interest in consistent construction, safety, signage, and maintenance standards. Major highways and roads passing through a city may be managed by county, state, or federal transportation agencies.

Federal transportation planning and funding programs strongly impact local transportation infrastructure. In 1962, the Federal-Aid Highway Act required cities of more than 50,000 people to establish a Metropolitan Planning Organization (MPO) in order to be eligible for federal highway funding (Dannenberg, Frumkin, and Jackson 2011; U.S. DOT 2017). The MPO policy-making board is generally comprised of local elected officials who approve regional plans (U.S. DOT 2017). If a municipality wants to improve a road or facility, it may be eligible for financing through the MPO's Transportation Improvement Program (TIP). Conversely, if a state or federal transportation agency seeks to upgrade roadways within a city's boundaries, the MPO process gives the city an opportunity to weigh in.

The federal government increased its support for active transportation projects through the 2005 transportation funding bill—the Safe, Accountable, Flexible, Efficient Transportation Equity Act: A Legacy for Users (SAFETEA-LU). Funding dedicated to biking and walking infrastructure was reduced in 2012 under the Moving Ahead for Progress in the 21st Century Act (MAP-21), but some states have maintained support for these initiatives (U.S. DOT 2018b; Georgetown Law 2012; Transportation for America 2017). Federal resources for active transportation infrastructure may not benefit all communities equally: One study found that lower-income areas were less likely to implement bicycle and pedestrian projects (Cradock et al. 2009).

Public transit systems like local buses are generally operated by independent "authorities." A local transit authority typically controls decisions about routes, stops, schedules, finances, and equipment. It may partner with city agencies to develop infrastructure that supports public transportation, such as dedicated bus lanes on roads, pull-outs at bus stops, bus shelters, traffic signals, road design, and signage.

Municipalities interact with state and federal funding, planning, and regulatory systems in ways that shape neighborhoods' built environment. These diverse policy arenas are not coordinated with the goal of promoting public health, nor are public health interests regularly represented in these decision-making systems. Indeed, many small cities do not have a city health department, but rather rely on the county or region for public health expertise. The cumulative impact of these disparate decisions over time has created inequitable access to health-supportive built environments. Implementing the strategies promoted by healthy living advocates to change these historical patterns requires coordinated action across many systems over a sustained period of time.

Summary

While everyone can benefit from more physical activity and better nutrition, physical environments are most likely to pose a significant barrier to healthier living in low-income neighborhoods. Healthy community advocates focus on creating strategies that are culturally, economically, and logistically appropriate for low-income communities. Doing so requires extensive community engagement. Therefore, implementing the vision for a "healthy city" involves not only new policy outcomes but also new processes to better engage stakeholders in developing policies, programs, and projects (Corburn 2009; Dannenberg, Frumkin, and Jackson 2011).

Although this chapter focuses specifically on physical activity and food access, it is important to remember that health determinants like access to retail stores, jobs, public services, health care, stable housing, transportation, and neighborhood safety are inter-related. Creating a bike path may provide both new transportation options and exercise resources. Improved public transportation may give people more time to exercise and a way to travel to a store with affordable, healthy food. Spending less money on food may enable people to rent higher-quality housing, reducing their exposure to lead, asthma triggers, pests, or safety hazards. Thus, improving environmental conditions to support healthy living in low-income neighborhoods may be a vital contributor to reducing both health disparities and poverty.

Emerging evidence suggests that action at all levels of the "public health pyramid" is needed to reduce health disparities (Frieden 2010). For built environments, this means connecting public health to a range of private, community, and government decisions. Significant built environment decisions are made at the local level, which increases the potential for community engagement. However, most local governments have limited financial, technical, and institutional resources for involving the public.

As well, low-income communities often lack capacity to engage in efforts to improve the health-supportive resources in their neighborhood. Thus, local initiatives to promote collaboration among diverse stakeholders hold potential for improving the equity of built environments.

Stakeholders in Duluth, Minnesota, leveraged federal, state, and local resources to improve the built environment conditions that shape residents' ability to live healthy lives with an explicit goal of reducing health disparities. Informed by state and national healthy living initiatives, they focused on changing policies, systems, and environments to improve food access and opportunities for physical activity. Their diverse efforts engaged multiple agencies, programs, sectors, and institutions. These efforts were informed and initially supported by external resources, particularly from the Minnesota Department of Health (MDH), but were coordinated, sustained, and led locally.

Connecting Environment and Health in Minnesota

Minnesota may seem like an improbable place to be a leader in health equity work, given the overall good health status of its population. However, Minnesota also has some of the worst health disparities by race and ethnicity in the nation. As the MDH's 2014 Advancing Health Equity Report states: "Minnesota ranks, on average, among the healthiest states in the nation. But the averages do not tell the whole story. Too many people in Minnesota are not as healthy as they could and should be, and the health disparities that exist are significant, persistent and cannot be explained by biogenetic factors. Minnesota has these disparities in health outcomes because the opportunity to be healthy is not equally available everywhere or for everyone in the state" (MDH 2014, 3). The report provides data on health disparities in the state, including that African American and Native American babies die at twice the rate of white babies. It correlates these disparities with social determinants including poverty, educational attainment, and incarceration rates. The analysis recommends that state agencies adopt a "Health in All Policies" approach to pursuing health equity, provide training and data to communities, and support local initiatives (MDH 2014).

Minnesota's health equity initiative built on a foundation of prior work to promote policies, systems, and environments supportive of health for all. Minnesota was an early leader in comprehensive, systems-based approaches to tobacco control (Public Health Law Center 2017). More recently, MDH leveraged funding from the CDC and the Health Impact Project, a collaboration of the Robert Wood Johnson Foundation and the Pew Charitable Trusts, to promote the practice of health impact assessment (HIA) in the state through grants, technical support, training, and a statewide HIA Coalition. As of 2018, the program had identified thirty-four HIAs conducted in the state (MDH 2018).

Minnesota benefited from years of work by community, not-for-profit, and private efforts to bring health considerations into nonhealth decisions. One early community effort to link built environment decisions to health was the 2010 Central Corridor Health Impact Assessment. A new "Central Corridor Rail Line" had been proposed to improve public transportation between the Twin Cities of Minneapolis/St. Paul and neighborhoods to the south. ISAIAH, a faith-based coalition of local congregations focused on racial justice, successfully applied for private foundation funding to do a HIA of this proposal.[1] The final "Healthy Corridor for All" report recommended changes in development policies, zoning, and planning around the new rail line to promote affordable housing, maximize job creation for local residents, and mitigate negative impacts on local businesses (Policy-Link 2011). This HIA helped community groups in the Twin Cities understand how powerful health arguments could be in public decisions and provided a model "for community engagement and analysis to help address community needs as (the region) plans for other transit corridors" (PolicyLink 2011, 4). Jeanne Ayers, a former leader of ISAIAH's Healthy Communities initiative, brought these experiences with her when she became MDH's Assistant Commissioner in 2011. A number of similar projects across the state increased the capacity of community groups and local governments to promote consideration of health in diverse policy arenas.

Building health equity into the state's public health infrastructure became a major focus of MDH. MDH focused on three foundational practices: (1) expand the understanding of what creates health; (2) implement a Health in All Policies approach with health equity as the goal; and (3) strengthen the capacity of communities to create their own healthy future (Ehlinger 2015). MDH Commissioner Edward Ehlinger called this the "triple aim of health equity" (Ehlinger 2015). In her role as assistant commissioner of health, Jeanne Ayers noted that the approach constituted a "theory of change to advance health equity. It blends an understanding of power and systems change. Power can be built through organizing the narrative, resources, and people. These three arenas are completely inter-related" (Ayers 2017).

One of MDH's primary tools for promoting community health was the State Health Improvement Program (SHIP, renamed the State Health Improvement Partnership in 2016). SHIP was a cornerstone of a major health reform law passed by the Minnesota legislature in 2008 (National Cancer Institute 2008). Between 2010 and 2017, SHIP provided over $130 million in assistance to partners in all eighty-seven counties and ten tribal nations in Minnesota (MDH 2017a). SHIP's goal was to invest in community-based primary prevention activities aimed at reducing the population's risk factors for chronic disease in order to reduce long-term health care costs. The program explicitly adopted the language of "policy, systems, and environment" changes and recognized that this was a major departure from public health's traditional focus on individual behaviors (MDH 2011). In 2009, a first round of SHIP grants was issued to help local health departments promote healthy eating, encourage active living, and reduce tobacco exposure in their communities. In subsequent iterations of SHIP funding, grant guidelines added a health equity focus.

Regional private foundations, including the Center for Prevention at Blue Cross Blue Shield Minnesota, the McKnight Foundation, Headwaters Foundation for Justice, and the Bush Foundation, among others, also provided support for built environment efforts (McKnight Foundation, 2019; Headwaters Foundation for Justice 2011; Bush Foundation 2018; Center for Prevention at Blue Cross and Blue Shield of Minnesota 2015a). These funders sought to enhance health equity through community-based work to change policies, systems, and environments. For example, the Center for Prevention's goal is to tackle "the leading causes of preventable disease—tobacco use, physical inactivity, and unhealthy eating—to increase health equity, transform communities, and create a healthier state" (Center for Prevention at Blue Cross and Blue Shield of Minnesota 2015a). It does so by promoting policy change, convening stakeholders to develop new approaches, providing technical support, and funding local initiatives (Center for Prevention at Blue Cross and Blue Shield of Minnesota 2015b).[2]

A diverse array of programs, policies, and projects emerged from these efforts to create neighborhood environments that support health equity. Within this vibrant statewide context, the diversity, durability, and impact of Duluth's efforts stand out. The Duluth initiatives are particularly remarkable given the small size, geographic challenges, and economic history of the city.

Duluth: Geographic, Historical, Economic, and Demographic Context

Located on the western shore of Lake Superior in the northeast corner of Minnesota, Duluth has a population of 86,000 (City of Duluth 2018a). It is the seat of St. Louis County, which despite being the largest county east of the Mississippi has just over 200,000 mostly rural residents. Duluth is comprised of communities stretching from affluent eastern neighborhoods through the downtown area and west into poorer neighborhoods abutting formerly industrial sites along the St. Louis River. The downtown area is hilly, and a steep escarpment limits development to the narrow area of shoreline west of town. The forested hills surrounding the town are a treasured recreational resource for hiking, mountain biking, and skiing.

Duluth emerged in the late 1800s as an international port where agricultural products, timber, and later taconite (iron ore) from the region were transported east across the Great Lakes (Bunnell 2002). Because of this location, Duluth's first newspaper nicknamed it the "zenith city of the unsalted seas" (Greater Downtown Council 2017). It eventually developed into an industrial center dominated by the steel industry (Duluth Area Chamber of Commerce 2017; Alanen 2007). Many of Duluth's buildings date to this period, with more than half of all housing built before 1950.

The U.S. steel industry declined after 1950, and U.S. Steel's Duluth operation closed in the 1970s, along with many associated businesses. Other industries that had been the mainstay of the economy, including agriculture and timber, also waned during this time period. Meanwhile, new transportation infrastructure elsewhere (including the Panama Canal and the expansion of East Coast ports) made cross-country shipping through the Great Lakes less attractive, reducing Duluth's importance as a port. Consequently, Duluth's population dropped 30 percent from 1960 to 1980. As of 1983, Duluth had an unemployment rate of 16 percent, more than double the statewide rate and among the highest in the country (Bunnell 2002).

As a result of its industrial history, the City of Duluth has a large number of "brownfields," sites of known or potential environmental contamination (U.S. EPA 2018g). Two former industrial sites totaling around 800 acres together comprise the largest Superfund site in Minnesota. The highly polluted St. Louis River was named one of forty-three Areas of Concern (AOC) under the Great Lakes Water Quality Agreement of 1987. As an AOC, the river has been the focus of cleanup efforts that improved water quality, restored aquatic ecosystems, and addressed contaminated sediments (Minnesota Pollution Control Agency 2016). These efforts boosted water-based recreation along Duluth's extensive waterfront, including kayaking, paddleboarding, and even surfing the waves of Lake Superior.

The Duluth economy has improved significantly over the past two decades. New manufacturing, aviation, technology firms, tourism, transportation, and services drove this growth (Duluth Economic Development Authority 2018b). Health care emerged as a major sector of the local economy. Duluth also grew as a launching point for tourism in northeastern Minnesota and was named the "Best Town Ever" in the United States by *Outside Magazine* in 2014 (Pearson 2014). Recent economic growth has spurred redevelopment of downtown Duluth with new restaurants, services, and businesses. This growth has increased demand to make productive use of former industrial sites in outlying areas. With the support of the city's brownfield and economic development programs, several new light manufacturing businesses have located on these reused sites in recent years.

The population of Duluth is 90.4 percent white (U.S. Census 2016). There are significant populations of racial and ethnic minorities, particularly African American (1,988, 2.3 percent), Native American (2,124, 2.5 percent), Latino (1,305, 1.5 percent), and Asian (1,293, 1.5 percent).[3] The Native American population in Duluth includes people from several tribes and bands, many of whom have close ties to reservations in the region.

The median household income in Duluth in 2014 was $43,518 (mean $60,682) (U.S. Census 2016) and the overall unemployment rate was low (5.1 percent). Continued growth of jobs in sectors including construction, aviation, health care, education, and professional services was expected (Duluth Economic Development Authority 2018b). The booming demand for housing as a result of this growth was reflected in a low (3.5 percent) vacancy rate for rentals in 2016. Just over 60 percent of the city's housing units were owner-occupied, with a median single-family house value of $145,900.

Despite the positive economic trends in Duluth, significant economic disparities existed within the population. The unemployment rate of African

Americans was 31.3 percent compared to 7.2 percent for whites (U.S. Census 2016). Similarly, the number of African Americans (65.9 percent) and Native Americans (49.3 percent) living below the poverty level greatly exceeded the percentage of whites below the poverty level (19.9 percent). Many of Duluth's racial and ethnic minority residents live in lower-income neighborhoods adjacent to former industrial sites.

These economic, demographic, geographic, and historical conditions were reflected in the health status of people living in Duluth. Community groups representing low-income and minority populations were well aware of the health disparities within the city. With the growing national recognition of connections between environmental, economic, and social conditions and health, local stakeholders explored the relationships between the built environment and health equity in Duluth and what could be done to change them. Community, government, and private efforts to promote health equity in Duluth have evolved over the past decade.

Shaping Duluth's Built Environment to Promote Health Equity

In the early 1980s, the Minnesota Department of Transportation (MNDOT) proposed to extend Route I-35 through downtown Duluth (Bunnell 2002). Community members organized in opposition to the plan, which would have demolished historic portside buildings, cut the city off from the waterfront, and destroyed a beloved park and rose garden. Former city planner Jerry Kimball said, "Leif Erikson Park was created by the WPA [Works Progress Administration] during the 1930s, and losing the Rose Garden was unthinkable" (Bunnell 2002, 341). The city convened a citizen's committee and began negotiations with MNDOT to modify the plan.

As part of the resulting agreement, MNDOT redesigned the project to maximize public access to the lake. A large section of the highway was built in tunnels below grade with bridges at street level, allowing better connection to the waterfront. A park constructed on top of the new highway replaced the old one, complete with a larger garden where the original roses were replanted. In addition, the project provided funding for the Lakewalk, a four-mile-long pedestrian walkway along the shore of Lake Superior. Built between 1986 and 1991, the Lakewalk became an anchor for redevelopment of the lakefront Canal Park as a tourist and recreational area (Bunnell 2002; Go Duluth MN 2018).[4]

The Lakewalk, Canal Park, and associated development marked the start of several decades of investment in outdoor recreation-based tourism that contributed to the city's rejuvenation. Trails surrounding the city earned Duluth a reputation as a mountain biking mecca. These natural resources attract year-round use despite the harsh winters—local tourism campaigns advertise the Duluth "winter experience" that includes fat-tire mountain biking in the snow as well as brewery tours and sled dog rides (Skihut 2018). Bike trails were also expanded within the city, with plans to eventually extend them the full twenty-six miles of the city's length (City of Duluth 2011).

Despite its image as a healthy, outdoor-oriented community, not everyone in Duluth was in good health. A 2013 St. Louis County Health Status Report showed that the mean life expectancy in Duluth was below the state average, and that there was a more than eleven year difference in life expectancy between wealthier and poorer zip codes (Gilley, Gangl, and Skoog 2011). Anecdotal observations by community service agency staff confirmed that many low-income and nonwhite residents faced significant health challenges. These disparities informed the efforts of a range of community agencies, government agency staff, and community leaders who sought to improve access to healthy food and opportunities for physical activity to support healthy living by all residents.

Stakeholders concerned about improving access to healthy food and physical activity first came together through the city's designation as a Minnesota "Fit City" in 2007. Over the next decade, efforts to create an environment that supported health for all residents of Duluth evolved through a wide range of activities. From an initial focus on encouraging individuals to make healthy choices, the initiative soon shifted gears to concentrate on changing policies, systems, and environments. Although many of the efforts were connected through Fit City Duluth's successor, the Healthy Duluth Area Coalition (HDAC), various initiatives were led by local agencies, community organizations, and private foundations. In addition to city, county, and regional government agencies, partners included the local YMCA, the Local Initiatives Support Corporation (LISC), Duluth's community action agency, local health systems, and many others. This collective body of work is referred to in this book as the "Healthy Duluth" initiatives.[5]

Many of the Healthy Duluth partners worked directly with low-income areas and communities of color. As well, many of the Healthy Duluth projects directly engaged residents. However, most individuals involved in the collaborations did so in a professional capacity. Through these varied spheres of activity, a cohort of professionals developed experience promoting health equity through policies, systems, and environmental (PSE) change. They sustained this vision by institutionalizing PSE concepts in their own organizations, supporting community coalitions, building systems for sharing data, and promoting health equity as a guiding principle for local policy-making. The ways in which Healthy Duluth partners promoted a health-supportive built environment became increasingly well coordinated. These efforts were not carried out by a single umbrella organization, but rather were interwoven actions led by different stakeholders at different times. The discussion that follows describes the health equity efforts organized through Duluth's brownfields redevelopment program, Fit City Duluth, the HDAC, the St. Louis County State Health Improvement Program (SHIP), and a series of three MDH-funded health impact assessments, among others (table 5.1). The final section summarizes ongoing efforts to sustain the Healthy Duluth work.

Brownfield Redevelopment and Healthy Living

Multiple public decisions, plans, and projects have a cumulative effect on the built environment in ways that impact community health. However, these decisions are usually made in isolation from each other. The process of brownfield redevelopment offers an opportunity to coordinate many of these forces. Because of Duluth's industrial legacy, most of the land available for potential redevelopment is a brownfield. Some of the earliest efforts to incorporate health into public decisions took place in the context of brownfield redevelopment projects. The city's Department of Business and Economic Development and the Duluth Economic Development Authority (DEDA) brownfield redevelopment work laid the foundation for the city's health equity work in other sectors.

Brownfields are properties where past land uses resulted in known or suspected environmental contamination of buildings, soil, or water (U.S. EPA 2018g; Minnesota Pollution Control Agency 2018). Government programs supporting brownfield redevelopment promote productive reuse of contaminated sites not eligible for the federal Superfund cleanup program. Because environmental remediation is so costly, developers are often wary

Table 5.1
Healthy Duluth timeline

2007	Duluth recognized as a "Governor's Fit City."
2008	Fit City Duluth forms as independent organization.
2009	Duluth team attends the CDC's "Pioneering Healthy Communities" conference.
	First State Health Improvement Program (SHIP) grants awarded.
	Safe and Walkable Hillside coalition begins.
2010	Health Duluth Area Coalition convenes.
2011	St. Louis County Health Status Report issued.
	Health impact assessment (HIA) conducted on the redesign of 6th Avenue.
2013	HIA of Gary-New Duluth Small Area Plan initiated.
2014	HIA of Lincoln Park Small Area Plan initiated.
	City receives U.S. EPA Brownfields Area-wide Planning grant for Irving Fairmount Brownfields Revitalization Plan in the Western Port Area neighborhoods.[6]
	St. Louis River Corridor initiative launches.
2015	"Grocery Bus" begins running.
2016	Mayor Emily Larson announces "health" and "fairness" as goals of city's new Comprehensive Plan.
	Zeitgeist Center for Arts and Community receives Center for Prevention grant to initiate Health Equity Collaborative.
	Bridging Health Duluth produces first integrated Community Health Needs Assessment in region.
2017	Team representing city, county, Metropolitan Interstate Council, and community attends National Association of Chronic Disease Directors' 3-day Walkability Action Institute.

of buying brownfield properties. The potential for contamination is a particular problem in low-income neighborhoods where the profit margin of development may not justify cleanup costs by private developers. Federal and state brownfield programs offer funding to assess contamination, determine appropriate cleanup strategies, and develop plans for uses that are compatible with any remaining contamination (U.S. EPA 2018g).

Brownfields are usually considered economic and environmental issues. They have underappreciated significance for public health (Minnesota Brownfields 2018b). Neighbors' concerns related to brownfields typically focus on *risks* of exposure to unknown toxicants. As well, the overall impact of redeveloping brownfields can provide long-term community health *benefits* by reducing blight, creating new businesses and parks or trails, and creating jobs. Local governments generally are motivated to participate in brownfield redevelopment efforts to pursue these potential economic, social, and environmental benefits.

Because Duluth is a fully built city, any new development will likely take place on land that is potentially contaminated by prior uses. The City of Duluth's Department of Business and Economic Development therefore has actively sought grants, technical support, and partnerships to facilitate brownfield redevelopment. U.S. Environmental Protection Agency (EPA) pilot assessment grants for brownfield sites in the early 2000s led to fifteen assistance packages between 2010 and 2018 (Timm-Bijold 2016). Since 2000, the city has received nearly $2 million in U.S. EPA site assessment grants, secured $15 million for site cleanup and redevelopment, and leveraged over $100 million in projects (Duluth Economic Development Authority 2018a; Timm-Bijold 2016).

These early cleanup projects often resulted in health-supportive changes in the built environment, although health equity was not an explicit aim. The ongoing efforts to clean up the St. Louis River decreased the potential for exposure to toxicants in surface waters, soils, and fish and expanded water-based active recreation opportunities. Several trails are located on former rail lines acquired and converted by the city. Between 2006 and 2010, the 10.2-acre Clyde Iron Works brownfield site was developed into an ice rink, sports complex, restaurant, and children's museum and is expected to serve as an anchor for additional sports and recreation facilities in the Lincoln Park neighborhood.

As part of receiving these grants, the city's economic development staff regularly attended U.S. EPA national brownfield meetings. These conferences emphasized the public health benefits of brownfield redevelopment. The U.S. EPA encouraged grantees to highlight potential community health improvements from their projects. With this guidance, Duluth's economic development program staff began seeking new ways to maximize health benefits of their work.

Interactions with brownfield programs created new opportunities for Duluth. For example, staff from the Agency for Toxic Substances and Disease Registry (ATSDR) Brownfield/Land Reuse Initiative became aware of Duluth's efforts and in 2010 invited the city to participate in a funding proposal to the Great Lakes Restoration Initiative. This project proposed to assess the public health benefits of cleanup and redevelopment of the St. Louis River and Lake Superior waterfront. As then-mayor Don Ness stated in his letter of support, "Our driving force in seeking [ATSDR's] assistance is in seeking to inform and engage the public in the public health benefits of land reuse" (Ness 2010). Although the full project was not funded, ATSDR and the City of Duluth convened a workshop in July 2012 to engage stakeholders in identifying community health indicators for restoration and redevelopment of the St. Louis River corridor. This interaction strengthened the Department of Business and Economic Development's connections with MDH, which in turn helped foster the subsequent MDH-city partnership to conduct HIAs in western Duluth (as described later in this chapter).

Another public health connection came through Minnesota Brownfields, a statewide nonprofit group formed in 2006 to "promote, through education, research, and partnerships, the efficient cleanup and reuse of contaminated land as a means of generating economic growth, strengthening communities and enabling sustainable land use and development" (Minnesota Brownfields 2018a). Heidi Timm-Bijold, Duluth's business resources manager, was a longtime board member of the organization. Duluth's health equity efforts benefited from its long-standing involvement with Minnesota Brownfields. For example, in 2012 the city was approached by the group's graduate student intern about developing a public health indicator tool for brownfield projects. Minnesota Brownfields and MDH later completed and publicly released this tool, which was piloted in Duluth's Lincoln Park HIA in 2014 and again in 2016 for the Irving Fairmount Brownfields Revitalization Plan (Minnesota Brownfields 2018b).

These experiences brought a health perspective into brownfield redevelopment, giving city staff new tools, ways of communicating with the public about the impact of their work, and relationships with diverse stakeholders. Eventually, these connections led the city to become the lead applicant on two HIAs, further developing its capacity to integrate health considerations into municipal decisions.

Fit City Duluth

In 2007, Duluth was recognized as part of the Minnesota "Governor's Fit City" program (Duluth News Tribune 2007). Fit City was a voluntary designation established under MDH in 2005 to highlight cities that had made a commitment to supporting healthy living (New Ulm Minnesota 2006). Duluth's application was written by the city's Parks and Recreation Department and focused on the city's extensive system of mountain biking trails, the Lakewalk, and other physical activity resources. After being awarded the designation, Parks and Recreation staff assembled a broad-based Fit City task force to explore expanding physical activity opportunities. Lacking resources or designated staff, however, the group soon dwindled.

Mimi Stender, a Fit City member and community volunteer, incorporated a nonprofit called "Fit City Duluth" to implement these goals after the city's task force stopped meeting. Stender became the executive director and members of original task force were invited to join the new Fit City Duluth board. As a nonprofit organization, Fit City Duluth was able to apply for grants to undertake substantive work to promote active living. Fit City Duluth's initial sponsors were St. Luke's Foundation, St. Mary's/Duluth Clinic Health System (now part of Essentia Health), the Local Initiatives Support Corporation (LISC), and Northland's News Center. These resources supported core staff, an AmeriCorps volunteer, expenses associated with convening meetings and conferences, and maintaining a website. Fit City Duluth coordinated several projects including a school wellness initiative, the Safe and Walkable Hillside neighborhood coalition, and workplace health assessments.

In July 2008, the St. Louis County health department received notice of a CDC-sponsored conference called "Community Approaches to Obesity Prevention" and shared this opportunity with Fit City Duluth. Stender, along with a local pediatrician who was a Fit City board member, attended the conference. This experience inspired them to focus Fit City's goals and strategies on policy change. According to Stender, "There were lots of different cities doing different things, but the ones that spoke most powerfully to us were those that were doing policy things. ... [We thought] 'this is it, now we know where we can really have an impact.'" She added, "This conference provided a renewed sense of confidence that PSE change can have a true and lasting positive impact on the health of community members" (Stender 2016).

After the CDC conference, Fit City Duluth began seeking support to pursue PSE work. Together with the local YMCA, Fit City Duluth applied for and received a Pioneering Healthy Communities (PHC) grant in 2009 (CDC 2011; Duluth News Tribune 2014). Pioneering Healthy Communities was a national partnership between the Centers for Disease Control and Prevention and the YMCA that had already enrolled dozens of communities. The grant required local stakeholders to attend the Pioneering Healthy Communities workshop in Washington, DC in December 2009 (Duluth News Tribune 2014). Ten people from Duluth attended, including Fit City board members, health professionals, county health department staff, the city schools superintendent, the Local Initiatives Support Corporation director, and a city council member. Participants learned about research on the built environment and health and about other communities' efforts to promote safer streets, build trails, and improve access to healthy food.

Soon after, Fit City developed an action plan to promote PSE changes. One of Fit City's first policy actions was to advocate that the city adopt a complete streets policy. As Stender said, "Mayor Ness understood right away … but it was hard to create a movement within city hall. … There were departments that were a big barrier at first. But then, after a while, they really got it" (Stender 2016). In March 2010, the city council passed a resolution directing the city to develop a complete streets policy. Although a final policy was never enacted, Stender noted, "They do now plan new street construction with the complete streets idea."

Fit City recognized the need to engage multiple stakeholders in policy advocacy and initiated an informal collaborative called the Healthy Duluth Area Coalition (HDAC). Over time, Fit City Duluth became less active as an organization and, in 2010, HDAC found a new home at the Zeitgeist Center for Arts and Community.[7] Despite its short duration as an organization, Fit City Duluth played a critical role in assembling local stakeholders, accessing national resources on built environment and health, and focusing Duluth's efforts on PSE approaches.

Healthy Duluth Area Coalition (HDAC)

After moving to the Zeitgeist Center for Arts and Community, HDAC worked to implement and broaden the scope of Fit City work plan. As Zeitgeist Center executive director Tony Cuneo said, HDAC realized that "if we can work on shared language and vision we should be able to bring together people interested in local food and healthy food to support equitable outdoor recreation and public transportation that works better for low-income people" (Cuneo 2016). Thus, HDAC strongly embraced a health

equity agenda. This focus was reinforced by the growing evidence of striking health disparities within Duluth (Bridge to Health Survey 2018; Gilley,
Gangl, and Skoog 2011).

Funding to support HDAC's project-based work and convening functions
came from a variety of sources over time. For example, the State Health
Improvement Program (SHIP) provided support for core staff who were able
to write grant proposals to other funders and coordinate the HDAC (Harala
2016). As of 2015, HDAC included seventeen local organizations and was
supported by two full-time staff members, an AmeriCorps volunteer, and
student interns (Healthy Duluth Area Coalition 2018).

HDAC's focused on promoting active living and healthy eating. The Fair
Food Access campaign was informed by a 2011 University of Minnesota-
Duluth study that identified the Lincoln Park neighborhood as a "food
desert" (Pine and Bennett, 2011). HDAC developed several efforts to improve
food access in this neighborhood, both through on-the-ground projects
and promoting policies to enhance future access. An early effort funded by
a $25,000 grant from State Farm involved community surveys to identify
barriers to accessing healthy foods, inform food access improvement projects, and monitor changes over time (French 2014c). Lisa Luokkala, former
director of HDAC, credits data from this survey with the success of a proposal to the Center for Prevention at Blue Cross Blue Shield of Minnesota
to support the Fair Food Access campaign's work in Lincoln Park (Center
for Prevention at Blue Cross and Blue Shield of Minnesota 2018a). The Fair
Food Access campaign also partnered with the City of Duluth and community groups to establish a new community garden in Lincoln Park and host
classes on cooking, gardening, and food preservation (French 2014a, 2015a;
Wilder Research 2014).

HDAC's second area of concentration, active transportation, focused
on promoting bus transit, biking, and walking. In 2012, HDAC hosted a
series of public meetings to get community input on transportation initiatives (Luokkala 2012). HDAC staff also participated in a number of direct
initiatives to support active transportation, such as a 2012 Hillside neighborhood bike and pedestrian survey, exploring designation of Duluth as a
"bike friendly city," and promoting a "Bus/Bike/Walk" month in May each
year (French 2014d; Luokkala 2013a, 2013b).

In addition to these campaigns, a key contribution of HDAC staff was convening, coordinating, and supporting communication among stakeholders

in Duluth. The Active Living and Fair Food Access campaigns both met monthly. Staff published updates on the HDAC website, communicated with members, and organized public outreach. According to HDAC, "individually, the organizations, initiatives and individuals we represent have limited capacity to advocate for public policy that supports their vision, but collectively we create a voice in the community and share resources to push policy and system changes that bring about better health" (Luokkala 2013c). Lisa Luokkala, who directed HDAC from 2011–2015, described HDAC as a "'plate,' not an umbrella, because we wanted to lift up everyone's great work and tie it to policy issues. So we became a platform to do that in Duluth." She added, "We kind of hunted as a pack for funding, which allowed us to go for larger, more comprehensive granting opportunities, then parts or portions were divvied out to organizations to complete certain parts but with a strong tie of always coming back to the table to work collaboratively" (Luokkala 2016).

Finding funding to support project-based staff who could also sustain the convening function of HDAC was an ongoing challenge. As Tony Cuneo noted, "You can get a wise funder and sell them on the need for convening but they are rarely willing to fund it long term, they want to start seeing projects again and distinct programs." He added, "To do this well you need coordination, and funding for coordination is the hardest to find" (Cuneo 2016). Recent efforts to identify new ways to sustain the HDAC are discussed in the section on Sustaining, Growing, and Evaluating Collaboration.

The Role of Public Health in Promoting Healthy Environments in Duluth

It may seem logical that the local health department would have a key role in community health promotion efforts. However, promoting public health through changes in the physical environment is not a traditional core function of local health departments. In Duluth, the county health department's role evolved along with developing community health equity initiatives.

Before 2008, Jim Skoog's work as a county health educator focused on changing individual health behaviors and increasing public awareness (Skoog 2016). One exception was his involvement with regional efforts to reduce exposure to tobacco smoke. Health departments and community groups including the local American Lung Association had worked together to successfully pass laws regulating smoking in indoor environments. This experience of working with a coalition to achieve policy change provided a foundation for envisioning a broader health department role in community efforts to address determinants of health. As Skoog said, "This tobacco work showed how you could be successful with policy change to impact health. ..." (Skoog 2016). Thus, by the time Fit City Duluth formed, health department staff had already had a positive experience working with community coalitions to achieve change outside of the traditional scope of the health educator's practice.

Around the same time that Fit City Duluth was forming, the Center for Prevention distributed copies of the DVD *Unnatural Causes* to local health departments across the state. It told the story of how physical, economic, and social determinants contribute to health inequities across the country (Unnatural Causes 2018). According to health department staff, "that documentary and its accompanying robust website stimulated much thought and action within PHHS (St. Louis County Public Health and Human Services) and in Duluth. It led directly to the decision ... to begin mapping health outcomes in St. Louis County" (Gilley, Gangl, and Skoog 2011, 26). *Unnatural Causes* presented a radically different way to think about the role of public health professionals in prevention. Rather than focusing on public education, delivering programs, and providing services, the video suggested a role for public health professionals in changing environments to achieve lasting health improvements for disadvantaged communities. As one health department staff noted, "I don't think the impact that *Unnatural Causes* had on us can be overstated" (Gangl 2016). This new way of thinking about the role of public health did not immediately resonate with health department leadership. However, with encouragement from Fit City Duluth members, staff eventually received permission to participate in the community initiatives.

Skoog joined the Duluth delegation to the Pioneering Healthy Communities conference in 2009, where he learned how local health departments were supporting PSE work in other communities. He recalled being advised by a conference speaker that reporting on the health status of different populations within the community could be a helpful contribution by a public health department (Skoog 2016). Although Duluth had been part of the seven-county "Bridge to Health" survey, which had been conducted every five years since 1995, this data was not at a fine enough geographic scale to show local disparities (Bridge to Health Survey 2018).[8] The health department hired an intern to undertake this project in 2010, but delays in obtaining data from the state meant that the report had to be completed by health department staff over the next several years. When the report was finally released in 2013, it documented striking differences in health status between wealthier and lower-income zip codes, as well as between whites and people of color (Gilley, Gangl, and Skoog 2011). It also highlighted obesity as a major community health problem, strengthening the rationale for promoting healthy eating and active living.

Meanwhile, these ideas about expanding public health's role in community change were being incorporated in the Minnesota Department of Health's expectations for local departments. In July 2009, the state issued two-year State Health Improvement Program (SHIP) grants to community health boards and tribal authorities totaling $47 million. SHIP's goal was to help communities address barriers to good health through PSE changes (MDH 2008). Healthy eating and physical activity initiatives were among several projects in Duluth that were included in the SHIP-funded program, which was administered through the Carlton-Cook-Lake-St. Louis Community Health Board.

One of the first projects undertaken was the Safe and Walkable Hillside Coalition. This coalition was initiated by Fit City Duluth's Active Living coordinator and transitioned to the St. Louis County health department with SHIP support. The coalition's goal was to "create an environment that is safe and welcoming for all pedestrians and bikers in the Hillside Community." The group identified three goals: (1) creating a safe and walkable Hillside for everyone; (2) creating a cleaner, greener, and more inviting Hillside; and (3) making certain that children can walk and bike safely to and from school (St. Louis County Health and Human Services 2011). Health department staff participated in bike and pedestrian counts in Hillside, laying the foundation for future active transportation planning. SHIP provided technical assistance through the Arrowhead Regional Development Commission, including a walkability assessment conducted with neighborhood residents near Hillside's Grant Elementary School. This led to implementing the national "Safe Routes to School" model to encourage children to walk or bike to school (National Center for Safe Routes to School 2018). The coalition also initiated a neighborhood street festival called HillFest to encourage community cohesion. In addition to these specific projects, the health department's work with residents around walkability provided a foundation for a HIA on the redesign of 6th Avenue in Hillside.

In 2012, a second round of SHIP funding (SHIP 2) was released. Starting with SHIP 2, St. Louis County was part of a regional application through Healthy Northland, a collaboration of local health departments that includes the Carlton-Cook-Lake-St. Louis Community Health Board as well as three additional rural counties (Aitkin, Itasca, and Koochiching counties) (MDH 2013; Healthy Northland Statewide Health Improvement Program 2018). With SHIP 2 funding, the health department continued its work in Hillside and established a second neighborhood coalition called Lincoln Park on the Move. It had similar goals to the Safe and Walkable Hillside, engaging community members in promoting a health-supportive built environment. Lincoln Park on the Move initiated a "Meet on the Street" event to promote social cohesion (Gorham 2016b). The health department also developed Safe Routes to School programs for a new middle school in Lincoln Park.

For the third round of SHIP funding in 2013, the state's guidelines changed significantly to emphasize engaging communities around health equity, consistent with the 2014 MDH Health Equity report (MDH 2014). The regional SHIP program embraced these new guidelines. After getting input from community groups, the St. Louis County health department focused on social determinants affecting low-income children. This work built on the school district's emerging interest in developing a comprehensive wellness program.

As the SHIP guidelines changed and the health department shifted its focus from community coalitions to schools, Safe and Walkable Hillside and Lincoln Park on the Move became less active. Nonetheless, residents continued to be involved in issues of community redevelopment, safety, access, and walkability projects. In addition, the health department partnered with HDAC to engage communities about planned road improvement projects. Health department staff also participated in HDAC projects including biking promotion events. The ongoing involvement of health department in community coalitions, advisory groups, and decision processes helped sustain those groups' energy and institutional knowledge. Staff also helped write proposals for additional funding to support related community efforts. Thus, MDH's efforts to promote a PSE approach through SHIP had significant impacts in Duluth (MDH 2017b). As Jim Skoog said,

"We finally figured out how to do stuff that is more permanent" (Skoog 2016). The health department has remained a consistent voice promoting health equity through PSE in the community.

Health Impact Assessments of Neighborhood Redevelopment

Concurrent to the SHIP program, MDH began exploring the potential of using health impact assessment (HIA) to integrate health into nonhealth decisions. MDH obtained several grants intended to build capacity for HIA throughout the state. Duluth received technical support and funding for three HIAs between 2010 and 2014. These opportunities allowed local stakeholders to develop greater familiarity with HIA, use health data to analyze how built environment decisions affect health disparities, and gather community input on improving environmental health equity. Because HIAs emphasize community input, these projects also supported resident engagement efforts. As well, the HIA process required input from multiple sectors, strengthening local stakeholder relationships. Finally, because the HIAs targeted timely decisions in key locations, their recommendations established an evidence base for future action. Each of the three HIAs built collaboration, capacity, and systems to improve health equity in Duluth's built environment.

6th Avenue Redesign HIA, January–June 2011

In 2010, an Arrowhead Regional Development Commission staff member identified an opportunity to apply to MDH for HIA funding. The MDH funding came through a grant from the Association of State and Territorial Health Officials (ASTHO) to conduct three HIAs in the state. The Arrowhead Regional Development Commission partnered with the St. Louis County health department to propose an HIA of a plan to redesign 6th Avenue, a busy roadway bisecting the Hillside neighborhood (St. Louis County Health and Human Services 2011). Begun in January 2011, the HIA project took around six months with an estimated total budget of $15,000 (Raab 2017). This project enabled many of the Healthy Duluth partners to work together for the first time on a transportation infrastructure project.

As noted previously, health department staff had been working with residents through the Safe and Walkable Hillside coalition for several years. Safe and Walkable Hillside had identified 6th Avenue as a major challenge

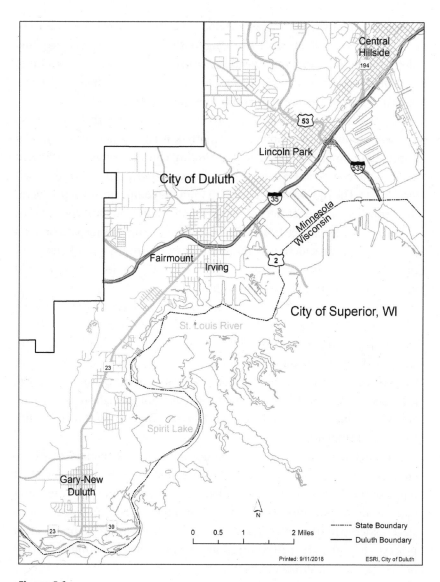

Figure 5.1
Map of Duluth neighborhoods where health assessments were conducted
Map credit: Richard Bunten

to the walkability of the neighborhood. The HIA took place in the wake of the 2011 consolidation of two neighborhood schools, which required many children to cross 6th Avenue to reach their new school. Because of the dangerous traffic on 6th Avenue, many of these children were being bussed to school, despite living only a few blocks away.

The HIA assessed the health impacts of the proposed 6th Avenue redesign with respect to accessibility, safety, physical activity, and livability, with a focus on vulnerable populations including children, older and disabled adults, and low-income residents (St. Louis County Health and Human Services 2011). The HIA team included staff from the county health department, the Arrowhead Regional Development Commission, and local consultants, with technical assistance from MDH staff. Because this HIA focused on road redesign, the team sought input from the city's engineers, but the city planning department was not extensively involved. The project also supported enhanced community engagement efforts.

The HIA's recommendations included increasing the number of bus stops to better accommodate people with physical limitations, adding a traffic signal, improving crosswalks, creating a designated bike lane, and better snow clearing. The team also recommended actions beyond the scope of the roadway project, including more affordable housing, improving the sidewalk network, and "adding amenities outside of the right-of-way to create greener, more neighborhood-friendly development" (St. Louis County Health and Human Services 2011, 5).

Although the roadway redesign has not yet been implemented, planning efforts continue. For example, a 2014 redevelopment strategy plan included many of the "livability" recommendations included in the HIA (Cunningham Group Architecture 2014). The 6th Avenue East HIA provided Duluth stakeholders with their first "hands-on" experience with HIA. Through this process, they strengthened connections and expanded the number of partners engaged in health equity work.

Gary-New Duluth Small Area Plan HIA, June 2013—June 2014

In 2012, MDH received another grant from the Health Impact Project, a partnership of Pew Charitable Trusts and the Robert Wood Johnson Foundation, to expand HIA capacity. In addition to supporting a statewide HIA collaborative, the project included support for three additional local HIAs. Having recently worked in Duluth on the 6th Avenue HIA, the state health department staff reached out to Duluth stakeholders. Together they identified two upcoming Small Area Planning (SAP) processes suitable for HIA. Duluth's comprehensive plan from 2006 called for SAPs to be developed for the economically challenged Gary-New Duluth and Lincoln Park neighborhoods. Although these projects involved different local stakeholders than the 6th Avenue HIA, MDH was encouraged to select Duluth because of the community's prior experience with HIA.

The Gary-New Duluth neighborhood was developed to house workers at the nearby U.S. Steel Duluth Works plant (Minnesota Department of Health Climate and Health Program 2014; City of Duluth 2006). Since the U.S. Steel Duluth Works plant closed in 1979, there had been little economic activity or residential investment in the area. The neighborhood is part of western Duluth, which lost 50 percent of its population between 1950 and 1980, a rate three times that of the rest of the city (Bunnell 2002, 362). As of 2010, the neighborhood had just over 3,000 residents, 99 percent of whom were white (Minnesota Department of Health Climate and Health Program 2014). Gary-New Duluth's poverty was higher (12 percent) than in Duluth as a whole (7 percent), with a median household income of $40,833. The neighborhood had only a handful of commercial businesses and many vacant houses. The nearest full-service grocery store is six miles away, a nearly twenty-minute bus ride. As Mayor Ness wrote in his letter of support for the Gary-New Duluth HIA, "The [U.S. Steel] site and the adjacent Gary-New Duluth neighborhood are representative examples of areas currently underutilized that are ripe for sustainable growth. In so doing, it will be critical to incorporate HIA components into the planning process. The planning and decision-making process will benefit greatly by a partnership amongst the City, the MDH, and the long list of stakeholders that include the U.S. EPA, the Minnesota Pollution Control Agency, neighborhood groups, the West Duluth Community Development Corporation, and the St. Louis River Alliance" (Ness 2012).

The Gary-New Duluth HIA was launched in June 2013, concurrent with the SAP process. The HIA grant provided approximately $15,000 to support local involvement in the project. The bulk of the HIA analyses were conducted by MDH staff, with input from a technical advisory committee (TAC) that included community members and representatives from the county health department, Arrowhead Area Agency on Aging, the Department of Parks and Recreation, transportation planners, and the local hospital.

Several members of the HIA TAC also served on the SAP steering committee to enhance coordination between the efforts. The HIA team conducted
several public meetings, focus groups, and a community survey to solicit
feedback from the public. The survey identified economic development,
crime, and access to goods and services as top community concerns.

The HIA team finalized the analysis in February 2014. The HIA suggested
recruiting high-job-density businesses and targeting workforce development efforts at young people in Gary-New Duluth. Similarly, the HIA noted
that the planned demolition of blighted properties should be combined with
appropriate lighting and streetscape design to maximize health and safety
benefits. The HIA also recommended developing convenient trail access
points "so that the trails do not simply cross through the neighborhood
but are accessible to neighborhood residents" (Minnesota Department of
Health Climate and Health Program 2014, 100).

It is difficult to evaluate to what extent the HIA will affect the process
of SAP implementation over time. Nonetheless, participants noted that the
HIA process broadened consideration of health, developed the capacity
of local residents to participate in planning, and laid the groundwork for
future collaboration among stakeholders. The HIA report also noted that
the process "increased the understanding of connections between health
outcomes and policy for city staff and other stakeholders, which will influence their work in the future" (Minnesota Department of Health Climate
and Health Program 2014, 6).

Lincoln Park HIA, January 2014—September 2015

A third HIA was supported under the MDH Health Impact Project grant
in connection with the Lincoln Park Small Area Plan. Lincoln Park is a
low-income neighborhood on the west side of downtown Duluth, closer
to the city center than Gary-New Duluth. The HIA team aimed to build
on the collaborations initiated in the Gary-New Duluth HIA: "The HIA
will promote sustaining discussion of health in policy-making; encouraging the city to be constantly intentional about the conversation of
health" (Minnesota Department of Health Climate and Health Program
2015, 4).

Lincoln Park is a "very dense, urban neighborhood with some of the
highest racial and ethnic diversity in the city. The area is a poverty pocket
and a food desert; has a poor walking environment; is adjacent to past

industry and current brownfields; has a neglected housing stock due to Duluth's 1 percent rental vacancy and high percentage of rental housing; has higher crime levels; and has limited transit access" (Minnesota Department of Health Climate and Health Program 2015, 3). The designated "study area" included a population of just over 2,500. In 2010, the median income was $19,825—less than half that of Duluth as a whole—and unemployment was high (20 percent), particularly among African American (50 percent) and Native American (39 percent) residents. Lincoln Park lies within zip code 55806, which had the lowest life expectancy in the city (73.44 years).

Nonprofit and government agencies had been actively pursuing community revitalization of the Lincoln Park neighborhood for many years. Significant developments included the Clyde Park athletic complex, a children's museum, a new middle school, expanded athletic fields, and construction of the Cross City bike and pedestrian trail through the neighborhood. In his second term, Mayor Ness promoted a vision of this area becoming Duluth's "sports corridor." One goal of the SAP process was to provide steps the city could take to build on these efforts. In contrast to the Gary-New Duluth HIA, which ran in parallel to the SAP process, the Lincoln Park HIA was fully integrated into the SAP.

The Lincoln Park HIA was initially scoped by the city planning and county health departments in January 2014. In addition to community representation on the advisory committee, public input was obtained through community events, one-on-one conversations between residents and staff, and two public meetings. Based on this input, the team focused its analysis on three health determinants: housing (availability, quality and affordability), community building/social cohesion, and access to healthy food. Looking at economic redevelopment through a "health lens," the HIA recommendations emphasized the creation of living wage jobs, increasing opportunities for social interaction, reducing crime and safety concerns, and creating a positive sense of place.

Reflecting on the process, the HIA team noted that the "integrated approach to the HIA was a very positive experience. ... The HIA coordinator was present to ensure health was discussed while SAP recommendations were formed. The advisory committee benefited by learning about the health process and reduced redundancy in meetings. ... It is possible that the HIA had more influence because it was discussed at almost every meeting and always on the forefront of participants' minds" (Minnesota Department of Health Climate and Health Program 2015, 133). City planning staff reported that, as the MDH had hoped, this HIA built their understanding of how their actions could promote health equity.

Summary: HIA and the City

These three HIA processes developed relationships and capacity in HIA among local stakeholders. Working together on the HIAs forged ties between city, county, and other agencies that had not worked closely together in the past. According to one city planner, "We were very separate in land use and planning activities—city and county—until recently. We have been meeting more with county planners and are actually working together now on several land use related issues. That is awesome. [It was] even the case in city hall with offices not working closely together in the past, but now these silos have come down and we are working together—it is a very exciting time" (Kelley 2016). At the same time, the Lincoln Park HIA cautioned that "city staff are very interested in incorporating health into the city's comprehensive plan update, but were concerned with how to go about that process—for example, if an HIA would be necessary and who would coordinate it?" (Minnesota Department of Health Climate and Health Program 2015).

The grant-funded efforts also exposed Duluth stakeholders to the practice of HIA in other communities. At least two city staff attended national HIA conferences and others participated in statewide trainings and the HIA collaborative. Although these three HIA projects built capacity to promote health through built environment decisions, several barriers remained. First, the HIAs informed plans, not decisions. Getting funding to implement these plans could be a challenge. Second, absent outside funding, the community does not have the capacity to support HIAs on future public decisions.

Sustaining Health Equity in Duluth

Stakeholders in Duluth recognized that significant inputs of external resources—including foundation and government grants and technical assistance—contributed to their PSE work. Support from external funders is unlikely to be sustained, raising the question of whether health equity has been institutionalized and will promote changes in the built environment over time. This section explores the sustainability of Healthy Duluth's work by examining impacts on key local decision-making processes, implementation projects, and emerging collaborative opportunities.

Health Equity in All Plans?

As described in chapter 3, the concept of "Health in All Polices" has been promoted as an overarching approach to improving health equity. Applying this idea to the built environment requires influencing local planning processes for land use, transportation, parks, and development. Although plans are not always implemented as intended, they provide a structure for coordinating decisions made across sectors, by multiple actors, over a long period of time. In other words, planning is necessary but not sufficient to implement visions of a healthier built environment. Nonetheless, there are promising signs that health equity is being integrated into local decision processes in a sustainable way.

Comprehensive Planning   When the Duluth comprehensive plan was updated in 2006 for the first time in decades, it called for SAPs for several neighborhoods, including Lincoln Park and Gary-New Duluth.[9] The SAPs were expected to be integrated into the 2016 plan update. HIA participants hoped that the health-informed provisions of the SAPs would become part of the city's comprehensive plan, but the mechanism to do so was not clear.

Soon after taking office in 2016, Mayor Emily Larson signaled that health equity was central to her overall vision for the city.[10] She announced in her first State of the City address in April 2016 that she was adding two new guiding principles to the comprehensive planning process: "1)— how does this increase fairness and opportunity across neighborhoods? And 2)—what are the health impacts of our decisions?" (Larson 2016). Healthy Duluth stakeholders viewed this as a commitment by Duluth's leadership to integrate health equity in all city decisions, not only those affecting the built environment.

In order to consider health in its ongoing decision-making processes, the city needed sustained partnerships with public health professionals. One early opportunity to do so came in 2016, when the city invited representation from the St. Louis County health department on the Irving Fairmount

Area-Wide Plan advisory team (Timm-Bijold 2016). The health department identified a staff person with the time and flexibility to participate in this short-term commitment. However, obtaining input, data, or analysis from a public health perspective on an ongoing basis may by limited by staff capacity.

Brownfield Redevelopment Planning in the Western Port Neighborhoods As described earlier, the city's Department of Business and Economic Development worked for many years to integrate health into redevelopment plans and projects. For example, redevelopment of the Universal Atlas Cement site in western Duluth is expected to create nearly 100 new jobs adjacent to the Gary-New Duluth neighborhood (Minnesota Pollution Control Agency 2011). Informed by HIA recommendations, city staff made sure that site plans included trails and street design conducive to active transportation. Recognizing the need to integrate health equity into brownfield redevelopment on an ongoing basis, city staff worked with Minnesota Brownfields to develop a streamlined brownfield health indicator tool, which they piloted during the Lincoln Park HIA.

In 2014, the city received a $200,000 grant from the U.S. EPA to develop a reuse plan for the western port neighborhoods of Fairmont and Irving, two small residential neighborhoods along the St. Louis River between Lincoln Park and Gary-New Duluth. These neighborhoods are bordered by a railyard, the 255-acre St. Lawrence River Interlake Duluth Tar Superfund site, and Route I-35. This area, originally referred to as the Western Port Area Neighborhoods (WPAN), suffered significant flood damage in 2012, including destruction of the community center. As Mayor Ness said in his support letter for the project, "Duluth's rising tide has not yet reached the WPAN. In order to foster economic growth and neighborhood stability within the WPAN, we must grapple with the brownfield sites that possess the potential for reuse and we must do so in harmony with its unique green spaces and precious water resources. ... We have no doubt that this [Area Wide Plan] opportunity is *THE* opportunity to move the collective vision of extant plans for the WPAN toward their much-needed implementation" (Ness 2014). Although the word "health" did not appear in the application, the twelve-page work plan guiding the project had many mentions of "human health," "public health," and "health impacts" (City of Duluth 2014a).

Without calling out health analysis as a separate process, as was done in the HIAs, the WPAN work plan expressed the city's intention to integrate public health in brownfield redevelopment. In addition, while emphasizing the health benefits of reducing exposure to environmental contaminants, the city made it clear that it aimed to address a broad range of health determinants based on community input (City of Duluth 2014a, 2014b; U.S. EPA 2015). Implementing Minnesota Brownfields' revised brownfields health indicator tool in this case contributed to a focus on social cohesion, connectivity, and economic stability in the final plan (Timm-Bijold 2016). Thus, Duluth's economic development office was a leader in bringing health into city plans and projects. As Heidi Timm-Bijold said, "We were not intentional about the health conversation [before], but now ... we are very clear about the conversation as it relates to food, safety, connectivity—it is just part of the discussion. So, as we move forward ... it is becoming normalized to think about health as part of the process" (Timm-Bijold 2016).

Bike Trail and Park Planning Duluth's comprehensive plan of 2006 recommended development of a Trail and Bikeway master plan, which was released in 2011. Responding to Mayor Ness's challenge that "Duluth should be the premier trail city in North America," the plan set forth a vision that "Duluth's trail and bikeway system has the potential to improve quality of life, foster economic development, preserve and enhance natural resources and enhance community and individual health and enjoyment" (City of Duluth 2011).

To help implement this plan, in 2014 the Minnesota state legislature approved a tourism tax ("the half and half tax") that allowed Duluth to raise up to $18 million over the next fifteen years for development of trails, parks, river access, environmental restoration, and recreational facilities around the St. Louis River.[11] The city planned to leverage other funding sources to generate a total of $50 million for twenty-five projects between 2015 and 2018 (City of Duluth 2016a, 2016b; Pioneer Press 2014).

When Mayor Larson took office in 2016, she affirmed her commitment to this initiative, calling it "an unmatched opportunity to extend the benefits of Duluth's success to all" (City of Duluth 2016b). In her first public update on implementation of the project, she emphasized community engagement, neighborhood parks, stimulating economic development and local jobs creation, and ensuring that the project benefited all Duluth residents. The mayor also indicated an awareness of the collaborative nature of this work by promising to "increase inter-departmental collaboration to give substance and cohesion to neighborhood revitalization and economic development goals." Several projects serving low-income neighborhoods were prioritized for early construction, including the Cross City trail, improvements in Lincoln Park, and the Gary-New Duluth Recreation Area (City of Duluth 2016b). These implementation priorities evidenced a continued commitment to support active transportation, economic development, and neighborhood cohesion consistent with the health equity-focused recommendations of the SAP HIAs.

Transportation Planning   The Duluth-Superior Metropolitan Interstate Council (MIC) is the Metropolitan Planning Organization (MPO) for Duluth. It provides regional transportation planning for a metropolitan area that spans two states, including Duluth, Minnesota, and Superior, Wisconsin, as well as several small urban areas adjacent to these cities (Duluth-Superior Metropolitan Interstate Council 2018). The MIC provides regional transportation planning services that bring together city, county, and state transportation engineers and other stakeholders on its technical advisory committee (TAC). Final plans and decisions are made by its policy board, which is comprised of local elected officials. The MIC has engaged in bike and pedestrian planning since the 1990s and formed a dedicated subcommittee including a public health representative in 2010. A staff member from the St. Louis County health department was appointed as a voting member of the TAC in 2015. Although transportation agencies are by law required to take health into consideration in their plans, health concerns are typically limited to traffic safety and air quality. Having a public health representative with a strong background in health equity ensured that consideration of broad health outcomes was a regular part of discussions.

Limitations and Challenges   These initiatives suggest that Healthy Duluth's goal of a built environment that promotes health equity has been institutionalized into local planning processes. Nonetheless, several stakeholders expressed concerns that without formally integrating health into implementation systems—such as project design, prioritization, and funding—these visions may not be realized in practice. Others cautioned that formalizing health equity as a decision-making criterion could lead to perfunctory mandatory review rather than meaningful collaboration and impact.

Where the Rubber Meets the Road: Implementing Health Equity in the Built Environment

Planning is necessary, but not sufficient, to shape the built environment. Therefore, Healthy Duluth partners have increasingly focused on opportunities to implement their vision. Notable are several recent projects aimed at promoting tangible health equity improvements in Duluth's built environment.

Food Access in Lincoln Park Healthy Duluth partners have worked for years to address poverty and food insecurity in Lincoln Park. The strategies developed through the Lincoln Park HIA spurred new initiatives and increased support for implementing projects. Three recent projects to improve food access in the area include the "Grocery Bus," a community garden/greenhouse, and a new Kwik Trip convenience store.

The Grocery Bus was an outcome of community conversations about the health impacts of poor transportation options and food access in Lincoln Park (Timm-Bijold 2016). Community members pointed out in the Fair Food Access door-to-door surveys and HIA public engagement meetings that there was limited bus service to the Super One, the nearest full-service grocery store. As well, the bus stop location was too far from the store entrance for people to easily carry bags of groceries. HDAC's Fair Food Access campaign worked with the Duluth Transportation Authority to institute the Grocery Bus—a special bus equipped with bins for groceries that runs once a week from Lincoln Park and Morgan Park (near Gary-New Duluth) directly to the Super One (Lundy 2016, 2017).

HDAC's Fair Food Access campaign also worked with Seeds of Success (an urban agriculture project of Community Action Duluth that works with unemployed community members) and other local groups to establish a farmers' market and community gardens in Lincoln Park. The Fair Food Access campaign enhanced these projects' contributions to health, neighborhood well-being, and economic development. For example, Fair Food Access provided a table for people to sign up for health insurance at the farmers' market. To highlight the gardens' potential impact on health and equity, Fair Food Access reported the monetary value, not just the quantity, of produce harvested. The city amplified these efforts by providing mulch, water, and compost for the gardens and was considering adding edible landscaping in trail and park projects. The city was also exploring the use of Community Development Block Grant funds for food access projects (Wilder Research 2014). These projects laid the foundation for the "Deep Winter Greenhouse," a collaborative effort of Seeds of Success, the Junior League, the City of Duluth, and a local architect that opened in 2018 (Community Action Duluth 2018; Timm-Bijold 2016).

In 2014, Kwik Trip announced its intention to locate its first Duluth store in Lincoln Park (Renalls 2014). Kwik Trip is a convenience store chain based in Wisconsin. Neighbors were initially concerned about the idea of a convenience store with high prices and unhealthy food. HDAC's Fair Food Access campaign invited Kwik Trip's chief financial officer to a community meeting about the proposed store (Wilder Research 2014). At the meeting, thirty-five residents gathered to ask the executive questions about Kwik Trip's business practices and were pleasantly surprised to learn that the stores carry a selection of fresh produce, baked goods, and staple foods (Renalls 2014). Residents were also pleased to hear that Kwik Trip is a family-owned business that sources the majority of its products from the region. Impressed with the executive's responses, they wrote a letter in support of Kwik Trip's application for a zoning variance to build the store (Wilder Research 2014). The year after Kwik Trip opened, the Fair Food Access campaign's door-to-door survey showed a noticeable improvement in residents' responses about access to food. Since then, two other Kwik Trips have opened in outlying western neighborhoods and more are planned for the future (Renalls 2015).

"Tactical Urbanism"   The Healthy Duluth partners recognized that public engagement was key to building support for implementation efforts. Around 2015, the HDAC Active Living group began promoting a series of high-visibility, creative events to engage the public's imagination about how streets in Duluth could better promote active transportation, social cohesion, and business development. Every May, they organized events for Bus/Bike/Walk month, including bike-themed movies, bike education, a "bike with the mayor" ride, and a bike art exhibit (French 2014d). A "parklet" program gave mini-grants to businesses to take over parking spaces and create temporary mini-parks with benches, tables, art, and landscaping (French 2015b). Most of these events were supported with small grants or event sponsorships.

Road Redesign   More concretely, Healthy Duluth sought opportunities to shape ongoing road redesign and construction projects. In 2014, health department and HDAC staff engaged in a proposed redesign of Superior Street, a major commercial street in downtown Duluth (French 2014b). They supported eliminating a section of diagonal parking in favor of parallel parking and a bike lane. Business owners successfully opposed the plan, citing concerns that reduced parking would harm their businesses. In another road construction project on 4th Street, HDAC's Active Living team successfully advocated for additional community engagement in the design process. The enhanced public input resulted in the inclusion of bike lanes, traffic-calming features, additional green space, and sidewalk buffers. Although there was no business opposition in this case, city engineers had raised concerns about the additional cost that the public support helped overcome. [12] On the western end of town, the city's Department of Business and Economic Development leveraged $3.3 million in grant funds to augment an ongoing highway repaving project with extra lighting, bus pullouts, new stoplights, and other safety improvements.

Summary   Healthy Duluth partners increased health equity considerations in many projects by engaging with implementing agencies. The relationship-building, technical assistance, and visioning processes that developed Healthy Duluth's capacity to promote such efforts was initially supported by outside resources, including MDH, the Health Impact Project, and private foundations. The examples demonstrate how this local capacity has impacted the practice of local decision makers. These projects all resulted from local stakeholders integrating health equity goals into programs whose primary objective was not health promotion. The potential to sustain such efforts absent external funding is explored in the next section.

Sustaining, Growing, and Evaluating Collaboration

Although many of the implementation activities described so far were carried out by a small subset of partners or by individual organizations, they were informed by nearly ten years of collaboration through Fit City Duluth, the HDAC, three HIAs, the city's brownfield program, and external training opportunities. As noted by several participants, these experiences developed partnerships between stakeholders, a "common language" around PSE and health equity, and a shared vision for a built environment that supports health for all residents.

Sustaining collaboration is challenging. Funders seldom support convening for the sake of developing collaborations for more than a few years at a time. These collaborations often decline without dedicated funding. However, there are several promising initiatives in Duluth that could help continue collaboration around these issues. These include the Zeitgeist Center's Health Equity Collaborative project, community health planning by local health systems, and the development of systems to track health data.

In 2016, the Zeitgeist Center for Arts and Community initiated a Health Equity Collaborative. This project was supported by a three-year grant from the Center for Prevention at Blue Cross Blue Shield of Minnesota's new Health in All Policies program (Center for Prevention at Blue Cross and Blue Shield of Minnesota 2018b). The Health Equity Collaborative aimed to build on past efforts of HDAC, engage new stakeholders at the community level, and implement at least eight policies to promote health equity in public institutions, private companies, and Duluth's two hospitals (Center for Prevention at Blue Cross and Blue Shield of Minnesota 2018b).

HDAC engaged health care institutions for many years, primarily as funding and technical support partners. However, the Affordable Care Act's requirement for hospitals to conduct a Community Health Needs Assessment (CHNA) provided impetus for health systems to take a broader role in prevention. In addition, it focused attention on the community benefits local hospitals must document to maintain their tax-exempt status (Keigley 2016). Healthy Duluth stakeholders worked to enhance community engagement in the CHNA and drive local health system investment in community health. Kayla Keigley, who led these efforts for Essentia Health in Duluth from 2014 to 2016, said: "It is a big culture shift for hospitals to think about population health. Now with the Affordable Care Act, it is so focused on what we can do before people come to the hospital, or better yet, keep them from coming to the hospital at all" (Keigley 2016). Initial efforts included funding support for "Together for Health," a school-based program to provide housing, economic development, and coordinating services for high-need families. Essentia Health also partnered with the health department to target prevention and clinical services to low-income housing developments where residents frequently visited the emergency department.

Building on this foundation, in 2016 the two major hospital systems in Duluth—Essentia and St. Luke's—collaborated to develop a joint CHNA. The planning group, later named "Bridging Health Duluth," included

Essentia Health-Duluth, Essentia Health-St. Mary's Medical Center, St. Luke's, the county health department, the Carlton-Cook-Lake-St. Louis Community Health Board, Healthy Northland, Generations Healthcare Initiatives, and the Zeitgeist Center for Arts and Community (Bridging Health Duluth 2016). The group was convened by Generations Healthcare Initiatives, a local foundation dedicated to promoting low-income communities' health. Health system staff undertook the majority of the analysis and writing. These partners analyzed available health data—including the Bridge to Health Survey—conducted community focus groups, and identified four priority areas. Two of these priority areas, "socioeconomic disparities based on race and neighborhood" and "obesity, including lack of access to healthy foods and physical inactivity," related directly to the Healthy Duluth work (Bridging Health Duluth 2016). In the words of one Bridging Health Duluth participant, "The goal and strategies selected were informed by foundational work and initiatives currently underway in our community, such as Health in all Policies" (Peterson 2017).

The participating hospitals committed resources to Bridging Health Duluth's implementation plan, including working with community groups "to address the social determinants of health such as housing, food access, safety, transportation, employment, and asset and income building" in low-income neighborhoods, supporting Health in all Policies (HiAP), and partnering with "local initiatives related to physical activity, multimodal transportation, and food access" to reduce obesity (Bridging Health Duluth 2016). The local health systems' growing focus on prevention and appreciation of the contributions of inequitable environmental conditions to health disparities created the potential for sustained support of healthy built environment initiatives.

Appropriate data are key to targeting, evaluating, and sustaining health equity work. Healthy Duluth initiatives made good use of available data, including the St. Louis County Health Status Report and the Bridge to Health Survey. However, these data sources were limited by scale, timeliness, and scope. Healthy Duluth partners recognized that in order to invest in community initiatives, health systems would need evidence that these efforts are effective in reducing health care costs at a fine geographic scale in real time. In 2016, Bridging Health Duluth brought together the local entities that collect or use health data to explore coordinating data systems. They continue to work on a publicly accessible tool to track community health status at a fine geographic and temporal scale to inform planning, decision-making, and program evaluation.

Initiatives such as the Health Equity Collaborative, the joint Community Health Needs Assessment, and efforts to improve geographically based population health data systems suggest that there is continued support for efforts to promote health equity through the built environment in Duluth.

Summary: The Future of Health Equity in Duluth's Built Environment

Health equity work in Duluth evolved in several loosely connected sectors including brownfield redevelopment, transportation, community food access, and land use planning (table 5.1). Shared experiences and coordinating groups like HDAC and Bridging Health Duluth facilitated networks across multiple sectors that developed strong personal relationships, a common vision, and shared language around health equity. As former HDAC director Lisa Luokkala said, health equity "has become a more common term that people can wrap their heads around, where four to five years ago we were really struggling to get people to grasp that concept. ... It is really interesting how that culture change happens." She added, "It was very intentional that we tried to spread the word. ... Now there is a broad group of professionals who use that term" (Luokkala 2016). The community is now seeing the concrete implementation of this vision through projects like community gardens, the Grocery Bus, and trail improvements in low-income neighborhoods.

Whether these sectors continue to collaborate remains to be seen. Reductions in external funding and staff turnover pose challenges for sustaining relationships and capacity in health equity analyses. Nonetheless, Duluth has made significant progress in creating a shared vision, intersectoral collaboration, and the institutionalization of a Health in All Policies approach.

Applying the Local Environmental Health Initiative Framework to Healthy Duluth

For more than a decade, Healthy Duluth efforts have promoted an equitable and health-supportive built environment (see table 5.2). Early work by the city's office of economic development to focus on the health implications of Duluth's brownfield redevelopment projects gained traction through the HIAs of two low-income neighborhoods. Meanwhile, efforts to promote

Table 5.2

Healthy Duluth and the Local Environmental Health Initiative Framework

Collaborative Function	Analysis of Healthy Duluth
Issue framing and problem definition	Reframed health disparities from a problem of individual behavior and health care to "Fair Food Access" and equitable active transportation.
	Defined problem as need for a health equity focus to prioritize, gain community input, and impact decisions affecting the built environment.
Resources for collaboration	Brought health stakeholders into new decision sectors. Generated and analyzed health data in new ways. HDAC obtained core support, new grants/projects (HIAs), and leveraged resources for partners' related projects. Grants, conferences, and agency staff provided technical information and supported community engagement.
Structure and decision-making process	Convened by multiple local organizations over time, including community, private, and government institutions.
	HDAC provided a forum for sharing information, coordinating, and developing strategy with consensus-based process.
	Community input provided by HDAC partner organizations and solicited through community-building, outreach, and survey efforts.
Impacts of collaboration:	
Outputs	County health status report, HIAs, brownfield plans, community surveys, HDAC newsletters/website, tactical urbanism projects.
Social outcomes	Relationships built through multiple projects over time facilitated ongoing partnerships and new city-county health department connections and developed a network of professionals committed to promoting health equity.
	Several HDAC members involved in new Health Equity Collaborative and Community Health Needs Assessment process.
Impacts on policies, systems, and environments (PSE)	Trail developments, community gardens, parks, and Grocery Bus have created more health-supportive environment in low-income areas.
	No evidence of population health improvements, but developing a system to track health outcomes.
	Incorporated health equity into comprehensive plan, Small Area Plans, and brownfields plans.
	Health representatives on transportation advisory committee.
	Informed MN Brownfield health indicator tool.

recreational physical activity evolved to focus on active transportation options for low-income communities. Fit City Duluth's first initiatives to encourage healthy eating developed into a wide menu of projects aimed at supporting local food production, neighborhood food sales, and public transportation to grocery stores. These efforts gained support from the public, community groups, professionals, and elected officials, as evidenced by the mayor's directive to incorporate health as an additional goal in the 2016 Comprehensive Plan update.

Issue Framing and Problem Definition

The initial focus of Fit City Duluth was on improving nutrition and increasing physical activity by "making the healthy choice the easy choice" (Public Health Law Center 2018). The group adopted a "policies, systems, and environments" approach to accomplish its goals. Its successor, the Healthy Duluth Area Coalition (HDAC) continued to coordinate, promote, and advocate for systems changes, particularly those that would improve food access and transportation options for low-income residents. Developing a common language and understanding of health equity helped professionals in diverse organizations coordinate around a wide range of projects, activities, and planning processes. Thus, the group reframed health disparities—which had been seen as largely an issue of access to health care and individual choices—as a community effort to provide equitable opportunities for everyone to live healthy lives. This reframing oriented health professionals and other partners away from individual education and services toward promoting policy, systems, and environmental changes.

Resources for Collaboration

Healthy Duluth was able to access both local and external resources. These initiatives tapped into an infusion of ideas, funding, and technical support from government agencies and private foundations committed to developing new local models for addressing the social determinants of health. As well, local stakeholders directed internal resources from their organizations toward efforts to promote healthier, more equitable built environments. These resources supported capacity building and specific projects.

Human Resources Many of the Healthy Duluth participants contributed "in kind" staff time with support from their employers, who saw connections between health equity efforts and their organizations' core goals. These included staff from the city, county, regional planning agencies, hospitals, and community groups. HDAC staff members were a key human resource, since they were responsible for organizing many of the meetings, facilitating discussions about strategies, proposals, and projects, and administering resources.

City staff involvement was supported by municipal leaders. Mayor Don Ness expressed how these initiatives fit in with his vision for growing Duluth: "Growth has to be sustainable, to include healthy neighborhoods, families, and individuals. Decisions made by the corporate city have a direct impact upon the community's health" (Ness 2012). Mayor Emily Larson also made it clear that she strongly embraced the idea of health equity. Thus, while many of the city's projects that promoted health equity leveraged outside funding, staff had clear mayoral support to write grants, partner with outside groups on projects, and prioritize city resources to promote built environment improvements in disadvantaged areas. Staff from city departments of business and economic development, planning, and parks were especially active in these efforts.

Another key source of human resources was the county health department. Former health educator Jim Skoog was an early leader in promoting systems changes in support of health. Subsequent funding through SHIP supported significant staff time devoted to related projects. Since 2009, there has been at least one full-time staff equivalent directed toward SHIP activities to improve determinants of health, primarily physical activity and healthy eating.

Staff from regional planning agencies serving Duluth also participated as part of their ongoing responsibilities. For example, an Arrowhead Regional Development Commission planner identified the first HIA opportunity and an MIC transportation planner contributed substantial time to the 6th Avenue HIA, as well as being longtime HDAC partners. As trained planners, these individuals understood the value of cross-sector collaboration and were personally supportive of these efforts.

Several staff from community and nongovernmental organizations were also active in HDAC. Leaders of community groups saw connections with their organizations' ongoing activities and directed human resources to aligned activities. For example, one of Community Action Duluth's organizers helped facilitate the Lincoln Park community survey in 2014. In recent years, hospital and health agency staff have become increasingly involved by encouraging a more community engaged and PSE-focused Community Health Needs Assessment process. The human resources they provided for convening, public engagement, analysis, and communication complemented HDAC's efforts.

Knowledge Resources   As noted throughout this chapter, Duluth benefited tremendously from conferences, training programs, and technical support provided by state and national government agencies and private foundations. Participation in these efforts built the capacity of Healthy Duluth partners. One of the first lessons local stakeholders learned was the importance of credible, detailed, timely local information. Fit City Duluth was inspired by its members' anecdotal information about the social and environmental health determinants affecting low-income areas and communities of color in Duluth. To quantify, support, and document these observations, the health department initiated the St. Louis County Health Status Report, which provided hard data about health disparities between zip codes in Duluth. The Bridge to Health Survey provided additional health-related information. Other organizations provided technical expertise, including regional health and transportation agencies. Although the HDAC did not have a consistent academic partner, the University of Minnesota-Duluth (UMD) food desert analysis was a valuable source of information, and the availability of interns from UMD provided ongoing assistance (Pine and Bennett 2011; Cuneo 2016).

Healthy Duluth drew on the emerging national consensus that the built environment impacts health and on Minnesota's strong support for environmental health equity. As the regional coordinator for SHIP, Annie Harala, said, "The state has historically provided some really solid technical assistance, and the state infrastructure is important. ... I feel like we are really spoiled living in Minnesota with all this support from MDH. MDH's Health Equity report has been foundational in helping change how we do our work. ... That gave us more power to come to the table saying, 'How you build the community affects health.' It wasn't just Los Angeles or San Francisco or New York City, it was that our commissioner of health believes this in Minnesota. So that helped get community on board" (Harala 2016). This credible regional support for their overall approach—in addition to the national perspective gained from conferences and training—boosted Healthy Duluth initiatives.

Financial Resources HDAC obtained financial resources to support convening the coalition on an uninterrupted basis since 2009. However, resources were often attached to specific projects, limiting staff time available for communications, strategy development, and coordination of partners' activities. In addition to grants, many organizations redirected existing funding sources to health equity priorities. External funding, like the HIA grants, paid for consultants, as well as for local staff, conferences, and public engagement efforts that contributed to building local capacity. SHIP funding supported local staff and some project costs. When asked if the infusion of outside resources had built sufficient capacity within Duluth to sustain this work, one regional planner said, "I feel [this work] needs to be sustained by federal agencies and foundations a bit longer to become sustainable at the local level. … As soon as these key players move on, I am concerned some of it could be weakened or watered down" (Herling 2016). Other conveners and partners obtained dedicated funding to pursue health equity work through grants, including the health impact assessments, brownfield planning efforts, and SHIP.

Group Structure and Decision-Making Processes

Duluth's small size provided opportunities for individuals to interact in multiple settings over time. HDAC was the most durable forum for collaboration around equity in the built environment. The former HDAC director described it as an "organization of organizations" that worked "at the grasstops" of groups representing at-risk community needs (Luokkala 2016). Its primary function was information-sharing, nurturing partnerships, and seeking project funding. HDAC's seventeen members met monthly, as did the major campaign work groups. HDAC committees made decisions by consensus.

HDAC did not have a direct role in all of the Healthy Duluth work. Many projects were conducted as partnerships of two or more groups, loosely coordinated with like-minded organizations, or communicated through blogs, public meetings, or individual relationships. Significantly, the City of Duluth was at no time a formal member of HDAC, yet city planning, funding, and policy decisions were crucial to progress (Healthy Duluth Area Coalition 2018). Despite not being members, city staff interacted with HDAC through its projects. Many of the Healthy Duluth efforts were grant-funded, so decisions within these projects were made by the lead agency according to the established work plan.

Community members and groups had significant input into the Healthy Duluth work. Several HDAC members directly served low-income communities and communicated their clients' needs to the coalition. The majority of these projects—including the ATSDR health analysis, the HIAs, and brownfield planning—were funded by programs that emphasized community engagement. Thus, although HDAC did not directly involve residents, its projects enhanced engagement in local decisions.

Collaborative Outputs and Outcomes

Because the health equity efforts in Duluth were diverse, diffused among multiple organizations, and interconnected, it is difficult to delineate all the Healthy Duluth outputs and outcomes. Fit City contributed to complete streets legislation. The brownfields planning efforts shaped land use and transportation design. Each of the HIA reports compiled data in an accessible way to guide SAP implementation. The county health department's reports and grant proposals were important products. The HDAC itself produced a wide range of communications materials, events, and public engagement efforts. For example, the HDAC Bus/Bike/Walk events, parklets, and blogs contributed to a community vision for healthier transportation and food access options. HDAC communications also sought to increase local decision makers' understanding of community benefits from promoting health equity through the built environment (Gorham 2016a). Going forward, integrating built environment data into the Community Health Needs Assessments will support project planning and evaluation. Thus, in addition to HDAC's direct products, many partners' outputs were influenced by this initiative.

Social outcomes were cited by many participants as important contributions to sustaining this work. Several partners also emphasized that Duluth's small size made it easier for professionals to connect across organizations and maintain individual relationships over time. As the leader of a local foundation said, "What has been great about Duluth is we do have a collaborative nature. I think we are the right size to be able to pull this sort of thing off. If we were the Twin Cities, there would be too many communities and too many players. We are small enough that we know each other and can build that trust and get something done. It is a scale that is manageable. ... There are complexities to our work, but there is a spirit of collaboration" (Peterson 2017). As one participant said, "The cool thing about Duluth is if you start a project that takes on a multisector approach to a problem, the table never gets smaller, it just keeps getting bigger, which is different than other places I have been" (Keigley 2016). Duluth's size also means that most of the professionals involved are city residents with a direct stake in the outcomes of efforts that affect their home neighborhoods, civic engagement, and personal lives.

Several projects promoted by Healthy Duluth have already impacted the physical environment. For example, the city prioritized constructing sections of the Cross City trail and parks improvements in low-income neighborhoods as part of the St. Louis Corridor Initiative. Documenting and linking health improvements to such environmental changes is likely to be a challenging long-term prospect. Bridging Health Duluth is developing a data system to track health outcomes at a temporal and geographic scale that may capture these impacts.

Policies and processes have also changed in significant ways. The mayor's commitment to include health as a goal of the 2016 Comprehensive Plan suggests a long-term commitment to these ideas. Inclusion of health interests in the Technical Advisory Committee of the Metropolitan Interstate Council has impacted transportation projects. The involvement of government staff, elected officials, and community leaders means that health equity concerns are more likely to be "top of mind" and given weight in public decisions. Although this has not been formalized in a Health in All Policies resolution or formal process between city government and the county health department, stakeholders noted that the shared understanding of how changes in the built environment can reduce health disparities has affected a wide range of decision processes. Outside of the Twin Cities, Duluth has performed the most HIAs in Minnesota and has been recognized by as a leader by the state (Raab 2017).

Conclusions

When Fit City began, Duluth already had made progress in reducing unemployment, stabilizing its population, and attracting new development. This upward trend increased optimism about the future yet also highlighted the disparities in who benefited from Duluth's improved fortunes and who did not. Since Duluth's designation in 2007 as a "Fit City," it has undertaken a range of efforts to improve access for all residents to health-supportive resources, particularly active transportation opportunities and healthy food. These efforts included development projects, community activities, planning efforts, and encouraging leaders' commitment to incorporate health equity considerations into local decisions affecting the built environment. The work involved community groups, service agencies, health care organizations, and multiple levels of government. Duluth has made significant progress toward Health in All Policies as a strategy for pursuing health equity. As Heidi Timm-Bijold said, "There has been a momentous but intentional aligning of the stars around this work" (Timm-Bijold 2016).

With its reputation as a postindustrial rust belt city with a recent history of high unemployment rates, observers often ask, "Why Duluth?" How did this small city develop such robust, diverse, and sustained efforts to promote health equity through decisions about its built environment? In response, local stakeholders credit the engaged and progressive spirit of Duluth, noting the robust university community, tradition of civic engagement, and the high level of voter turnout. Several interviewees stated that they originally came to the city—many as students at UMD—because of access to outdoor activities. Indeed, the story of Duluth's recent economic growth is peppered with tales of entrepreneurs and small business owners who moved to Duluth for the quality of life.[13] Former mayor Don Ness was quoted by *Outside Magazine* as saying, "Despite the weather, or maybe because of it, Duluthians are super passionate about this city" (Pearson 2014). This commitment to community was cited as a motivating and bonding force among Healthy Duluth stakeholders.

City leaders supported Healthy Duluth efforts as consistent with their vision for Duluth's future, but for the most part specific projects were initiated by staff. Recent efforts to use Community Development Block Grant (CDBG) funds and city land for urban agriculture, prioritization of St. Louis Corridor projects in low-income neighborhoods, and the directive to incorporate health in the comprehensive plan indicate growing commitment by local leaders. This commitment bodes well for the sustainability of these efforts. However, the HDAC has experienced difficulty sustaining support for convening functions over time. Given the multisectoral nature of the effort and the important roles of diverse community and government institutions, finding ways to continue this convening function is key.

The financial, technical, and human resources enjoyed by health equity efforts in Duluth over the past decade, its small scale, and the progressive cultural environment begs the question of whether its experience is replicable in other communities. Other communities may be able to borrow some of Duluth's approaches, but there may be differences based on their local resources, organizations, and culture. Duluth's experience also suggests that the process of learning together, identifying local needs, and building cross-organization relationships is a key to success. Opportunities to work together on pilot projects, interact with residents, and convene diverse groups may be essential for collaborative initiatives to identify the most productive ways to pursue equity in their local environment.

6 THE Impact Project: Trade, Health, and Environment around Southern California's Ports

Case Summary

In our globalized world, most consumer products are shipped from where they are made to their final user through a complex "goods movement system" of container ships, trains, warehouses, and trucks. More than 40 percent of all goods imported into the United States enter through the ports of Los Angeles and Long Beach in Southern California, making that area a major hub of freight transportation (figure 6.1). The emissions, noise, light, and traffic from goods movement activities pose health risks to surrounding communities and workers. In 2001, the University of Southern California's Environmental Health Sciences Center, which has a major focus on air pollution research, and community partners hosted a town hall meeting in which participants highlighted these concerns. Subsequently, academic and community partners formed the "Trade, Health, and Environment Impact Project"—or simply THE Impact Project—to elevate health equity as a central concern in goods management decisions. THE Impact Project supported community-based science, built capacity within communities and among academic researchers to knowledgeably participate in decision-making, and translated emerging health research to inform goods movement planning. This case focuses on the resources, approaches, and strategies local stakeholders used to protect community health from the cumulative impacts of a complex system of decisions made in multiple sectors at the local, regional, state, national, and international level.

Introduction: People, Ports, and Public Health

We use goods produced in other countries every day—cars, clothing, technology, food, and countless other consumer products. These products travel to us through a network of ships, planes, trains, and trucks. Most goods arrive in the United States at a deepwater port in container ships. These containers may then be trucked to railyards, taken by train or truck to warehouses, and eventually transferred to trucks or vans for local delivery. This goods movement system creates negative externalities—unintended health and environmental impacts—including air pollution, traffic accidents, noise, and dangers to workers. Despite extensive federal and state regulations, these externalities may significantly affect the health of communities located near goods movement operations. According to Cummings (2018), "Ports are spaces where the unequal costs and benefits of trade and consumption see their most immediate and palpable distribution." People living near the ports of Los Angeles and Long Beach have long been concerned about the health impacts of goods movement activities on their communities. Since around 2001, environmental organizations, academics, and community groups have increasingly worked together to address these concerns through systems change. This chapter focuses on a community-academic collaborative, THE Impact Project, which aimed to reduce the health impacts associated with goods movement from the ports in Long Beach and Los Angeles, California. It examines the resources, strategies, and processes the partners used to overcome political, economic, and institutional barriers to change at the local level. Although THE Impact Project was just one of many ongoing efforts to promote environmental health and justice in port-adjacent communities, it had a significant impact on local systems-change efforts—even in the context of powerful state, national, and global economic and political forces.

The U.S. economy depends on a global transportation system that continues to grow rapidly. Roughly 40 percent of the goods imported to the United States pass through the ports of Los Angeles and Long Beach, totaling over a billion dollars in cargo each day (Cummings 2018; McDonnell and Kitroeff 2016). Trade through these ports more than doubled between 1995 and 2017 (Port of Long Beach 2018b; Port of Los Angeles 2018a). A total of 16.8 million twenty-foot containers (twenty-foot equivalent units, or TEUs) entered the two ports in 2017, representing a major sector of the

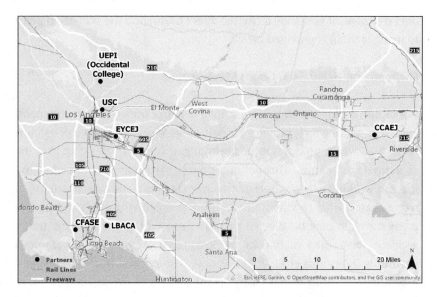

Figure 6.1
Map of Southern California ports region and locations of THE Impact Project partners
Map credit: Karl Korfmacher

Southern California economy. Despite the 2016 expansion of the Panama Canal that allowed larger ships to pass through to East Coast ports, the ports of Southern California are expected to continue growing for the foreseeable future (McDonnell and Kitroeff 2016; SUNY 2016). This projection has spurred expansion of railyards, railways, highways, and warehouses in the region. Many of these infrastructure improvements are subsidized by public funds, including $1.2 billion in transportation projects supported by the American Recovery and Reinvestment Act (ARRA) stimulus starting in 2009 (Matsuoka et al. 2011).

Although individual parts of the goods movement system (e.g., emissions from trucks, locomotives and oceangoing ships) are regulated by state, federal, and in some cases international law, their cumulative environmental impacts can cause significant health problems for those who live nearby. These impacts are concentrated around "intermodal" facilities—including ports, railyards, and warehouses—where goods are moved from one form of transport to another. Air pollution is the primary environmental health concern, but water pollution, noise, traffic, bright all-night lighting, and safety hazards can also affect the health of workers and nearby communities. A brief overview of how these activities affect health and the systems in place to manage them is provided below.

Environment, Health, and Goods Movement

Goods movement activities at ports involve trains, trucks, heavy equipment, and ships, all of which produce air pollution. Many of these vehicles burn diesel fuel, which produces more harmful gases and particles than gasoline or natural gas engines. This pollution poses particular risks to people living and working near goods transportation facilities and can contribute to regional air quality problems. In addition, people living near goods movement activities may be affected by noise, constant bright lighting, traffic accidents, pedestrian safety risks, traffic congestion, and spills of hazardous chemicals (Matsuoka et al. 2011). People who operate trucks, trains, and machinery, work in warehouses, or unload containers at the ports face health risks from air quality, heat, and other safety hazards.

Air Pollution and Human Health

Historically, air pollution was considered a local problem resulting from combustion for cooking and small-scale commercial activities. With increasing industrialization in the twentieth century, larger factories with tall stacks contributed to regional air pollution concerns. In 1948, more than twenty people died after an industrial air pollution buildup around Donora, Pennsylvania (Davis 2003). This event was followed closely by the infamous London fog of 1952, during which mortality rates tripled, then remained elevated for months, killing an estimated 12,000 people (Bell, Davis, and Fletcher 2003). These lethal air pollution events, along with increased understanding of the health impacts of chronic exposure to air pollution, were primary motivators for federal air quality regulations implemented in the United States in the 1960s and 1970s (Andrews 2006). Although these policies drastically reduced pollution, regional air quality problems persist, particularly in major metropolises. At the same time, research on the health impacts of air pollution has led to greater concern about long-term exposure to even low levels of air pollution. Air pollutants commonly associated with goods movement activities contribute to a wide range of health problems.

Air quality varies constantly, which makes understanding the health impacts of air pollution challenging. Local air quality depends on weather (temperature, sunlight, precipitation, mixing of the atmosphere by wind, etc.), geography, emissions from both stationary (e.g., industrial) and mobile (e.g., vehicle) sources, and the types of chemicals emitted by these sources. The effects of pollutants on people vary based on how long they are exposed and their individual vulnerabilities.

Environmental health concerns related to goods movement focus on diesel exhaust from trucks, trains, ships, and heavy equipment at ports. As a foundation for understanding the health concerns surrounding goods movement, it is important to have an overview of the chemical components of diesel exhaust, the health effects of inhaling these chemicals, the extent to which goods movement activities contribute to overall air quality in urban areas, and who is most susceptible to this pollution. Diesel exhaust consists of gases and particulate matter. The gases include nitrogen oxides (NO_x), sulfur dioxides (SO_2), carbon monoxide (CO), and volatile organic compounds (VOCs). Especially in urban areas, diesel exhaust can be a significant contributor of nitrogen oxides, which in turn are the primary precursor of ground-level ozone (Dallmann and Harley 2010; Kota et al. 2014). Ozone is a constituent of smog and has a variety of health effects (Olivieri and Scoditti 2005; Bernstein et al. 2004).

Diesel combustion is also a major source of particulate matter in urban environments (California Air Resources Board 2018; Rosenbaum, Hartley, and Holder 2011; Hasheminassab et al. 2014; Kim and Hopke 2008; Kim et al. 2010). Particulate matter is categorized by size because smaller particles may penetrate the lung more deeply, enter the blood, and have more severe health effects (Oberdorster et al. 2004; Araujo et al. 2008; Weuve et al. 2012; Li et al. 2003; Li et al. 2016; Bernstein et al. 2004). The smallest particles, called ultrafine particles (UFP), may even enter cells and cause DNA damage (Li et al. 2016). Exposure to fine particulate pollution has been associated with respiratory, neurologic, and cardiovascular effects (Pope et al. 2004; Pope and Dockery 2006; U.S. EPA 2009b; Utell and Frampton 2000).

Research suggests the combined effects of particles and gases comprising diesel exhaust can contribute to cognitive impairment, diabetes, and chronic obstructive pulmonary disease (COPD) (Ranft et al. 2009; Liu et al. 2013; Kramer et al. 2010; Andersen et al. 2011). Pregnant women who breathe diesel exhaust may have pregnancy complications and low-birth-weight babies (Wilhelm and Ritz 2005; Basu et al. 2014; Wu et al. 2009; Green et al. 2009). Based on studies of workers exposed to diesel exhaust, the U.S. Environmental Protection Agency (EPA) categorized diesel as a "likely human carcinogen" in 1999, and the International Agency for Research on Cancer (IARC) classified it as a "known human carcinogen" (IARC 2012; Benbrahim-Tallaa et al. 2012; Garshick et al. 2012; Attfield et al. 2012).

Air quality can vary significantly across small distances. For example, one study found elevations of ultrafine particles (UFPs), nitrogen dioxide, and elemental carbon within 150 meters of busy roads (Zhu et al. 2002; Boothe and Shendell 2008; Greco et al. 2007). Studies have also detected higher rates of certain cancers among people living near known sources of diesel emissions or who are exposed in the workplace (Silverman et al. 2012; Mack 2004; Crouse et al. 2010). Models suggest that cancer risk from diesel emissions is much higher for people living close to these facilities (Hricko et al. 2014; Hand et al. 2004; NEJAC 2009; Pingkuan Di 2006).

In many urban areas, diesel is the largest source of NO_x and small particulates (U.S. EPA 2002). In 2005, the Los Angeles and Long Beach ports produced around 25 percent of the region's air particulate matter and 25 percent of diesel emissions (Port of Los Angeles 2007; Matsuoka 2014). While there have been significant reductions in emissions from vehicular sources since 2007, goods movement activities still significantly impact air quality in Southern California (Hasheminassab et al. 2014). The ports remain the largest fixed sources of air pollution in the region, emitting more pollution every day than the region's 6 million cars (South Coast Air Quality Management District 2018b).

Certain people are more vulnerable to air pollution than others because of their age, genes, or health status. Research shows that children are particularly affected by air pollution. Children who grow up in areas with air pollution from traffic have reduced lung function (Gauderman et al. 2004; Gauderman et al. 2007). Uncertainty remains about the role of air pollution in the development of asthma (Eder, Ege, and von Mutius 2006; Sarnat and Holguin 2007; McConnell et al. 2010). However, several studies have found that children who live or go to school near high-traffic areas are more likely to develop asthma and to have more frequent asthma attacks (McConnell et al. 2010; Gauderman et al. 2005). In addition, ambient air pollution can trigger asthma attacks in both adults and children who have asthma (Peel et al. 2005; Jacquemin et al. 2015; Sunyer et al. 1997).

Thus, a wide range of health effects are associated with air pollution from goods movement activities. Communities near transportation activities recognize that the health of their residents may not be adequately protected by the complex system of federal, state, and regional policies, regulations, and programs that have been implemented to control air pollution. The next section provides a brief overview of this system and the gaps that leave certain communities at risk of exposure to harmful levels of pollution.

Air Pollution and Goods Movement: The Policy Context

The extreme air pollution events of the 1950s heightened the public's awareness of air pollution. The United States responded to the growing public concern by passing the Clean Air Act (CAA) of 1963. This law had a weak role for the federal government; most implementation and enforcement was left to the states. Differing state air quality standards encouraged polluting industries to locate in the states with the weakest regulations. Air quality was eventually recognized to be a regional problem, since air pollution crosses state lines and states with weaker controls could "export" their pollution to downwind states. To address such problems, the CAA was strengthened in 1970, setting national standards for air quality. Although it has since been revised several times, the structure of the 1970 Clean Air Act remains the guiding framework for air quality management today (U.S. EPA 2017f).

The goal of the CAA was "to protect and enhance the quality of the Nation's air resources so as to promote the public health and welfare and the productive capacity of its population" (U.S. Congress 1970). Under the CAA, the EPA was directed to set National Ambient Air Quality Standards (NAAQS) for six "criteria pollutants"—sulfur dioxide (SO_2), nitrogen oxides (NO_x), particulate matter (PM_{10} and $PM_{2.5}$), carbon monoxide, ozone, and lead (U.S. EPA 2016b). Each state must submit a State Implementation Plan (SIP) for review by the EPA specifying how it will meet NAAQS requirements (U.S. EPA 2016d). The EPA was directed to set the NAAQS to "protect public health with an adequate margin of safety" based on the best available science, to be reviewed every five years. For example, in 2015 the EPA lowered the NAAQS for ozone from 75 to 70 parts per billion (ppb) (U.S. EPA 2018j).

Despite the health concerns noted previously, there currently is no separate standard for ultrafine particles (RTI International 2015). Although there is no NAAQS for diesel pollution, California regulates it as a toxic air contaminant (California Air Resources Board 2018).

Because air quality fluctuates constantly, the EPA sets multiple standards for several pollutants based on different time periods. For example, the primary NAAQS standard for $PM_{2.5}$ is set at 12 µg/m^3 (micrograms per cubic meter of air) averaged over an entire year and 35 µg/m^3 for any twenty-four-hour period (U.S. EPA 2016b). If air quality monitoring shows that pollution exceeds NAAQS standards, the area is designated a "nonattainment area" for that pollutant and is subject to stricter regulations (U.S. EPA 2017a).

The Clean Air Act addresses mobile sources of pollution by directing the EPA to set national standards for allowable emissions from different kinds of consumer vehicles, heavy-duty vehicles (trailer trucks and buses), and non-road engines (locomotives and aircraft). Because of its persistent air quality problems, California has been allowed to adopt more stringent vehicle emissions (U.S. EPA 2013a). In addition, the 2007 Highway Rule required new bus and truck diesel engines to meet lower emissions standards and burn ultra-low-sulfur diesel (ULSD) fuel, reducing per-vehicle emissions of sulfur by 90 percent (U.S. EPA 2017d). To support implementation of this rule, the federal government established a program of grants to support the retrofitting and replacement of existing diesel engines (U.S. EPA Agency 2017d, 2018h). Air quality was expected to improve significantly as older engines were replaced over time. However, increases in the number of engines operating in an area, weak implementation or rollback of these rules, or new sources of pollution could reverse these trends.

Emissions from ships burning marine diesel pose an additional health hazard. In 2007, researchers estimated 60,000 annual cancer deaths from the global diesel emissions of oceangoing ships (Corbett et al. 2007). Although the CAA sets standards for marine engines, these do not apply to ships from other countries. Container ships burn marine diesel fuel or "bunker fuel," which is less expensive but produces more pollution than other types of diesel. Under rules adopted by the EPA in 2009, all ships operating within 200 miles of the U.S. coast must meet stricter standards (U.S. EPA 2017e). Implementation of this requirement is expected to greatly reduce pollution from oceangoing ships in U.S. ports (U.S. EPA 2018d). New rules by the International Maritime Organization will expand those controls to ports around the world by 2020 (Gallucci 2018; International Maritime Organization 2018).

Major expansions of goods movement facilities usually must be reviewed under the National Environmental Policy Act (NEPA) and similar state laws (Port of Long Beach 2018a). As described in chapter 2, an environmental impact statement (EIS) under NEPA must predict the environmental impacts of the project, compare them to alternatives including a "no-build" (baseline) scenario, and allow for agency and public review. The process of deciding which goods movement projects require EISs, what impacts are analyzed, and to what extent impacts are mitigated in final plans is frequently controversial (U.S. EPA 2016c).

Thus, multiple policies, programs, and regulations manage the environmental impacts of goods movement activities throughout the United States. Implementation of this system in Southern California is unique in several ways. The region has struggled with poor air quality for decades. In addition to being home to a large number of industrial, freight, and traffic sources of pollution, mountain ranges surrounding Los Angeles trap pollution over the city. These factors, as well as abundant sunshine, contribute to the area's infamous smog. The South Coast Air Quality Management District (SCAQMD) is responsible for managing air quality in Southern California. To address its persistent air pollution problems, Southern California has some of the strictest air emissions controls in the country. Implementation of these restrictions has led to a 75 percent reduction in ozone since the 1950s, despite a tripling of the local population (SCAQMD 2018a). Nonetheless, the region is still a nonattainment area for $PM_{2.5}$ and ozone (SCAQMD 2017).

Transportation continues to be a significant contributor to air pollution in the region, despite Southern California leading the United States in vehicle-based air pollution reduction efforts. Around three-quarters of the pollution contributing to ozone in the Los Angeles region is attributed to mobile sources (SCAQMD 2018a). Many of these vehicles are associated with goods transport: On the I-710 freeway, over 25 percent of the vehicles are heavy-duty diesel freight trucks (Human Impact Partners 2011). Despite California's strong air quality protection programs, there are limits to how much it can regulate emissions. For example, in 2010 a federal judge ruled that California could not restrict trains idling on the basis that the regulation interfered with interstate commerce (Williams 2010).

Even with the multitude of health-based regulations that have significantly improved air quality, air pollution continues to pose a health threat to people in Southern California, particularly those living and working near transportation facilities (Brown et al. 2014; Boothe and Shendell 2008). As well, emerging research on health impacts of fine particulates shows significant acute and chronic health effects of $PM_{2.5}$ exposure at levels below the current U.S. EPA standards (Shi et al. 2016). Thus, increasingly stringent ambient air quality standards, emissions standards for new industrial facilities, programs promoting cleaner engines, and environmental impact reviews of major new activities have significantly improved air quality, but risks remain for communities located near hubs of goods movement activities.

Health Impacts of Noise, Light, and Traffic

Other major concerns of people living near goods movement operations include noise, twenty-four-hour lighting, and traffic. Sometimes called "nuisance" concerns, these issues are typically addressed by local laws or private legal actions but are not generally regulated as "environmental" hazards.

The cranes, machinery, trains, trucks, and traffic associated with goods movement can produce high levels of noise around the clock. Research in both community and occupational settings shows that noise can significantly affect health. In a residential setting, the primary concern is usually sleep disruption and stress (Lercher et al. 2002; Evans 2006). Studies have associated chronic noise exposure with cognitive problems, heart disease, and stroke (Babisch 2006; Stansfeld et al. 2005; Sorensen et al. 2011).

Noise standards for transportation activities are set by the federal government. Non-transportation sources, such as industrial activity, may be regulated by local government through noise ordinances (SCAQMD 2012). Noise regulations apply to planning, constructing, and assessing the impacts of new projects. For example, noise standards from the U.S. Department of Housing and Urban Development (HUD) are used to assess what kind of noise abatement measures need to be built into new public housing constructed near roadways, railyards, or airports (HUD 2018b). Similarly, environmental impact reviews of transportation projects must model noise impacts to show they do not exceed standards. In practice, however, it has been challenging for residents to act on existing sources of noise (e.g., the increased traffic around a port or the frequency of train horns) or address the cumulative impacts of multiple sources. The U.S. EPA's Office of Noise Abatement and Control, established under the Noise Control Act of 1972, was stripped of its funding in 1981 and has not received congressional budgetary support since that time, limiting noise abatement actions by the federal government (Shapiro 1992).

Many port facilities are lit by stadium lighting to facilitate twenty-four-hour operations and promote safe working conditions. This light often spills over into adjacent neighborhoods. Human and animal research suggests that bright nighttime lighting has negative health effects, including disruption of sleep, hormones, and immune function (Chepesiuk 2009; Pauley 2004; Cho et al. 2015). California has no policies in place to regulate light pollution (National Conference of State Legislatures 2016). However, there are standards for lighting at industrial facilities, and some municipalities, including Los Angeles, have ordinances restricting spillover lighting or "light trespass" (Municipal Research and Services Center 2016; County of Los Angeles 2018). Technical solutions such as light shields, height restrictions, and lighting designed to illuminate only the ground may reduce these problems. Nonetheless, neighbors of port facilities frequently mention spillover lighting as a negative impact on their quality of life (Matsuoka et al. 2011).

Growth in goods movement activities frequently results in increased traffic, which can create the potential for bike, pedestrian, or car collisions in adjacent residential neighborhoods. Accidents involving trucks or train derailment also pose the risk of spilling hazardous materials. Neighbors frequently report that truck traffic negatively affects their quality of life because it brings more traffic jams and excessive noise, makes it less safe to exercise outdoors, and reduces the "walkability" of neighborhoods.

When a new transportation facility is proposed, or an existing facility is being expanded, the impacts of increased traffic are part of the environmental review process. Regional transportation planners model increases in traffic in order to develop routes that do not adversely affect residential streets (U.S. DOT 2018a). However, incremental expansion of operations that do not require environmental review may result in additional traffic on existing roadways. In such cases, municipalities may work with industries to develop voluntary truck-routing agreements; however, local communities' ability to control ongoing increases in traffic associated with existing facilities are limited.

Thus, "nuisance" factors like noise, light, and traffic associated with goods movement developments can negatively affect the health of adjacent communities. Research increasingly shows that cumulative environmental exposures such as air pollution and stress can multiply health effects (Payne-Sturges et al. 2015; Clougherty et al. 2007). Residents may face challenges in addressing these problems including limited resources for advocacy, absence of conclusive local data supporting their concerns, and lack of policy tools to mitigate the impacts of goods movement activities.

Worker Health

The health impacts of goods movement are also significant for workers, including dock, rail, and warehouse workers and truck drivers. Overall, the transportation and warehousing sector is one of the riskiest occupational sectors (Bureau of Labor Statistics 2018). Workers may be exposed to heat stress, poor air quality, and high levels of noise (Landon, Breysse, and Chen 2005). The limited staff of the federal Occupational Health and Safety Administration (OSHA) and related state agencies cannot regularly inspect these workplaces to make sure regulations are being followed. Many workers in the transportation sector do not belong to unions that can advocate for better protections (Cummings 2018). Most port truck drivers are classified as "independent contractors," which limits their ability to access worker protections and to complain about conditions without losing their jobs (Smith, Bensman, and Marvy 2010). Independent contractor status may exacerbate pollution exposures because driver-owners may not be able to afford to maintain emissions controls on their trucks (Cummings 2018). Many people employed in goods movement activities are low-wage, temporary, or contract workers, which means they are likely to have additional health challenges such as poor health care and may themselves live in highly polluted neighborhoods (Matsuoka et al. 2011; Murphy 2017).

Other Health and Environmental Concerns

In addition to these direct health impacts resulting from goods movement decisions in Southern California, there are many additional indirect health and environmental consequences. For example, the diesel fuel emissions and discharge of sewage from container ships may pollute coastal waters. The noise of ship engines can harm marine mammals, and ships sometimes strike and kill them. Discharged ballast water from ships may transport invasive species that can damage local marine ecosystems. The current system of goods movement also has significant climate change implications. The transportation sector comprises nearly 30 percent of all greenhouse gas emissions in the United States (U.S. EPA 2018i). Global shipping currently contributes around 3 percent of total annual anthropogenic greenhouse gas emissions (Matsuoka et al. 2011; Bouman et al. 2017). Finally, global trade has implications for people living in countries like China, where regulations may be less protective of environmental health. Although these are not "local" community health issues, they may be significant concerns for local, regional, or national stakeholders engaged in goods management decisions.

Environmental Justice and Goods Movement

People living or working near goods movement hubs may be impacted by multiple environmental health hazards. Ports and railyards are often located adjacent to other polluting industries. The communities surrounding these industrial and transportation facilities tend to be lower-income and are home to many immigrants, refugees, and people of color. Hricko and colleagues (2014) found that there was a significantly higher percent of families in poverty living adjacent to California railyards compared to those living in the surrounding county. For most of these sites, the proportion of Latino residents was similarly elevated. For example, they analyzed demographic data from communities surrounding the Union Pacific railyard in Los Angeles, which was constructed in 1980. At the time of construction, the adjacent neighborhoods had a higher proportion of racial minorities (68 percent versus 47 percent in the county) and less than half the average income. By 2005, the percent of minority residents in the neighborhood had increased from 68 percent to 89 percent (versus 69 percent in the county). Based on analysis of other recent railyard expansion proposals, the authors suggest that goods movement facilities continue to disproportionately affect lower-income areas and communities of color (Hricko et al. 2014). This pattern is not unique to California. A national study of port communities found that the proportions of lower-income black or Latino residents living near ports were higher than in the overall U.S. population, sometimes by a factor of two to three (Rosenbaum, Hartley, and Holder 2011).

In response to these concerns, in 2007 the U.S. EPA asked the National Environmental Justice Advisory Committee (NEJAC) to "provide advice and recommendations about how the Agency can most effectively promote strategies, in partnership with federal, state, tribal, and local government agencies, and other stakeholders, to identify, mitigate, and/or prevent the disproportionate burden on communities of air pollution resulting from goods movement" (NEJAC 2009, 1). NEJAC appointed a Goods Movement Work Group (GMWG) to research the issue and develop recommendations. The GMWG recommendations emphasized the need for strong community participation and collaborative governance, as well as additional research, regulation, and funding (NEJAC 2009).

Goods Movement in Southern California

Given Southern California's history of air quality problems associated with transportation, it is not surprising that it is a hub for research, community action, and policy to address the health impacts of goods movement. At the same time, global trade's importance to the economy poses a political challenge to those who hope for stronger regulations. Many of the neighborhoods adjacent to the ports of Los Angeles and Long Beach are home to communities with limited political power and economic resources. In contrast, the power of industries involved with goods movement in Southern California is formidable: It includes the world's largest shipping agencies and the nation's largest railroad companies, as well as major trucking and logistics corporations, real estate developers, and retail giants. Nonetheless, community groups in Southern California have succeeded in increasing awareness of the health impacts of goods movement. Not only have these groups advocated for health considerations in related decisions, but they have also reached out to support other port-adjacent communities across the country. Many groups have contributed to these efforts. This case study focuses on THE Impact Project, an initiative that leveraged the resources of community and academic partners to influence the systems governing goods movement. The discussion explores the evolution of these efforts over the past fifteen years, the resources that supported them, their impacts on goods movement decisions, and implications for other communities living near intermodal transportation hubs.

Case Overview: THE Impact Project

In 2001, the Natural Resources Defense Council (NRDC) partnered with homeowner and environmental groups to sue the Port of Los Angeles for failing to conduct an environmental impact report (EIR) on the expansion of container-handling facilities leased to the China Shipping Holding Company as required under the California Environmental Quality Act (CEQA) (Natural Resources Defense Council 2002a, 2002b). The suit ended with a $50 million settlement that funded pollution prevention and mitigation efforts around the port (Cummings 2018). The China Shipping suit was the culmination of years of efforts to force the Port of Los Angeles to address the health and environmental concerns of homeowners from the port-adjacent San Pedro and Peninsula neighborhoods (Natural Resources Defense Council 2002a). The settlement has been hailed as the start of a comprehensive effort to address environmental health impacts of port-related activities in the region.

Other communities abutting goods movement infrastructure in Southern California were also becoming increasingly concerned about port expansion and attendant air pollution, traffic safety, and noise issues. Neighborhood, environmental, and community health groups organized around different aspects of good movement decisions in the region. For example, in the late 1990s the Center for Community Action and Environmental Justice (CCAEJ) began fighting construction of inland warehouses to store freight from the ports. Other groups focused on individual rail, port, and highway projects. The projected rapid growth of the ports added urgency to these efforts.

At the same time that community concern about the health impacts of the ports was growing, local academic researchers were publishing disturbing findings about air pollution's effects on children (Kunzli et al. 2003; Gauderman et al. 2004; Gauderman et al. 2005). Because of the region's infamous air quality problems, Southern California was a hotbed of research on the health effects of air pollution. One hub for this research was the University of Southern California (USC). USC researchers initiated the Children's Health Study in 1993 to investigate the impacts of air quality on children's health with initial funding from the California Air Resources Board and subsequent support from the National Institute for Environmental Health Sciences (NIEHS), the U.S. EPA, and the Health Effects Institute.

The Children's Health Study eventually enrolled 12,000 children (Southern California Environmental Health Sciences Center 2018b).

With NIEHS funding, USC established an Environmental Health Sciences Core Center in 1996 (Southern California Environmental Health Sciences Center 2018a). The Core Center provided support for administrative costs, pilot research projects, outreach, and other programs to foster environmental health research. The environmental health center included researchers from USC and the University of California, Los Angeles (UCLA) and was administered by the USC Keck School of Medicine. Subsequent funding of an NIEHS/EPA Children's Environmental Health Center (CEHC) at USC brought additional resources for environmental health research and outreach.

The NIEHS-funded Core Center at USC had a dedicated budget of $100,000 per year to support community engagement around issues of environmental health. Its Community Outreach and Engagement Core (COEC) "shares research findings with the public and functions as a bridge to inform researchers about community concerns" (Southern California Environmental Health Sciences Center 2018c). From 1997 to 2016, the COEC was led by Andrea Hricko, a public health professional with experience in government and media. Hricko also led the CEHC's outreach program and obtained additional foundation grants that supported community engagement around goods movement issues, particularly air pollution. Staffing levels for outreach varied but usually included at least one full-time program manager and administrative support.

In 2001, the COEC hosted a town hall meeting in Inglewood, California, on environmental health issues ranging from lead poisoning to air pollution. This event brought together a number of the COEC's existing partners, as well as additional community groups, researchers, and government officials. During the open mic portion of the meeting, attendees from the ports region highlighted health concerns related to rapid expansion of port facilities, with some speakers saying their communities were being "smothered" by truck emissions. Coalition for a Safe Environment (CFASE) Executive Director Jesse Marquez told the crowd that the emissions from ships delivering containers from other countries were not regulated by U.S. or California air pollution authorities, which shocked most attendees (Hricko 2016). After the meeting, one participant commented that many in attendance "realized that we'd been working on all these air pollution issues, and the ports were such a significant part of this, and they had completely escaped our attention" (Minkler et al. 2012, 36).

In light of these community concerns, COEC staff explored how they could leverage their research to support ongoing community efforts related to port expansion. The COEC staff started by systematically reaching out to the groups that had spoken at the town hall meeting to learn more about their concerns, activities, and goals. These included two groups the COEC had worked with previously on air pollution issues: the Center for Community Action and Environmental Justice (CCAEJ), which focused on pollution related to warehouses in Riverside, and the Long Beach Alliance for Children with Asthma (LBACA). The COEC also reached out to two recently formed groups, Coalition for a Safe Environment (CFASE), which was based around the Port of Los Angeles in Wilmington, and East Yard Communities for Environmental Justice (EYCEJ) in the City of Commerce, which focused on the impacts of train and truck traffic on communities located near railyards, warehouses, and the I-710 freeway in the southeastern part of Los Angeles County.

In 2002, Hricko learned that Interstate 710 (I-710) from Long Beach to downtown L.A. was going to be expanded (figure 6.2). As she recalled: "I was taking a group of students on a port tour in 2002 and thought I should find out what the daily truck volume was on the I-710 freeway that we would be traveling down. I was shocked to read that government agencies and the transportation industry had been meeting for more than a year to develop ways to expand the freeway so that three times as many trucks from the ports could travel on it. ... None of the environmental justice groups along the I-710 had heard about the expansion or [was] asked to be involved in what seemed to be secret meetings" (Hricko, 2016). Hricko wrote a letter to the Gateway Cities Council of Governments, which represents communities along the I-710, asking that minutes of the meetings be made public. With the release of the minutes, environmental justice groups learned of the potential destruction of 700 homes as part of the proposed project.

Many environmental justice groups in the area were particularly concerned about the impacts of rail transport, but they had not worked together previously. After being introduced through the COEC, several groups including EYCEJ, CCAEJ, and CFASE joined together to form the Modesta Avila Coalition (MAC) to coordinate regional efforts to fight railyard expansion proposals. The MAC was named after a young woman who was jailed in 1889 for allegedly obstructing a railroad that had been built through her mother's property in San Juan Capistrano (Modesta Avila Coalition 2006). This group served as a structure for amplifying local organizing efforts to reduce air pollution from railyards in Wilmington/Long Beach, Commerce, and San Bernardino. The Modesta Avila Coalition solidified the trust and connections among the key environmental groups that later joined in forming THE Impact Project.

Through these efforts, the COEC staff and partners came to understand that goods movement activities disproportionately impacted the health of low-income urban areas and communities of color. They concluded that federal and state policies did not effectively protect local communities from the cumulative environmental impacts of goods movement activities. Southern California is rich in community and environmental justice groups. Many local community groups across the region were concerned about health effects associated with trade, but they were not connected with each other. However, no one group had the broad technical knowledge, staff capacity, coordination, and skills needed to engage in the multiple projects, plans, and proposals associated with the growing goods movement activities in the region.

After consulting with environmental health center faculty and external advisers, the COEC decided to partner with residents, community environmental justice groups, and an asthma alliance to address the wide-ranging health effects of port activities. The COEC and these community partners soon realized that a more comprehensive collaboration was needed to support their regional engagement in goods movement decisions. They also recognized the need for expertise in environmental policy processes, and so engaged Professor Robert Gottlieb and colleagues from Occidental College's Urban Environmental Policy Institute, who brought expertise in community organizing, social justice, and policy change.

Together, these academic and community partners formed the Trade, Health, and Environment Impact Project—or simply THE Impact Project—in 2005 (table 6.1). The goal was "to ensure that reducing health, environmental and community impacts becomes central to the transportation and goods movement planning and policy process. THE Impact Project also seeks to shift the nature of the debate about ports and freight movement to elevate community voices in the policy arena, while also using

Table 6.1
THE Impact Project partners

Organization Name	Description of Organization
Center for Community Action and Environmental Justice (CCAEJ)	Founded by Penny Newman in 1978, CCAEJ led community efforts to fight the warehouses built throughout Riverside and San Bernardino Counties beginning in the 1990s. At the 2001 town hall meeting, Executive Director Newman spoke about how these warehouses increased truck traffic and pollution in formerly agricultural/rural/suburban communities roughly 70 miles northeast of the ports. CCAEJ's participation highlighted the regional health effects of truck and rail traffic associated with the growth of the ports. CCAEJ left THE Impact Project in 2014 because of the burden of travel from Riverside to Los Angeles.
Coalition for a Safe Environment (CFASE)	CFASE was founded in 2001 by Jesse Marquez to address the environmental problems facing Wilmington, a predominantly Latino community in Los Angeles. Executive Director Marquez participated in the 2001 town hall and became a longtime member of THE Impact Project. CFASE developed particular expertise in commenting on environmental impacts of new infrastructure projects.
Community Outreach and Engagement Core (COEC), University of Southern California (USC)	Part of USC's Environmental Health Sciences Center, which formed in 1996 with a focus on the health effects of air pollution, the COEC's role is to promote bidirectional communication between communities and researchers. COEC director Andrea Hricko had a background in journalism and occupational/environmental health. The COEC staff provided THE Impact Project's fiscal and administrative home, as well as access to USC researchers' expertise.
East Yard Communities for Environmental Justice (EYCEJ)	EYCEJ was cofounded in 2001 by Angelo Logan and Gilbert Estrada to focus on the environmental health threats facing residents in Commerce/East Los Angeles, in particular a massive railyard in Commerce and the region's major truck route to and from the ports—the I-710. EYCEJ later began organizing efforts in Long Beach around another railyard proposal.
Long Beach Alliance for Children with Asthma (LBACA)	LBACA was founded by Dr. Elisa Nicholas in 1999 to provide direct services to children with asthma and promote policy changes to reduce environmental contributors to asthma. LBACA worked closely with USC to educate residents about the latest findings on the relationship between air pollution and lung problems. Its A-Team volunteers counted trucks and documented pollution levels near schools and along highways with port truck traffic.
Urban Environmental Policy Institute (UEPI), Occidental College	UEPI was founded by urban environmental policy scholar and activist Robert Gottlieb in 1997 to support Occidental College programs that promote social and environmental justice in the region. UEPI faculty provided policy expertise to THE Impact Project. UEPI is now the home of the Moving Forward Network.

the science and policy work of the academic partners to strengthen those voices" (NIEHS 2018c).

THE Impact Project was facilitated by COEC and USC staff members who also administered project funding. Of the community partners listed in table 6.1, one—the Center for Community Action and Environmental Justice (CCAEJ)—withdrew in 2014 because of the logistical challenges of traveling from Riverside to Los Angeles for meetings. THE Impact Project received multiyear grants from private foundations (primarily The California Endowment and The Kresge Foundation) totaling over $2.2 million between 2006 and 2012 that supported the six partners' activities (Hricko 2016). Grants were split evenly between the academic and community partners, after accounting for costs of joint workshops and conferences. Work plans for the grant proposals were developed jointly, then were submitted and administered by USC staff. Ongoing funding from a variety of foundation and government sources also supported the USC outreach core's work on goods movement.

THE Impact Project faced many challenges in trying to protect community health from activities associated with goods movement. Most significant were the strong political and economic forces involved in goods movement decisions. As EYCEJ's Angelo Logan said, "We're up against huge forces. The railroads, the shippers, the Wal-Marts, companies with money and lobbyists and PR firms" (Roosevelt 2009). Because of the scope of goods movement activities, THE Impact Project aspired to inform a multitude of decision-making contexts such as local land use decisions, state planning committees, EIR processes, and even national air pollution policy. Finally, the neighborhoods most directly affected by these forces were generally lower-income communities of color with little political power. Although effective community organizations existed, they often had limited staff and multiple competing priorities. Making a difference despite these challenges necessitated diverse strategies, resources, and actions over a long time horizon.

THE Impact Project has been variously characterized as a way of "leveraging" resources to engage researchers in local problems, as a vehicle for supporting community engagement in a public participation process, and as community-based participatory research (Garcia et al. 2013; National Academies of Sciences Transportation Research Board and Strategic Highway Research Program 2011; NIEHS 2013). Regardless of how its activities are described, the project's goal was to support the efforts of community groups to reduce health disparities by influencing regional goods movement decisions. It provided a collaborative structure for bridging the experience of powerful local environmental justice groups with the scientific expertise of environmental health researchers.

One of the challenges of analyzing THE Impact Project's accomplishments is the complexity, scope, and scale of decisions in which its partners engaged. Each member organization had a rich portfolio of work in environmental health research, community organizing, or policy engagement. Their collaboration through THE Impact Project produced new materials, forged relationships, and supported engagement in multiple decision arenas that complemented these ongoing efforts. As well, many groups that were not part of THE Impact Project worked on these issues simultaneously. By one count in 2011, there were more than fifteen organizations with full-time staff working on these issues, as well as numerous volunteers (Matsuoka et al. 2011).

The rest of this chapter highlights how THE Impact Project advanced, complemented, and enhanced efforts to protect community health from the externalities of goods movement activities. It focuses on the products, activities, and events directly supported by THE Impact Project's funding and collaborative structure. However, it also strives to illuminate "ripple effects" through which this collaboration enhanced efforts outside the scope of THE Impact Project.

THE Impact Project's range of activities was extensive. In the period from 2005 to 2016, key efforts were focused in three areas: public communication, capacity building, and engagement in policy processes. The examples given here highlight how partners' activities grew from their experiences with THE Impact Project. These examples provide a basis for discussion of how this partnership shaped goods movement decisions in Southern California.

THE Impact Project's Collaborative Efforts

THE Impact Project's diverse strategies fell within three broad categories: public communication, capacity building, and engagement in policy processes. These three functions closely supported each other. Public communication activities raised the awareness of residents, community leaders, and elected officials that individual goods movement proposals like port developments, new railyards and warehouses, and highway expansions were not just economic development decisions, but also had regional health implications for communities living near goods movement hubs. In order to focus growing public awareness on influencing specific decisions, THE Impact Project's community partners required dedicated staff time, technical resources, and communication tools.

Public Communication

Increasing public awareness of the health consequences of goods movements was a key strategy. Throughout its messaging, THE Impact Project emphasized the economic, demographic, and geographic disparities of the negative externalities of goods movement. The project developed multimedia communication tools and organized public events appropriate to diverse local communities. Members also wrote articles, blogs, and short editorials for the mainstream news media and for the local groups' newsletters and websites to keep issues of goods movement and health in the public eye (THE Impact Project 2010a).

Media

Before 2002, Los Angeles news outlets had not devoted significant coverage to the health effects of pollution resulting from ports. THE Impact Project partners supported a significant increase in media attention as part of its efforts to build public awareness of these issues (Garcia et al. 2013). After emceeing the 2001 USC town hall meeting, National Public Radio reporter Warren Olney produced a series of radio stories on ports and air quality. In 2002, Gary Polakovic wrote the first significant story in the *Los Angeles Times*, calling the ports "LA's worst polluter" (Polakovic 2002). Between 2003 and 2007, *Los Angeles Times* reporter Deborah Schoch wrote nearly 200 articles on goods movement, most of which addressed health, safety, and pollution-related issues. COEC staff and community partners worked closely with journalists, helping them access scientific information, hear local community members' perspectives, and understand events unfolding around new proposals. Sometimes THE Impact Project members were quoted; other times they assisted reporters "on background" or took journalists on "toxic tours" of the ports (Ostrov 2012).

THE Impact Project partners also informed journalists of upcoming decisions, hearings, and issues of concern to community groups. This contributed to frequent coverage of organizing efforts and public hearings on development projects. Other times, partners worked closely with journalists investigating community concerns. For example, in 2003 USC COEC director Andrea Hricko spent hours talking with *Los Angeles Times* reporter Deborah Schoch about the lack of community input into the Major Corridor Study for the I-710. Schoch's related articles contributed to growing concern about the proposal and contributed to a reset of the public participation process (Schoch 2003a; 2003b; Hricko 2016).

Communications Tools

THE Impact Project produced communications tools appropriate for diverse audiences. These included short video clips, interactive maps, policy briefs, and infographics. These products were used by staff members in their various outreach and training activities but were also available to the public on THE Impact Project's website, which served as a hub for research-based environmental health information related to goods movement. Some of these tools translated emerging scientific findings from academic journal articles into readable summaries. Others synthesized the state of knowledge on issues such as air pollution and asthma. Photographs captured the impacts of ports on neighborhood residents—such trains passing behind school playgrounds and truckyards visible from a child's bedroom. Short videos documented the stories of residents affected by truck traffic associated with the ports (THE Impact Project 2018).

Partners used these communication products to enhance understanding of the health equity impacts associated with goods movement activities. As THE Impact Project community partner Angelo Logan said, "Providing research, collating fact sheets, infographics, a whole bunch of information related to the environmental health impacts of a proposed project, really debunking the arguments the port was making ... [and] having the resource of USC being able to dig into the data to come up with answers was really important" (Logan 2016).

Organizational Capacity Building

In addition to its communication efforts, THE Impact Project initiated a number of projects that built capacity in organizations serving affected neighborhoods. For example, grant subcontracts to the community partners supported staff, funded events, and provided small stipends to community members engaged in community-based science (THE Impact Project 2012a). Ongoing outreach by the project's partners to new community groups, government officials, and professionals engaged additional stakeholders. These activities helped diverse groups translate public awareness into policy action and developed a core of expertise within partner organizations that could sustain this work in the future.

A-Teams

THE Impact Project supported neighborhood-based teams of community members called A-Teams (short for "Neighborhood Assessment Teams") through education, capacity building, and technology for community-based data collection (Truax et al. 2013). Starting in 2012, THE Impact Project partners recruited A-Team members from four neighborhoods and trained them to use P-Trak particle counters to measure trends in air pollution and compare the ultrafine particle concentrations in different communities (Truax et al. 2013; THE Impact Project 2010a, 2011). Later, A-Team members counted trucks to document the extent of traffic affecting residential neighborhoods near schools.

A-Team members also received training on the health effects of air pollution, video production, and public speaking techniques, which increased their ability to present scientific findings and personal stories in public settings. Each A-Team used its monitoring capacity to raise awareness in its community in different ways. At one point, CCAEJ A-Team members "measured pollution at a highly impacted neighborhood and compared that to a neighborhood where key elected officials live. This highlighted the disparity in exposures between the decision-makers and the people who live in the community" (Truax et al. 2013, 14).

Technical Reports, Summaries, and Research Presentations

THE Impact Project leveraged the technical expertise of USC researchers and the COEC staff's ability to analyze, synthesize, and communicate environmental health information. Perhaps the most direct way in which technical expertise was leveraged was by identifying opportunities for USC researchers to share research findings that linked port-related air pollution with health effects on local populations. Researchers' testimony on the health effects of air pollution helped make emerging science accessible and meaningful to decision makers. In addition, THE Impact Project translated these new findings into a range of communication products. For example, the project produced a number of infographics designed to communicate the negative effects of traffic on health and well-being.

In 2011, the project issued a report funded under a separate grant from the Kresge Foundation to Occidental College. The report, called "Global Trade Impacts: Addressing the Health, Social, and Environmental Consequences of Moving International Freight through Our Communities," provided an overview of port-related health impacts, trends, and predictions for increased goods movement activities and case studies of seventeen goods movement hubs throughout the country (Matsuoka et al. 2011). This report served as a resource to groups around the country and framed an agenda for future action.[1] Its recommendations highlighted the need for community groups in different regions to share information, organize strategies, and promote national-level policy changes.

In 2012, THE Impact Project partners produced four policy briefs about the health impacts of goods movement activities, respectively called "Driving Harm" (trucks), "Tracking Harm" (railways), "Storing Harm" (warehouses), and "Importing Harm" (ports) (THE Impact Project 2012a, 2012c, 2012d, 2012e). All members of THE Impact Project worked on these briefs, which were edited by the partners from Occidental College. The policy briefs helped community partners educate their members and staff, as well as local officials and other stakeholders, about the needs for policy change (Southern California Environmental Health Sciences Center 2012).

"Moving Forward" Conferences

Starting in 2005, THE Impact Project organized a series of meetings that came to be called the "Moving Forward" conferences. These meetings focused on supporting community engagement in addressing health impacts from goods movement activities. Each of these meetings was successively larger (350 attendees in 2005, 400 in 2007, and 550 in 2010) and attracted participants from other port communities in the United States and around the world (THE Impact Project 2010b). A fourth conference was held by the Moving Forward Network in 2017 with 500 attendees (Moving Forward Network 2018).

Through these initiatives, THE Impact Project interacted with groups organizing around transportation hubs in other regions nationally and internationally. Participants expressed a desire to share lessons learned, technical resources, and strategies and to explore the state and national-level policy implications of their work. To address this need, THE Impact Project partners helped create the Moving Forward Network (MFN), a national network of groups working to address health impacts of international trade on disadvantaged communities (Moving Forward Network 2018).

In 2014, the Moving Forward Network received a two-year, $900,000 grant from the Kresge Foundation through the Urban Environmental Policy Institute (UEPI) at Occidental College. Its website, meetings, and campaigns facilitated information sharing and it provided direct support (through small subgrants) for community groups from seventeen port communities, including THE Impact Project. USC continued to lend technical support, for example, by providing updates on new research related to air quality and health for the MFN website. Two former members of THE Impact Project were hired by UEPI as MFN staff members—Angelo Logan as campaign director (formerly with EYCEJ) and Jessica Tovar as policy director (formerly with the LBACA) (Moving Forward Network 2018). THE Impact Project remained involved in the Moving Forward Network as a regional member, with several of its partners serving on the MFN Advisory Board.

THE Impact Project's Engagement in Goods Movement Policy Decisions

THE Impact Project's goal was to help affected communities influence decisions about the operation, development, and expansion of goods movement activities to better protect public health. Its activities were designed to support effective engagement in local decisions, which was achieved by increasing awareness of health information, participation by community members, and the transparency of decisions being made in multiple arenas.

The partners' roles in these decision processes included commenting on environmental impact reports, testifying at hearings, serving on committees and task forces, organizing community members to participate in these processes, educating decision makers, and developing alternative proposals. Different partners played different roles—for example, academic partners could not advocate for policy but could provide information that enhanced the effectiveness of community partners' advocacy efforts. When scientific credibility was needed, the academic partners could tap faculty to testify about the findings of relevant research. The partners used multiple approaches in different decision sectors, and their strategies evolved over time. The focus here is on THE Impact Project's engagement in conducting environmental impact reviews of proposed projects, developing new policy initiatives, influencing state and federal policy change, and promoting more inclusive planning for the I-710 freeway expansion. These policy processes spanned more than ten years (table 6.2), and many were ongoing simultaneously. The sections that follow (1) describe THE Impact Project's evolving engagement in infrastructure development proposals; (2) trace how the partners were involved with local planning and policy processes; (3) give several examples of how the partners engaged at the state and federal level in efforts to better protect community environmental health; and (4) highlight their decade-long involvement in the planning process around expanding an eighteen-mile section of the I-710 freeway through southeast Los Angeles. Taken together, these examples showcase how the partners' efforts evolved from reacting to development proposals, to changing how the planning process integrated public input, to creating more health-protective development alternatives.

Involvement in Environmental Review of Goods Movement Expansion Proposals

As described in Chapter 2, the National Environmental Policy Act (NEPA) requires major federal actions with significant environmental impacts to produce an environmental impact statement (EIS). Many states have a parallel process of review for state and local government actions. California's Environmental Quality Act (CEQA) requires lead agencies to produce an environmental impact report (EIR). For federal actions within California, the NEPA and CEQA processes are combined under the authority of the California Natural Resources Agency and referred to as an EIR/EIS (Council on Environmental Quality 2014). This process provides for public comment on the draft EIR and outside parties may sue in court if they believe the process was conducted improperly.

Before 2004, homeowner, community, and environmental groups had accumulated years of experience fighting specific proposals for port expansion, new railyards, and warehouses. As early as 1997, the Center for Community Action and Environmental Justice (which became an Impact Project partner), fought a proliferation of warehouses and truck traffic from the ports. In 2001, the Natural Resource Defense Council (NRDC), the Coalition for Clean Air, and homeowner groups near the Port of Los

Table 6.2

Timeline of THE Impact Project engagement in goods movement decisions

2001	Natural Resources Defense Council and the Port of Los Angeles settle China Shipping lawsuit.
	USC and partners sponsor town hall meeting on environmental health in Inglewood, CA.
	I-710 Major Corridor Study (MCS) initiated.
2004	Modesta Avila Coalition forms to coordinate regional efforts on community impacts of railyards.
	Academic and community partners begin meeting to discuss formation of a broader coalition.
2005	Environmental impact review initiated for the Southern California International Gateway (SCIG) railyard project of the Burlington Northern Santa Fe Railway (BNSF) and Port of Los Angeles.
	Formation of THE Impact Project.
	THE Impact Project hosts first Moving Forward Conference (350 attendees).
2006	Clean Air Action Plan issued by the ports of Los Angeles and Long Beach; four members of THE Impact Project appointed to Implementation Task Force by the mayor of Los Angeles.
	THE Impact Project receives $600,000 grant from The California Endowment.
2007	THE Impact Project members from USC and EYCEJ appointed to 6-member USEPA Environmental Justice Advisory Council's Goods Movement Work Group (GMWG).
	Environmental review process initiated for expansion of the I-710 freeway.
	THE Impact Project hosts second Moving Forward Conference (400 attendees).
	Coalition for Environmental Health and Justice (CEHAJ) forms to focus on community impacts of I-710 freeway, develops "Community Alternative" (CA7).
2008	Los Angeles Harbor Department adopts Clean Truck Program (CTP).
2010	Health Impact Assessment of I-710 expansion project conducted. THE Impact Project hosts third "Moving Forward" conference (550 attendees).
	THE Impact Project releases four policy briefs on goods movement.
2013	Metro decides to conduct a Recirculated Draft Environmental Impact Report (RDEIR/SDEIS) for I-710 expansion that included new Alternative 7.
2014	Moving Forward Network forms with a $900,000 grant from Kresge Foundation.
2015	City of Commerce Green Zones ordinance passes.
2016	Clean Up, Green Up (CUGU) ordinance passed by the City of Los Angeles.
	California Superior Court upholds challenges to the BNSF SCIG EIR from the National Resources Defense Council and the City of Long Beach, requiring reanalysis of air quality impacts.
2017	Moving Forward Network sponsors fourth Moving Forward Conference (500 attendees).
	Metro releases I-710 RDEIR/SDEIS for public comment.
2018	Metro selects Alternative 5c as preferred alternative for I-710 project.
	Port of Los Angeles announces plans for REIR of BNSF SCIG project.

Angeles successfully argued that the port had failed to conduct an EIR for the China Shipping Terminal, blocking the project until environmental concerns were addressed and winning $50 million in mitigation benefits for the community (Matsuoka et al. 2011). According to NRDC, this was a "precedent-setting settlement that dragged the Port into the 21st century in terms of environmental compliance" (Pettit 2008). The Coalition for Clean Air's policy director summarized the decision's significance saying that "for the first time, the Port of Los Angeles, not the workers or the communities, will be required to shoulder substantial costs to correct its illegal development practices of favoring shipping tenants over public health. ... The Court's decision today tells the Port Authority that its operational health will depend on its ability to protect people who live, work and breathe in and around the harbor area" (Natural Resources Defense Council 2002a).

This lawsuit was hailed as a turning point for how port development projects were reviewed. It helped launch the Port of Los Angeles' Clean Air Action Plan (CAAP) (Pettit 2008; Port of Long Beach and Port of Los Angeles 2017). Despite these efforts, the need to engage in EIRs of new development proposals continued. Soon after it formed, THE Impact Project partners engaged in the EIR process for a proposed railyard expansion. This experience set the stage for its future policy work.

In 2005, an EIR was initiated for the Southern California International Gateway (SCIG), a 153-acre, $175 million railyard proposed by the Burlington Northern Santa Fe Railway (BNSF) (Schoch 2005; Los Angeles Harbor Department 2018; Port of Los Angeles 2013). The site for the proposed railyard was located immediately south of the existing Union Pacific Intermodal Container Transfer Facility (ICTF) in Wilmington, which is four miles north of the ports of Los Angeles and Long Beach (Port of Los Angeles 2013). At the time, 750,000 containers per year were trucked from the ports to be transferred onto trains at the ICTF, which was also slated to double in size. The proposed SCIG would accommodate an additional 1.5 million containers per year, with an estimated 2 million annual truck trips impacting lower-income communities of color in Wilmington (part of the City of Los Angeles) and Long Beach (Port of Long Beach and Port of Los Angeles 2006b; Parkin 2016).

Proponents of the project argued that it would significantly improve regional air quality by removing 1.5 million truck trips per year from the I-710 freeway (Port of Los Angeles 2013; Parkin 2016). With the new railyard, trucks that currently carry containers from the ports twenty miles north to BNSF's Hobart railyard in the City of Commerce would instead have to travel only four miles to the SCIG (Weikel 2012).

This reasoning suggested that construction of the SCIG would reduce regional air pollution. However, there were concerns about local community health impacts. Residents of the diverse neighborhoods of West Long Beach, located across the Terminal Island Freeway from the proposed SCIG, were concerned that the prevailing winds would carry the pollution from the additional 2 million trucks arriving at the SCIG into their communities. This area also contains numerous "sensitive receptors," including five schools, day care centers, and a homeless veterans' center (Schoch 2005).

Local residents soon organized to oppose the SCIG proposal based on community health and environmental concerns. At the first hearing about the SCIG in 2005, community groups mobilized more than 200 attendees (Hricko 2016). THE Impact Project partners, including the Wilmington-based Coalition for a Safe Environment (CFASE), East Yard Communities for Environmental Justice (EYCEJ) (which later set up a satellite office to help organize the West Long Beach communities), Long Beach Alliance for Children with Asthma (LBACA), and the USC COEC, along with local residents and the NRDC, were active in the SCIG review process. Several of these groups later joined the "Stop the SCIG" campaign to focus on the effects of this particular proposal (Green L.A. Port Working Group 2018). As with the China Shipping project, the public's primary opportunity to engage in the decision was through the EIR process under the CEQA.

THE Impact Project enabled all of its members to be more effective participants in the SCIG deliberations. For example, the community partners documented the proximity of schools, playgrounds, football fields, homeless veterans' centers, and other "sensitive receptors" that would be impacted. USC analyzed the BSNF SCIG Draft EIR by "looking at the traffic baseline, the claims that the new railyard would reduce traffic congestion and air pollution, and the claims that by building a new massive railyard near West Long Beach the region's air would be made cleaner" (THE Impact Project 2018). USC research helped LBACA make the case that, despite the claims that the SCIG would improve overall air quality, it could worsen conditions for local children with asthma by increasing emissions near residential neighborhoods. In 2010, EYCEJ and LBACA gave a presentation to the Long Beach city council about the potential local health impacts of SCIG and that same year the USC COEC director made a presentation about the project to the Long Beach Unified School Board (THE Impact Project 2010b). CFASE and LBACA and EYCEJ organized local protests against the project. Based on these and other interactions with local policy makers, the City of Long Beach moved from initial support of the proposal to joining the lawsuit against it (Hricko 2016). In addition to extensive policy engagement by the communities around the SCIG site, THE Impact Project's connections provided a regional perspective to this proposal. In 2009, the San Bernardino–based CCAEJ group gave a press conference naming BNSF "Polluter of the Year," which generated media coverage of the cumulative regional health impacts of railyard growth (BNSF declined the award) (Snibbe 2010).

The SCIG EIR was released for public comment in September 2011. It was revised and released for additional comment as a Recirculated EIR in 2012 (Los Angeles Harbor Department 2013). Despite community concerns about the project (including a candlelight vigil in front of the mayor's mansion and a twenty-four-hour hunger strike by community organizers including CFASE and EYCEJ), the Port and City of Los Angeles voted to certify the final EIR of the SCIG in 2013 (Parkin 2016; Green L.A. Port Working Group 2018). The EIR found that the facility would have a net positive impact on air quality by incorporating green technology and reducing truck traffic on the I-710 freeway. Multiple lawsuits were filed challenging the EIR. Plaintiffs included the City of Long Beach, the Long Beach School District, the South Coast Air Quality Management District, local community and environmental justice groups (including THE Impact Project partners CFASE and EYCEJ), and the Natural Resources Defense Council, with support from the California Attorney General's Office. In 2016, the California Superior Court ruled that that the EIR was insufficient. Among the concerns were that the EIR underestimated air pollution and noise impacts on local neighborhoods, failed to account for impacts on existing railyards, and assumed full implementation of unenforceable mitigation measures (Parkin 2016). Contrary to the EIR findings, the court suggested that the project could actually worsen air quality in the region. This ruling blocked the project until a revised EIR could be completed (Mongelluzzo 2016). In the fall of 2018, the Port of Los Angeles and BNSF announced their intention to reanalyze the air quality impacts sections, circulate a revised EIR for public comment, and reconsider the project (Chirls 2018).

THE Impact Project enhanced community groups' ability to bring their concerns into the EIR process. Nonetheless, this case highlighted the inadequacies of the EIR process as a framework for protecting community health. In addition to the time and expense required to participate effectively in the EIR process, community groups can only react to existing proposals, alternatives set forth by the lead agency, and narrowly defined health analyses, with limited consideration of cumulative effects. Litigation is costly and time-consuming. In addition, even when legal action leads to a settlement, there is no effective way for communities to ensure compliance. As well, community groups' faith in settlements had been undermined when the ports allowed delayed implementation of several provisions of the China Shipping settlement without informing the public (Barboza 2016b). Through experience in the SCIG and other EIR processes, THE Impact Project partners recognized the limited efficacy of participating in the EIR process. They therefore sought other opportunities to shape the way goods movement systems were planned, reviewed, and implemented to more proactively and effectively promote health considerations.

Local Planning and Policy Processes

The China Shipping lawsuit and subsequent experiences like the BNSF SCIG EIR process underscored the failure of existing policy processes to adequately address the cumulative health impacts of good movement decisions. THE Impact Project had several early opportunities to address the health impacts of goods movement issues more comprehensively. One effort was through the Los Angeles Clean Air Action Plan (CAAP), which was adopted in 2006 (Port of Long Beach and Port of Los Angeles 2006b). The CAAP included a Clean Trucks Program that aimed to phase in cleaner diesel engines ahead of federal timetables (Cummings 2018). THE Impact Partners were active participants in these local planning efforts. In addition, they explored tools that local governments could use to shape the development, expansion, and operation of goods movement activities. A common theme of the project's local policy engagement was increasing transparency in decision-making processes. Increased transparency was expected to allow nongovernmental partners to participate earlier and more effectively.

Clean Air Action Plan

After the China Shipping settlement, the ports of Long Beach and Los Angeles began developing a plan to address air pollution from the ports (Port of Long Beach and Port of Los Angeles 2017). The plan was finalized in 2006 following the election of Los Angeles Mayor Antonio Villaraigosa, who supported efforts to address the ports' environmental health impacts (Garcia et al. 2013). In 2006, the Ports of Los Angeles and Long Beach adopted the San Pedro Bays Clean Air Action Plan, committing to reduce the ports' emissions by 45 percent over a five-year period (Port of Long Beach and Port of Los Angeles 2006b; Hricko 2008; Minkler et al. 2012). The plan "ushered in a slew of anti-air pollution strategies including the ports' Clean Trucks Programs, vessel pollution reduction programs, and advanced new technology, such as the world's first hybrid tugboat"(Port of Long Beach and Port of Los Angeles 2006a).

Although the CAAP adoption coincided with the establishment of THE Impact Project, the partners had already begun to collaborate during development of the plan. Following the passage of the CAAP, five of six Impact Project partner groups were invited to serve on the CAAP implementation task force (Garcia et al. 2013). While time-consuming, holding such appointments allowed project members to act as watchdogs over implementation of the plan and mobilize against efforts to dilute the plan (Garcia et al. 2013; Hricko 2008). Although the committee did not continue to meet regularly, THE Impact Project partners remained involved in implementation of the CAAP.

The Clean Trucks Program (CTP), adopted by the L.A. Harbor Department in 2008, was a cornerstone of the CAAP (Matsuoka et al. 2011; Cummings 2018). It aimed to replace or retrofit older trucks to reduce diesel emissions. THE Impact Project's materials on the Clean Trucks Program emphasized health benefits both to communities living near the ports and workers at the ports. They also recognized the economic burden of these measures, advocating for a Clean Trucks Mitigation Fund and for trucking companies to hire truckers as employees (rather than as independent contractors) so these lower-income workers would not bear the brunt of emissions control costs (THE Impact Project, 2012a; Cummings 2018).

According to the ports, diesel emissions from trucks at the port were reduced 90 percent over three years, ahead of the CTP schedule (Port of Long Beach and Port of Los Angeles 2018). Other parts of the CTP did not go as smoothly: In 2010, THE Impact Project partners worked with port officials to ensure that penalties were assessed on shippers who engaged in "container switching" (moving containers from new trucks to older, noncompliant vehicles after leaving port property) (THE Impact Project 2010a).

In 2012, the final step of the CTP banned all trucks that did not meet the 2007 federal Clean Truck Emission Standards (Port of Long Beach and Port of Los Angeles 2018, 2006a). The CAAP was updated in 2010, and the ports continue to hold periodic public meetings to give updates on progress (Port of Long Beach and Port of Los Angeles 2006a; U.S. Supreme Court 2013; Matsuoka et al. 2011). Nearly ten years after adoption of the plan, concerns came to light about failures to comply with emissions reduction timelines (Port of Los Angeles 2018b; Times Editorial Board 2016). This highlighted the importance of remaining involved in implementation.

Local Land Use Planning, Practices, and Policies
THE Impact Project partners' focus on the risks to people living nearest to these pollution sources led them to explore tools to buffer and mitigate environmental harm from goods movement. Partners worked in their own communities on diverse efforts that encompassed regulation, planning, incentives, enforcement, land and transportation policy, and design standards.

For example, California passed a state law in 2003, Senate Bill No. 352 (SB 352), that prohibited building new schools within 500 feet of a busy road or freeway (NIEHS 2012b). However, SB 352 did not prohibit expanding highways or railyards near an existing school. In 2005, the Center for Community Action and Environmental Justice worked with the Riverside County planning agency to incorporate a 1,000-foot buffer zone in "good neighbor" guidelines, which planning commissioners used to deny new warehouse proposals near homes, schools, and hospitals (Matsuoka et al. 2011). Riverside County also passed truck routing and no-parking/idling regulations to reduce the impacts of trucks on residential neighborhoods (Matsuoka et al. 2011).

The City of Commerce's 2015 Green Zones ordinance was a comprehensive local effort to promote environment and health. Although the ordinance did not explicitly target goods movement industries, it provided for incentives, support, and promotion of greening all businesses in the area to mitigate the impacts of the four railyards and other transportation infrastructure in Commerce. East Yard Communities for Environmental Justice (EYCEJ) was a leading advocate for the ordinance. The Green Zones ordinance is an example of how THE Impact Project partners' work evolved from fighting specific proposed developments to a more comprehensive, proactive approach. An EYCEJ brief on the effort noted that "rather than considering specific uses or developments one-on-one as they emerge or are proposed, the policy recommends defining a buffer zone around the City's established sensitive uses, coupled with limitations on the future siting of sensitive uses that could create conflicts with existing or future businesses" (EYCEJ 2018b). As Angelo Logan of EYCEJ said, "We have to fight things— all kinds of things—but we also have to have a vision for something better" (Bogado 2015).

A similar ordinance called "Clean Up, Green Up" (CUGU) was passed by the City of Los Angeles in 2016 targeting three "toxic hot spot" neighborhoods (Clean Up Green Up 2018; Barboza 2016a; Sylvia 2016). The Coalition for a Safe Environment (CFASE), an Impact Project member, was among the community groups that championed this policy. In addition to supporting green businesses, the ordinance set standards to minimize spillover lighting, require landscaping vegetation to conserve water and filter air particulates, evaluate noise impacts of additions and improvements, and install signage to inform residents of health risks of near-roadway air pollution (City of Los Angeles 2015).[2] At the same time, the city council passed a rule requiring that all new housing built within 1,000 feet of a freeway include a high-efficiency air filtration system (Barboza 2016a). THE Impact Project members from USC provided testimony noting the potential health benefits of this provision. The community partners emphasized broad community benefits, including creation of green jobs that would create economic opportunities for residents. These local laws reflect implementation of a vision for local efforts to protect public health in areas cumulatively impacted by goods movement and other industries (EYCEJ 2018b, 2010).

Increasing Transparency and Participation in Local Policy Processes

The initiatives described thus far are just a few examples of the ways partners in THE Impact Project directly engaged in local decision processes. Through this work, they recognized the need to increase transparency and expand public participation opportunities in ongoing policy and planning efforts. For example, partners successfully encouraged the Ports' Harbor Commission to begin publishing agendas, videotaping hearings, and posting searchable transcripts of meetings online (Matsuoka et al. 2011). The proceedings of port authorities in many other regions remain much less accessible to the public (NEJAC 2009). THE Impact Project partners pushed for expanded opportunities for public input and community representation on policy advisory committees. THE Impact Project reported in 2010 that "one unexpected success is that SCAG (Southern California Association of Governments) opened their Goods Movement Steering Committee to Impact Project members as a response to our advocacy about environmental justice and environmental health" (THE Impact Project 2010a, 7). The growing number of meetings to attend and issues to follow challenged the capacity of the partners, who needed to make strategic choices about which opportunities represented the most effective use of their limited resources.

State and National Policy Engagement

Although the primary focus of THE Impact Project was on the local impacts of goods movement, participants recognized that many of the decisions driving goods movement in this region were shaped by state, federal, and in some cases international laws and agencies. For example, in 2003, California passed a bill limiting to 30 minutes the time trucks could be left idling off port property. However, this law did not limit idling on port property, despite the fact that on-site truck emissions can significantly affect air quality in fenceline communities. Community groups advocated for the South Coast Air Quality Management District to adopt anti-idling rules applying to both trucks and trains on port property, which it did in 2006. In 2010, however, a federal judge ruled that the South Coast Air Quality Management District's rail idling restrictions interfered with interstate commerce (Matsuoka et al. 2011). In this case, federal action was needed to address concern about trains idling at railyards. Martha Matsuoka (2008, 27) called these efforts using a "social movement regionalism" approach, and as THE Impact Project partners uncovered legal constraints to local action, they took steps to address the gaps in state and federal policy.

National Environmental Justice Advisory Council Because of their national leadership on the community health impacts of goods movement, in 2007 two of THE Impact Project members were appointed to serve on the EPA's six-member National Environmental Justice Advisory Council's newly formed Goods Movement Work Group (GMWG) (Matsuoka et al. 2011; U.S. EPA 2011). The GMWG final report included many examples from Southern California and references to work of THE Impact Project partners.

Although the GMWG report did not directly change any policies, it set forth recommendations for consideration by federal agencies to address environmental justice issues in their planning, funding, and policies. Local groups could also point to this document in their own work. For example, the report advocated for the use of health impact assessment (HIA) in goods movement decisions. This recommendation supported THE Impact Project's promotion of an HIA of the I-710 expansion. The U.S. EPA later published an "environmental justice primer" for communities around ports that incorporated the GMWG's work (U.S. EPA 2018a).

Moving Forward Network and National Policy   THE Impact Project's Moving Forward conferences gave rise to the Moving Forward Network (MFN). MFN became a vehicle through which THE Impact Project and other local partners could collaborate to change federal policy that would benefit all communities. In 2015 the MFN initiated a "zero campaign" asking the EPA to hold ports to Clean Air Act standards for industrial emission sources. As the MFN campaign director, Angelo Logan, said, "Part of the mission and goal is to build an infrastructure for groups across the country to help them have resources to influence national policy—but at the same time we support local" (Logan 2016).

THE Impact Project members' participation in these efforts contributed their experiences in Southern California to national policy campaigns. In addition, participating in these national forums provided the local partners with new knowledge, visibility and credibility, which enhanced their ability to obtain support for their local initiatives.

Broadening Consideration of Health in I-710 Expansion Planning

Interstate 710 (the I-710, also known as the Long Beach Freeway) is an eighteen-mile stretch of freeway that connects the ports of Long Beach and downtown Los Angeles with rail, truck routes, and warehouses on the east side of the city (figure 6.2) (National Academies of Sciences Transportation Research Board and Strategic Highway Research Program 2011; Matsuoka 2014). The I-710's eight general traffic lanes have been notoriously overcrowded for decades, and growth of the ports has significantly increased the number of trucks carrying goods to warehouses and railyards (Matsuoka 2014). The I-710 is under the jurisdiction of Caltrans, the state transportation agency, which partnered with local agencies including the Gateway

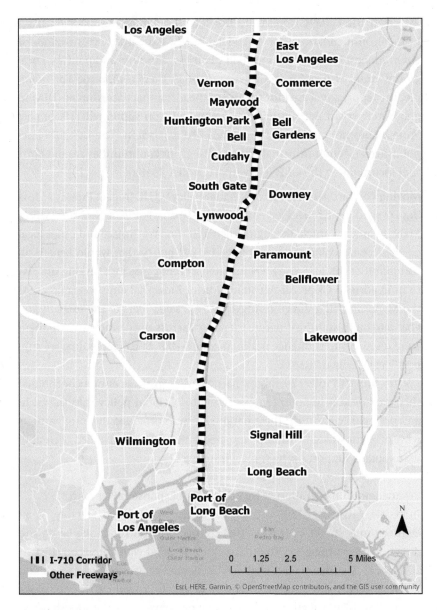

Figure 6.2
Map of I-710 corridor
Map credit: Karl Korfmacher

Cities Council of Governments (GCCOG), Southern California Association of Governments (SCAG), and the Los Angeles County Metropolitan Transit Authority (Metro, formerly known as MTA) to plan for the future of the freeway (Gateway Cities Council of Governments 2018; Southern California Association of Governments 2018; National Academies of Sciences Transportation Research Board and Strategic Highway Research Program 2011; LA Metro 2018d). THE Impact Project and other community groups advocated for greater consideration of health in planning for this $6 billion project over a period of nearly fifteen years.

Government agencies began planning for expansion of an eighteen-mile section of the I-710 around 1999. The first step was a $3.9 million Major Corridor Study, which was launched by Metro in 2001 and completed in 2005 (National Academies of Sciences Transportation Research Board and Strategic Highway Research Program 2011; Schoch 2003a). Although the effort claimed to include a significant commitment to public outreach, few residents in the corridor were aware of the study until 2003, when the *Los Angeles Times* reported that plans for expansion of the I-710 could result in destruction of up to 700 nearby homes (Schoch 2003b). Community groups criticized the outreach efforts for not posting minutes of planning committee meetings, holding meetings primarily during the work day, misleading public materials, and minimal attendance at public meetings (Schoch 2003b). In addition to the loss of homes, concerns included air quality, noise, traffic safety, and disproportionate impacts on low-income communities and communities of color (National Academies of Sciences Transportation Research Board and Strategic Highway Research Program 2011).

According to COEC director Andrea Hricko (2016), the resulting public outcry from the *Los Angeles Times* story "stopped completion of the I-710 Major Corridor Study in its tracks. Environmental justice groups demanded a completely new structure to gain true public input and transparency in the freeway expansion process and to more carefully consider the air pollution impacts." Six new local Tier 1 Community Advisory Committees (CACs) and an overarching Tier 2 Community Advisory Committee were formed. Several future Impact Project members (USC's Professor Ed Avol, LBACA's Dr. Elisa Nicholas, and EYCEJ Executive Director Angelo Logan) were appointed to the Tier 2 Citizens Advisory Committee, which met over thirty times in nine months to develop recommendations to the Oversight Planning Committee (OPC) (National Academies of Sciences Transportation

Research Board and Strategic Highway Research Program 2011; LA Metro 2018b; Gateway Cities Council of Governments 2018; Gateway Cities Council of Governments 2006). Whereas the initial public outreach structure ran parallel to, but separate from, the planning and decision-making committees, the new structure integrated community participation into analyses, recommendations, and decisions. In its final report, the Tier 2 CAC stated that "health is the overriding consideration" and that "major infrastructure improvements must be conditioned on achieving air quality goals to protect public health" (Human Impact Partners 2011; I-710 Major Corridor Study Tier 2 Community Advisory Committee 2004). The "locally preferred solution" (LPS) that was endorsed by the Major Corridor Study report in 2005 included ten general traffic lanes separated from four lanes for trucks and minimized the number of homes that would be removed. One analysis of the Community Participation Framework for the Major Corridor Study described it as "collaborative, bottom-up decision making"—a far cry from the criticisms of the study's initial participation structure (National Academies of Sciences Transportation Research Board and Strategic Highway Research Program 2011).

After the Major Corridor Study's locally preferred solution was identified, an environmental review process for the expansion was initiated in 2007. An environmental impact report (EIR) was required by California's Environmental Quality Act process (CEQA), as well as an environmental impact statement (EIS) under the National Environmental Policy Act (NEPA). Caltrans had overall responsibility for the joint EIR/EIS process, which was paid for by Metro and managed by the Gateway Cities Council of Governments (GCCOG). The EIR/EIS process examined five alternatives, including a "no build" scenario (LA Metro 2011; Gateway Cities Council of Governments 2018).

The participation process for the EIR/EIS was based on the MCS Community Planning Framework (National Academies of Sciences Transportation Research Board and Strategic Highway Research Program 2011). It provided for up to eighteen Local Advisory Committees to ensure strong community representation (Matsuoka 2014). Although these committees were set up for the EIR/EIS process, they provided input on related planning discussions as well.

This structure provided multiple opportunities for input, but the sheer number of meetings and complexity of the process challenged THE Impact Project partners' resources to engage in all of them (Matsuoka 2014).

Nonetheless, their membership on standing committees gave them timely access to information about the process and opportunities to provide input to formative decisions. In addition to participating directly in the committee structure, the project members lobbied successfully for local health department staff to be appointed to committees (Hricko 2016). Partners also met regularly with elected officials and others who sat on the Local Advisory Committees to increase their understanding of health concerns (THE Impact Project 2009). They also attended public meetings, organized residents to attend hearings, submitted documentation of potential health impacts, and commented on draft documents. Matsuoka (2014, 21) described participation by THE Impact Project - simultaneously sitting on working committees while also organizing public advocacy and engagement- as an "inside-outside" strategy.

The partners also pushed for the EIR/EIS to include both a health risk assessment (HRA) and a health impact assessment (HIA). Based on their past experiences, they were not convinced that the standard EIR/EIS process would sufficiently protect health of people living near the I-710. They pointed out that people living in the fifteen communities within the I-710 corridor already had poorer health status than others in the region, and that there were ten schools and six day care centers within a quarter mile of the I-710 (Coalition for Environmental Health and Justice 2009). The partners hoped that conducting both a HRA and a HIA would enhance consideration of cumulative impacts on these vulnerable populations.

In 2008, the partners in THE Impact Project successfully advocated for a health risk assessment to be conducted as part of the EIR/EIS. The HRA process already existed under CEQA, but this was the first time it was used for a transportation project (SCAQMD 2018c; Sausser et al. 2009). The HRA process focuses on air quality, particularly the cancer risk from toxic air contaminants (Lester 2008). The HRA report predicted that by 2035, all alternatives under consideration would improve air quality and reduce cancer risk, with exceptions in some areas within 300 meters of the freeway (ENVIRON International Corporation 2012). Despite expectations of increased traffic over this time period, decreases in pollution were predicted because of the phase-in of cleaner engines under new state and federal regulations (Yeung 2012).

Although the HRA provided additional health analysis of the project alternatives, it assessed only a narrow range of health impacts from air pollution (Human Impact Partners 2011; NEJAC 2009). After one member of THE Impact Project attended a local training on HIA in 2008, the group began to explore the idea of doing an HIA of the I-710 as part of the EIR/EIS process (NEJAC 2009). The partners realized that an HIA of the I-710 project proposal had the potential to bring new health information into the process. Soon after, THE Impact Project partners met with local officials who were on I-710 Local Advisory Committees to advocate for an HIA. They also organized groups of residents, local health departments, and experts to speak at public meetings in support of HIA (Heller 2016). In October 2009, the I-710 Project Committee voted in support of doing a HIA (EYCEJ 2009, 2017). Partners continued to push for the HIA to be included as an official part of the EIR/EIS process. In 2010, the GCCG contracted with Human Impact Partners, a nonprofit consultant from Oakland, to conduct an HIA and specified that their findings should be part of the final EIR/EIS. As Matsuoka noted (2014, 21), "Caltrans and Metro agreed to adoption of an HIA as part of the formal EIR/EIS process, but community organizations and advocates had to continually push for integration of the HIA findings in the [Draft] EIR/EIS analysis."

The HIA assessed a broader range of health effects than did the HRA, including the effects on air quality, jobs, noise, access to neighborhood resources, and mobility issues such as safety, travel time, physical activity, and stress involved in commuting for work (Human Impact Partners 2013). The HIA integrated community members' concerns, observations, and perceptions with quantitative data. It found that all alternatives under consideration would likely improve human health through better air quality and employment opportunities, but that negative impacts from noise might be expected. The I-710 HIA used the air quality models developed for the EIR/EIS, which ensured consistency with the rest of the analyses, but did not test the implications of alternate assumptions, such as higher future traffic projections. Safety impacts were found to be mixed, with the potential to improve safety in some areas and decrease it in others (Gateway Cities Council of Governments 2018). The HIA also noted that the expansion plans missed an opportunity to promote health through improved public transportation, walkability, and bikeability (Human Impact Partners 2011). The HIA recommended options to improve each health determinant and promote health equity.

The final HIA was submitted to the GCCOG in November 2011 (Human Impact Partners 2011). The HIA was forwarded along with the EIR materials to Caltrans, which declined to consider it as part of the final EIR (Human Impact Partners 2011). Although the HIA was not part of the final EIR, these efforts helped to raise awareness of health issues in the I-710 planning process in several ways. For example, stakeholders believed that the HIA contributed to Caltrans' decision to consider a new alternative for the I-710 expansion (Human Impact Partners 2011). In addition, according to EYCEJ's Angelo Logan (2016), "The HIA made people who were making recommendations to Caltrans realize that public health is much broader. ... Building a freeway is not just about what happens on that freeway, it is about what happens in the community."

Meanwhile, several of THE Impact Project partners joined other community and public interest groups including Physicians for Social Responsibility and the Natural Resources Defense Council to form the Coalition for Environmental Health and Justice (CEHAJ), which aimed to develop an alternative for expansion of the I-710 that better promoted community health and equity (EYCEJ 2017, 2018a). Because this was an advocacy coalition, USC was not an official member but provided technical support as needed. CEHAJ proposed "Community Alternative 7" (CA7), which it described as "an alternative vision of how goods movement projects, like the I-710 Corridor Project, can protect community health, improve quality of life, improve air quality, and effectively and safely plan for the region's goods movement growth" (EYCEJ 2017). CA7 included elements such as mandating zero-emissions vehicles, promoting public transportation, improvements in bike and pedestrian infrastructure, protecting the nearby Los Angeles River, and community benefits in the form of training and hiring local residents. As Angelo Logan (2016) said, "Within the environmental justice community, this was a shift in approach—becoming more proactive and less reactive, less 'let's stop the project' [and] more like 'let's promote a different project.'"

The Draft EIR/EIS was released for public comment in 2012. The California Endowment provided $25,000 to CEHAJ to hire a technical consultant to help the group comment on the DEIS/DEIR. Although Matsuoka (2014, 19) referred to this as a "David and Goliath battle" (referencing the over $30 million paid to the DEIS/EIR consultants), these resources contributed significantly to the effectiveness of the community responses. In September

2012, CEHAJ submitted 832 pages of comments on the existing alternatives and detailed its CA7 proposal. CEHAJ then encouraged local officials and other members of EIS/EIR committees to advocate for consideration of CA7. In addition, CEHAJ worked with California State Senator Ricardo Lara to propose legislation that would require Caltrans to evaluate broader considerations of community health, such as those embodied in CA7. Although the bill (S.811) passed both houses, the governor did not sign it (Matsuoka 2014). After reviewing comments and new information, in March 2013 the project committee produced a Recirculated Draft Environmental Impact Report/ Supplemental Draft Environmental Impact Study (RDEIR/SDEIS) (LA Metro 2018c). This process included a review of new alternatives, including Alternative 7, which was based on CA7 (LA Metro 2015; EYCEJ 2017). Alternative 7 fell short of CA7, however, because the I-710 Project Committee noted that mitigation provisions could not be considered under the CEQA process (LA Metro 2014). Nonetheless, according to Matsuoka (2014, 6), "Not only does CA7 reflect a major organizing win, it represents an alternative vision of how goods movement projects, like the I-710 Corridor Project, can protect community health, create jobs, improve quality of life, improve air quality, and effectively and safely plan for the region's goods movement growth."

Technical studies in support of this RDEIR/SDEIS were released for public comment in the spring of 2017. In spring 2018, Alternative 5c (expansion of general purpose lanes, safety improvements, and community health program funding but no designated freight corridor) was identified as the "preferred alternative" (LA Metro 2018a). Although the I-710 expansion project is not yet underway, it is clear that THE Impact Project partners, along with NRDC, CEHAJ, and others, shifted the decision process toward greater consideration of community health (LA Metro 2018c). THE Impact Project engaged through partners sitting on I-710 committees, briefing local officials and other committee members, and organizing community members to effectively participate in public meetings. The partners' knowledge of both the policy process and environmental health research led them to effectively advocate for additional analysis—the HRA and HIA—to inform the decisions. On the other hand, their influence in policy outcomes was still constrained by the structures, alternatives, and baseline assumptions determined by the government agencies. Nonetheless, this environmental review process included more robust opportunities for participation and set a new standard for engagement in goods movement planning (National Academies of Sciences Transportation Research Board and Strategic Highway Research Program 2011). As Matsuoka (2014, 23) wrote, "Winning change has not been easy but with smart and relentless advocacy and funding support for leadership development, technical assistance, and community organizing to expand and deepen regional community leadership, the campaign to transform the I-710 corridor is changing the way transportation planning and major infrastructure projects can help not harm communities."

Overview: The Impact Project's Engagement in Decision-Making Processes
THE Impact Project aimed to inform an entire local policy system, which necessitated interacting in a wide range of sectors, from land use to transportation to air quality at the local, regional, state, and even national levels. Although there were no government agency representatives in THE Impact Project, the partners interacted with policy actors and institutions regularly. These interactions included commenting on proposed actions as part of established processes (e.g., EIR/EIS), proposing local laws, enhancing participation in existing decision-making processes, and building networks to change the state and federal policy environment. THE Impact Project's most significant outcome was indirect: building its partners' capacity to engage in issues on an ongoing basis. As a result, it is difficult to evaluate the full effect of the initiative. Nonetheless, partners and observers agreed that the collaboration fostered by THE Impact Project promoted consideration of community environmental health concerns in goods movement policy (NIEHS 2013). According to Cacari-Stone and colleagues (2014, 1621), "The formalization of THE Impact regional partnership was described as a key change in the policy landscape, enabling ongoing regional dialogue and increased procedural justice." How the partnership leveraged resources to create this change is examined next.

Applying the Local Environmental Health Initiative Framework to THE Impact Project

THE Impact Project's dedicated funding ended in 2012, but it continued to receive some support as a regional member of the nationwide Moving Forward Network. As of 2018, partners continued to meet every other month to share information and coordinate activities. In addition, the experience, capacity, and connections forged through THE Impact Project laid the groundwork for the partners to continue promoting consideration of health in ongoing goods movement decisions.

The project contributed a multisectoral, regional, scientifically informed, community health and environmental justice perspective to goods movement decisions in Southern California. In retrospect, the partners believed that their collaboration contributed to change beyond what they might have accomplished individually. As USC's Hricko noted, "Without THE Impact Project and the close connections we at USC built with community and environmental justice groups around port and goods movement issues, our outreach program could never have fully understood the cumulative impacts of air pollution and traffic in these disproportionately impacted communities." EYCEJ's Logan (2016) added: "Working with USC and Occidental College allowed our community members to better grasp exactly how air pollution was impacting their health and to come up with policy solutions to address the issue."

Table 6.3 uses the conceptual framework for local environmental health initiatives to clarify the unique resources leveraged by THE Impact Project and how its collaborative structure contributed to changes in goods movement decisions.

Issue Framing and Problem Definition

Before THE Impact Project was formed, numerous groups had opposed port, railyard, and highway expansion projects based on community concerns including health. Most of these efforts, such as the China Shipping lawsuit, focused on specific proposals and their local impacts. THE Impact Project reframed the entire range of plans, projects, and decisions relating to goods movement as a regional environmental health and justice issue. THE project's explicit goal was "to change how the global trade and freight transportation issues are being framed" (Matsuoka et al. 2011, 60). The media attention, new decision processes, and initiatives described throughout this chapter speak to their success in doing so.

In addition to increasing attention to the health externalities of goods movement, the project specifically focused on the cumulative impacts of good movements on communities already burdened by excessive environmental pollution. By emphasizing the multiple sources and health

Table 6.3

THE Impact Project and the Local Environmental Health Initiative Framework

Collaborative Function	Analysis of THE Impact Project
Issue framing and problem definition	Reframed issue of goods movement as a regional phenomenon with environmental health and equity consequences.
	Broad regional scale required involvement of multiple communities.
	Targeted diverse scope of decisions by multiple decision makers.
Resources for collaboration	Human resources included 6 partner groups and their staff.
	Leveraged time, skills, and credibility of researchers.
	Supported by foundation grants and partner groups' core funding.
Structure and decision-making process	Brought existing community groups into new issues, areas, and roles; consensus decision-making, shared convening responsibilities, and equitable funding distribution.
	Fiscal management/administration of project funding by USC.
	Met frequently during period of robust project funding (2006–2012); monthly meetings continued 2013–2016; semi-monthly post-2016.
	Stable partnership of 6 groups (one partner withdrew in 2014 due to logistical challenges).
Impacts of collaboration:	
Outputs	Diverse communication tools and strategies to build general public awareness and support partners' advocacy efforts (policy briefs, videos, website).
	A-Teams (community based science)
	Hosted workshops and large conferences.
Social outcomes	Increased partners' capacity (scientific knowledge, partnerships, credibility) to engage in goods movement decisions.
Impacts on policies, systems, and environments (PSE)	Close working relationships between partners supported ongoing collaboration outside of THE Impact Project.
	Served on planning and advisory committees.
	Greater transparency, public involvement, and consideration of health in a wide range of goods management decisions.
	Informed local "green" ordinances.
	Gave rise to national Moving Forward Network.

determinants associated with goods movement, the project provided a basis for collective action by geographically disparate groups. Highlighting the common concerns of multiple groups and the regional scope of the problem assisted communities' efforts by capturing media attention, attracting financial resources, and disseminating technical information. Communicating the cumulative impacts of multiple ports-related activities and types of hazards also increased the public's understanding that although each individual new activity might comply with existing regulations, the additive effects of these activities had significant negative health implications.

THE Impact Project emphasized disparities in impacts on neighborhoods that already suffered from multiple environmental exposures and poorer health status. The partners also promoted awareness of vulnerable populations within communities, particularly children. This reframing highlighted the ethical implications, health costs, and community impacts on already overburdened communities. This focus also helped legitimize and give moral standing to port-adjacent community members as participants in decision processes.

Resources for Collaboration
Compared to many areas of the country, the greater Los Angeles area is rich in community groups, local foundations, and scientific expertise. However, when THE Impact Project first started, these groups were focused on their local communities' concerns rather than the wide-ranging health impacts of regional goods movement decisions as a whole. By providing a scientific basis for these arguments and coordinating among established groups in new ways, THE Impact Project was able to access significant human, technical, and financial resources over time. The partners were all involved in seeking, prioritizing, and applying these resources, with fiscal administration provided by USC.

Human Resources   The collaborative's primary human resources were its paid staff, both at USC and in the partner groups that received subcontracts. Each of these partners leveraged additional human resources. THE Impact Project's relevance to USC's environmental health center's research justified devoting the majority of staff time at the Community Outreach and Engagement Core (COEC) to goods movement issues for most of the period between 2001 and 2014 (Hricko 2016). In addition, the COEC leveraged the efforts of researchers themselves to speak at hearings, talk with journalists, review reports, and contribute to technical summaries. Engagement in these activities increased environmental health researchers' skills and interests in future policy engagement. For example, USC Professor Ed Avol participated in the I-710 Major Corridor Study, served as consultant to the Port of Los Angeles Community Advisory Committee, and was appointed to the Harbor Community Benefit Foundation, among other public advisory roles. Avol (2018) noted, "It has been critically important to get public health and air pollution impacts a seat at these discussions, and we pushed to do just that."

Although the project's core team included neither government agency staff nor elected officials, the partners worked with policy makers in a variety of capacities. For example, partners frequently reached out to local elected officials and health department staff to educate them about health impacts and community concerns. These individuals within government were then able to bring THE Impact Project's information to bear in decision-making settings in which partners were not directly involved.

Knowledge Resources   THE Impact Project accessed both community and scientific knowledge to support its partners' engagement. One of the most significant resources available was the technical expertise of USC researchers and its staff's ability to analyze, synthesize, and integrate scientific information to make it accessible to communities. The National Institute of Environmental Health Sciences (NIEHS) core center program encourages researchers to study environmental health problems identified by the COEC. The geography, poor air quality, and population density of Southern California made this an ideal community in which to study the impacts of air pollution on health.

THE Impact Project also leveraged local knowledge from residents about their needs, experiences, and observations living and working near goods movement hubs. It documented and disseminated this knowledge through its communication materials and video storytelling and by helping residents participate in hearings. As well, THE Impact Project generated new knowledge through community-based science. For example, A-Teams collected particulate concentration readings and truck counts that they reported in public hearings. Thus, the project facilitated a two-way exchange of information in which the community partners shared their knowledge of residents' concerns and researchers provided relevant technical expertise.

Financial Resources   THE Impact Project received several grants from private foundations to support its work. Grant proposals were generally written by COEC staff in partnership with the community group members and were submitted by, awarded to, and administered by USC. Financial resources were then divided equally among the partners to support staff and direct costs of their work. While USC officially controlled the majority of financial resources, the collaborative process gave all partners a role. Although this system took the burden of grant administration off the community partners, it did somewhat restrict the work plans. For example, some USC researchers were initially concerned about being the hub for the A-Teams, whose monitoring was not considered "fully scientific" because the P-Trak particle monitors they used were not up to research standards (Hricko 2016). Additionally, as a research institution USC could not be directly involved in advocacy, so grant proposals had to clearly distinguish partners' roles in THE Impact Project related to education, capacity building, and translating knowledge from their advocacy work. USC administrators required that at least one proposal involving THE Impact Project be reworked because it was too advocacy-oriented (Hricko 2016). Thus, being hosted by an academic institution both facilitated the group's access to and somewhat constrained its use of financial resources.

Group Structure and Decision-Making Processes
Although the fiscal administration of THE Impact Project was based at USC, it was a partnership in which all members shared decision-making power. The group met monthly to discuss plans, projects, and proposals. Project membership was stable over time, although CCAEJ withdrew in 2014 because of the challenges of traveling seventy miles from Riverside to meetings. All major decisions about how to prioritize issues, what activities to undertake, and what projects to seek grant support for were made by consensus.

Collaborative Outputs and Outcomes
Outputs included communication products, trainings, and policy engagement. Many of the communications outputs of THE Impact Project are easily identified: The project's website included a comprehensive collection of videos, research summaries, and policy briefs. The project also hosted a wide range of events, including workshops and the Moving Forward conferences.

The various forms of policy engagement (attending hearings, participating on committees, promoting local policies, shaping decision processes, etc.) may also be considered collaborative outputs.

The initiative's "social outcomes"—the impacts on capacity, relationships, and roles of members—continue to shape the partners' involvement in goods movement decision-making. Even after the project's major funding ended, partners met regularly to share information about ongoing issues.

As with any collaborative systems-change effort, it is difficult to conclusively identify THE Impact Project's outcomes in the policy arena (Cacari-Stone et al. 2014; Korfmacher et al. 2016). Because of the breadth of decisions relating to goods movement, the diverse approaches to influencing these decisions (e.g., legal action, negotiation, organizing, testifying, etc.), and the multiplicity of organizations involved in goods movement in Southern California, it is clear that THE Impact Project's contributions were just one factor. However, the trends in decision-making prior to and outside the scope of THE Impact Project strongly suggest that the initiative had significant policy outcomes. In addition, several studies in which decision makers were interviewed about THE Impact project attested to the widespread perception that it had a long-term impact on policy change (Cacari-Stone et al. 2014; Garcia et al. 2013).

In addition to impacts on policy outcomes, THE Impact Project helped change policy processes by creating new ways of participating in goods movement decisions. Prior to the project's formation, various community groups involved in areas heavily impacted by goods movement lacked a structure through which they could advance their collective interests. THE Impact Project successfully pushed for greater transparency and opportunities for participation, built community capacity to testify in public hearings, and gained positions on relevant committees. The diverse technical, human, and financial resources of THE Impact Project contributed to these lasting changes.

At the same time, it is important to note that while some goods movement decisions have been influenced by health concerns in recent years, changes in large-scale plans and policies have been limited. As Matsuoka and colleagues (2011, 50, 57) noted, "Despite the ever-growing evidence about the nature of these widespread health, environmental and workplace issues, these findings have not been widely incorporated into policy

decisions about expanding the size of ports and the freight transportation system in the United States.... Because the goods movement policy
debates are framed primarily as economic development and job creation
approaches, negative impacts on health, labor, community and environment continue to be seen only as externalities." In the context of such
enormous national and international forces, the procedural, educational,
and mitigation accomplishments of THE Impact Project are significant, and
are likely to lead to long-term improvements.

THE Impact Project was a leader in redefining goods movement as a
driver of environmental health inequities. Through the Moving Forward
conferences and outreach to other communities nationally, partners were
able to share their experiences and build greater public awareness of the
issue. These efforts continue to support related activities in port-adjacent
communities across the country.

Conclusions

THE Impact Project facilitated collaborative efforts to promote more health-
protective goods movement decisions in Southern California. Unique contributions from academic, community, and funding partners made this
possible. The community organizing and problem-solving experience of the
partners formed a strong foundation for policy engagement. The resources
of the USC COEC were essential for coordinating, developing, and expanding efforts to bring new perspectives from both communities and researchers into local decisions about goods movement. Private foundation funding
enabled the project's outreach, translational, and participatory efforts.
Government agencies responded by enhancing opportunities for public
participation and consideration of health in new projects. This tapestry of
human, technical, and institutional resources provided a unique context
for reframing how concerned communities responded to the encroach-
ment of goods movement infrastructure throughout the region.

Some of the changes influenced by the project, such as the Clean Air
Action Plan, local laws, and a new model for participation in Environmental Impact Review processes, were durably institutionalized. The USC COEC
had ongoing NIEHS funding that supports continued commitment to these
efforts. In addition, community groups continue to engage in goods movement decisions with the knowledge, tools, and connections gained through

THE Impact Project. Nonetheless, the capacity to sustain these efforts depends largely on the ongoing priorities of the community groups.

Can this local initiative to address goods movement be disseminated elsewhere? As already noted, THE Impact Project helped launch the nation-wide Moving Forward Network to promote health protection for communities around other parts of the country. What worked in Southern California may not be appropriate in other areas facing similar challenges. Matsuoka and colleagues (2011, 49) acknowledge that "in regions with fewer organizations and/or less developed attention to health, ports, and freight transportation, strategies are geared towards education and identifying opportunities for establishing coalitions and networks." On the other hand, MFN provides an opportunity for other communities to learn from each other's experiences.

THE Impact Project's capacity to sustain collaborative relationships, access credible health information, and work across diverse issue areas reframed the conversation around goods movement in ways that are likely to have a lasting impact on decision-making in Southern California. Thus, although there are great challenges in confronting the growth of such a powerful and important economic force in the region, according to Minkler and colleagues (2012, 37), "The community-driven movement built by THE Impact project has dramatically influenced and changed how policy decisions about goods movement are made."

7 Local Environmental Health Initiatives: The Impacts of Collaboration

Each of the local environmental health initiatives described in this book used different resources, structures, and approaches to change diverse systems that managed environmental and public health in its community. This chapter uses the Local Environmental Health Initiative Framework to analyze how these collaborative efforts promoted environmental health equity. This framework emphasizes the process of issue framing and problem definition, the resources for collaboration (human, knowledge, and financial), the initiatives' structures and decision-making processes, and the impacts of the collaborative efforts. These impacts include outputs (products), social outcomes (capacity and relationships), and impacts on policies, systems, and environments (PSE).

Issue Framing and Problem Definition

Each local initiative redefined a longstanding health issue as a problem of environmental health inequity, emphasizing that lower-income communities and people of color were disproportionately affected. This reframing introduced new stakeholders into existing decision-making arenas. These initiatives also identified gaps in existing environmental management systems that contributed to the problem. These new problem definitions shaped the scope, scale, and approach of the initiatives.

In many ways, the portrayal of lead as a "health issue with a housing solution" was a straightforward reframing of a problem by the Rochester Coalition to Prevent Lead Poisoning (CPLP). However, there were actually several elements of this problem definition. First, lead poisoning was highlighted by an elementary school principal, Ralph Spezio, as an issue of children's overall well-being, particularly with respect to their success in school. Thus, the initiative's definition of "health" was very broad. Second, CPLP emphasized how lead's impacts on children contributed to the city's social problems. The coalition presented a long-term vision for a lead-free city with better-educated citizens, less criminality, higher earning potential, and fewer long-term medical issues—all problems that were central concerns to the larger community. Third, CPLP advocated that changing local lead policy was an "achievable win" that would give the community hope and confidence to make progress in other issues. Solving the lead problem, they argued, would yield improvements in community morale. Identifying housing—particularly low-income rental housing—as the driver of childhood lead poisoning put the focus squarely on the city rental housing inspection process, but it also necessitated public education, landlord training, county health department funding, and coordination with public housing programs. CPLP acknowledged the economic challenges of Rochester's housing market and accordingly emphasized the potential for cost-effective solutions. Because it promoted less-costly lead hazard controls rather than permanent lead removal, CPLP stressed the need to sustain efforts over time.

The effort in Duluth to connect decisions about the built environment to health equity required framing a complex problem in a clear and consistent way. Decisions affecting the built environment occur in many sectors of local government, including transportation, land use planning, economic development, and parks and recreation. Private-sector development decisions, multiple state and federal agencies, community preferences, and economic forces also shape land use. Healthy Duluth leveraged the emerging national consensus that improving food access and active transportation opportunities can advance health equity. The partners reframed Duluth's vision for sustainable growth around a green economy as an opportunity to create healthy built environments for all residents. Healthy Duluth focused on low-income neighborhoods but recognized that long-term sustainability would depend on a citywide commitment to "Health in All Policies." This problem definition required engaging multiple policy actors and targets for action.

THE Impact Project arose from community concerns about the health impacts associated with shipping, railyards, trucking, and warehousing around the ports of Southern California. The project argued that the multiple existing policies regulating goods movement activities did not sufficiently protect the health of people living closest to intermodal transportation hubs from cumulative harms. This problem definition encompassed several related insights. First, it broadened the consideration of health concerns from a focus on air quality alone to include multiple impacts (e.g., noise, traffic, and light pollution) on community health. Second, it highlighted how existing regulatory systems, with their focus on regional environmental quality, did not effectively protect fenceline communities from concentrated hazards close to highways and transportation facilities. Third, it emphasized that the heaviest burdens fell on children, low-income residents, and communities of color. Finally, it framed goods movement as a regional phenomenon in which decisions made in one locality were likely to have unanticipated, unassessed, and unregulated effects on other communities in the region. THE Impact Project encompassed the largest scale and scope of the cases. Because it implied such broad targets for action, the project's strategy was to help affected communities better advocate for their own health protection, engage in multiple decision-making arenas, call attention to the regional environmental justice implications of decisions on specific local projects, and shape how community health concerns are integrated into future decision processes.

All three initiatives reframed long-standing environmental issues in terms of health equity. Their diverse problem definitions inspired new approaches to old issues. The way each initiative reframed the problem had important implications for who it involved, what resources it could access, how it was structured, and what it accomplished.

Leveraging Resources for Collaboration

By definition, these collaborative initiatives operated outside the scope of existing programs, agencies, and organizations. This situation required marshaling new resources and redirecting existing resources to support their efforts. It is typically more difficult to obtain support for convening, strategic planning, and analysis than for programs, products, and activities. Therefore, resources are often a limiting factor for collaboration. As noted in chapter 3, collaborative resources may be categorized as "human," "knowledge," and "financial," although there is significant overlap. Table 7.1 recaps the types of resources leveraged by each initiative.

Table 7.1
Summary of resources for collaboration

	Coalition to Prevent Lead Poisoning	Healthy Duluth	THE Impact Project
Human	1–3 paid CPLP staff; 15–70 volunteer committee members (health care, education, community, legal, city/county government, housing agencies).	1–3 staff; health impact assessment (HIA) consultants; staff from local health department, city, community group partners.	Project partners (staff and members of 2 academic and 4 community groups) shared convening tasks (organizing meetings, notes, etc.); USC staff administered grants.
Knowledge	Expertise, data access, analytic capacity of committee members; experience of community partners; public relations partners' skills; federal agencies and national lead groups' input.	Health department and city data, maps, and analyses; transportation planners' technical knowledge; Bridges to Health survey; community surveys.	Academics' expertise in environmental health research, policy analysis, and communications; community partners' experience with organizing and understanding of community concerns.
Financial	Grants from insurers, local government, United Way, private foundations, donation of services by public relations partners.	State health department funding (SHIP); HIA grants; brownfield planning grants; private foundation grants.	Private foundation grants (Kresge, California Endowment); NIEHS funding for USC core functions supported staff time.

Human Resources

These local environmental health initiatives involved diverse stakeholders who brought skills and perspectives needed to address complex problems in new ways. However, collaborative efforts take energy, time, and resources, and so many potential participants—particularly those engaged in programs targeted by the initiative for change—may have strong disincentives to participate. It can therefore be challenging to sustain involvement by all key stakeholders. As summarized in table 7.2, the three initiatives accessed and leveraged human resources from different constellations of community, academic, government, and private-sector organizations to support their respective efforts.

Table 7.2

Contributions of human resources from different sectors

	Coalition to Prevent Lead Poisoning	Healthy Duluth	THE Impact Project
Community	Series of community agencies hosted CPLP; community groups served on committees, educated and organized residents to support lead law.	Community organization (Zeitgeist Center) hosted Health Duluth Area Coalition; community groups/service agencies served on campaigns and participated in projects to engage residents.	4 local community groups were key partners; they educated, organized, and involved their members and residents of impacted communities in policy processes.
Government	Local, state, and national agencies participated as (non-decision-making) members of CPLP committees.	City of Duluth led 2 HIAs and brownfield plans; local health department and transportation agency staff participated in HDAC.	No direct participation in THE Impact Project structure.
Academia	UR environmental health sciences researchers, outreach program, and clinicians served on committees, reviewed materials, conducted analyses, gave community talks.	Limited involvement: UMD faculty wrote food access report; provided interns.	USC environmental health sciences researchers provided technical knowledge, testimony, review; USC hosted project; Occidental College partners provided environmental policy expertise.
Private sector	Health care professionals, risk assessors, lead trainers joined CPLP. Early involvement by property owners declined over time.	Health care sector provided data and staff analysis capacity.	No direct participation in THE Impact Project structure.

Coalition to Prevent Lead Poisoning   The human resources mobilized by the Rochester Coalition to Prevent Lead Poisoning were primarily the individuals who contributed time to the working committees. At the height of activities, this included around seventy people. These committees involved diverse organizations that saw the goal of reducing childhood lead poisoning as closely aligned with their missions. Coalition committee members included staff from a public interest law firm, the local community action agency, the county health department, various city departments, neighborhood group leaders, and many others. The health sector—including researchers, clinicians, public health professionals, and health insurers—was well represented, adding to the credibility of the organization. Most committee members attended meetings as part of their jobs, but several volunteers participated as interested community members.

There was limited involvement from the private sector whose business was most likely to be affected by CPLP's efforts: landlords and rental property managers. Several property owners and real estate professionals participated early in CPLP's history but dropped off over time. However, a number of individuals involved in lead hazard control work, including risk assessors and trainers, remained involved for many years. In addition to the time contributed by committee members, CPLP had staff members who supported the work of the committees, developed public communications, and conducted community outreach.

Healthy Duluth   Local government agencies contributed significant, sustained staff resources to the efforts to advance health equity in Duluth's built environment. City staff involvement included the parks department staff who initiated the original Fit City designation, city planners who participated in the health impact assessments (HIAs), and the economic development officials who integrated health equity into brownfield redevelopment projects. Regional and county health department staff helped launch the Pioneering Healthy Communities project, supported active living and food access projects, and participated in the HIAs. Transportation planning agency employees engaged in active and public transportation projects. Community groups contributed staff time to attend meetings, hosted AmeriCorps volunteers, and dedicated existing resources to related projects. Staff at health care organizations also contributed time to collaborative efforts. Academic institutions were not extensively involved, with the exception of University of Minnesota-Duluth (UMD) providing several applied analyses and a regular stream of student interns. Many but not all of these stakeholders participated in the Healthy Duluth Area Coalition, which also hired staff to support convening the coalition and managing related projects.

THE Impact Project   Although its core membership was small, THE Impact Project coordinated closely with a many organizations, agencies, and coalitions, which in turn leveraged additional human resources. The University of Southern California (USC) Environmental Health Sciences Center provided staff support through its Community Outreach and Engagement Core (COEC). The COEC dedicated significant staff time to goods movement issues, writing grants to support the project, conducting related outreach, and summarizing research findings related to the health impacts of goods movement activities. Staff and faculty from the Urban Environmental Policy Institute at Occidental College contributed environmental policy expertise. THE Impact Project community partners facilitated the engagement of additional staff, members, and residents in their organizations' related activities, programs, and events. Government agencies and the private sector were not directly involved in the partnership.

Human Resources Summary   One measure of success is whether the collaborative efforts involved people who had not been previously engaged in addressing the identified environmental health problem. Before the CPLP formed, health professionals were the core actors involved in childhood lead poisoning efforts in Rochester. CPLP engaged a wider range of community, education, housing, and other interest groups in the issue. Before the formation of Fit City Duluth, the primary effort to promote healthy environments was the work being done by public health professionals on smoke-free indoor air. Healthy Duluth engaged many other agencies and community stakeholders. THE Impact Project, which had the broadest range of targets for change, directly involved the narrowest range of stakeholders—academics and community leaders. Although many of these partners were already focused on specific aspects of goods movement, THE Impact Project broadened their engagement. It also leveraged additional human resources through the staff and membership of its partner groups. The Moving Forward conferences brought in hundreds of attendees from across the country. Thus, all three initiatives mobilized a wide range of new human resources to address an existing problem of environmental health equity.

Each initiative drew on human resources from many groups that had not previously been involved in addressing the identified environmental health problem. However, it is also important to note which stakeholders were *not* involved in each collaborative. Notably, none of the initiatives depended on human resources from groups that were targets for systems changes. For example, rental property owners had a minor role in the Rochester CPLP and goods movement industries were not partners in THE Impact Project. Many "target" organizations—particularly government agencies—provided information and technical resources but were not responsible for convening, strategic direction, or decision-making functions.

Knowledge Resources

Each initiative leveraged knowledge through its members, who provided access to data, analysis capacity, community experience, and professional expertise. This makes it difficult to distinguish human resources from knowledge resources. In fact, some argue that human resources *are* knowledge resources, since all participants contribute based on their training, skills, and experiences (Ascher, Steelman, and Healy 2010). Diverse members provided different types of knowledge—for example, health data, environmental science, community values, and insight into systems-change approaches. As well, all of the initiatives procured technical services using their financial resources.

The main knowledge function of the initiatives was to synthesize multiple kinds of information. They relied primarily on existing data, but strategically generated new data to fill identified gaps. They complemented national research with local information and worked to translate this knowledge in policy-relevant ways. All three initiatives emphasized that their positions were science-based, bolstering their credibility. They all leveraged knowledge about public health, environment, and community experiences to advance systems change.

Public Health Expertise   Each effort accessed public health expertise in different ways. CPLP had such extensive involvement by clinicians, public health professionals, and researchers that the coalition's co-chair, Bryan Hetherington, quipped: "No one could afford to buy the expertise that we got for free" (Hetherington 2016). In Duluth, clinicians helped establish Fit City Duluth, local health department staff played sustaining roles throughout Healthy Duluth efforts, and health system staff developed the Bridges to Health survey, conducted data analysis, and convened the community health needs assessment. THE Impact Project partners included clinicians and USC's environmental health scientists.

The availability of health data varied from case to case. Predictably, more health surveillance data were available in the larger cities. For example, THE Impact Project could draw on local studies of near-road pollution and community-level health effects. Childhood lead poisoning data were available at the zip-code level in Rochester, but most health outcomes data were available only at the city or county level in Duluth. Lack of fine-scale local health data made it difficult to connect environmental determinants with health disparities at scales meaningful to communities.[1]

Thus, each initiative tapped health expertise that informed its understanding of the problem, helped develop effective solutions, and bolstered credibility. CPLP and THE Impact Project directly accessed nationally known researchers whose work suggested that the environmental exposures were of greater health concern than previously thought. Health professionals in all three cases expressed enthusiasm about the opportunity to inform local solutions by collaborating with environmental and community stakeholders. As USC Professor Ed Avol said about his involvement in THE Impact Project, "We all had a commitment to improving the public health and reducing the environmental exposures, and THE Impact Project provided opportunities to do so" (Avol 2018). Similarly, community physician Dr. Richard Kennedy noted that working with CPLP gave him "a sense of empowerment because we had so many bases covered. We had so many smart people coming together, I felt like we could do this, and was willing to put the time into it" (Kennedy 2018). Former Monroe County health director Dr. Andrew Doniger agreed, saying that "it was clearly the beginning of a community movement, and our staff were thrilled to be part of that. They felt like they were being listened to after all of the frustration they had felt; now there was a chance that things were going to change. ... I don't think we felt threatened. I think that we felt appreciated" (Doniger 2017).

Environmental Knowledge All three initiatives also had the capacity to access, analyze, and create knowledge about environmental conditions.

CPLP members included housing agencies and lead inspectors who educated the group on how to prevent, identify, and address residential lead hazards. The 2002 Needs Assessment produced models and maps identifying high-risk neighborhoods. The Get the Lead Out (GLO) project generated information about hazards in high-risk neighborhoods. Healthy Duluth included transportation and land use planners, brownfield experts, and parks and recreation staff with expertise in managing the built environment. Healthy Duluth also generated new environmental knowledge through HIA consultants, community surveys, and the University of Minnesota-Duluth food access report. All partners in THE Impact Project started with a baseline understanding of environmental health, which was enhanced by interacting with USC air quality researchers. As well, the A-Teams generated knowledge about air quality, truck traffic, and other environmental conditions in their communities. Thus, in all cases, environmental knowledge came from the participation of technical experts who recognized that collaborating with new stakeholders could elevate solutions to environmental problems they had been working on for years. As Duluth transportation planner James Gittemeier said, "Urban planners have espoused livable communities for decades ... but when we tried to talk about this, it wasn't as powerful as when public health convened everybody, then the community realized it was a public health issue" (Gittemeier 2018).

Community Experiences, Values, and Preferences Each initiative integrated residents' experiences, values, and preferences. CPLP's bylaws required 30 percent of the members of its board to be from or represent affected communities; these members brought community knowledge into the coalition's work. In addition, the GLO project documented the challenges facing low-income families, such as the widespread fear that complaining about lead hazards could lead to eviction. This input from community members informed CPLP's support of policy approaches that did not rely on tenant complaints about lead hazards. Although Healthy Duluth efforts did not directly involve residents, community service agencies represented their clients' needs. In addition, Healthy Duluth projects elicited community input through development of neighborhood coalitions, conducting food access surveys, and public meetings on HIAs and brownfield planning efforts. THE Impact Project had a strong structure for accessing community knowledge through its four community-based partner groups. Community members' experiences were documented through the short video storytelling projects, A-Teams, and testimony at public meetings. While all three initiatives accessed community knowledge, their different contexts resulted in varying strategies for doing so. In CPLP and Healthy Duluth, professional members of the coalitions elicited community input because environmental health equity was not initially at the forefront of local community groups' agendas. THE Impact Project, by contrast, was driven by community groups' concerns about the environmental health implications of goods movement; these groups initiated and directly informed all its efforts.

All three initiatives harnessed members' knowledge about systems change and advocacy approaches. Some made focused efforts to further develop these skills. CPLP's board included many professionals with extensive experience in policy engagement as community organizers, public interest lawyers, and civil servants. It established a Leadership Development subcommittee to build the skills and roles of affected community members. The Healthy Duluth efforts were inspired by members' experiences passing tobacco control policies. Watching *Unnatural Causes* and attending national conferences enhanced their policy advocacy skills. Healthy Duluth grew to include members from community organizations with advocacy experience, government agency staff, and former elected officials. THE Impact Project community partner members were steeped in community organizing experience. The academic members included individuals with strong policy backgrounds. The project also worked with others such as the Natural Resources Defense Council (NRDC) with extensive knowledge of California's air regulatory system. All three groups built on their core members' past experience in systems change.

Generation, Transmission, and Use of Knowledge   As social scientists who study the role of science in environmental policy have found (Ascher, Steelman, and Healy 2010), three "knowledge functions" are necessary for producing well-informed decisions: generation, transmission, and use. Each initiative was able to access multidisciplinary knowledge, data, and experience in different ways. As modestly resourced collaborations, their ability to generate new knowledge was limited. Each initiative filled gaps in local environmental health data by collecting community-based information (e.g., CPLP's Get the Lead Out project, community surveys in Duluth, and THE Impact Project A-Teams) and analyzing existing information in new ways. Although these knowledge-generating tasks were important, they did not take a significant portion of the groups' resources. Rather, the initiatives' goal was to use existing information more effectively to advance solutions to environmental health equity problems. In order to use such multidisciplinary data, the initiatives needed the capacity to access and analyze it. For example, a public interest lawyer combined existing health department data on lead poisoning by zip code with U.S. Census data to analyze the distribution of lead risk in Rochester by race and ethnicity. This simple geographic analysis fundamentally recast the issue of lead as one of environmental justice.

Information on health and the environment often resides in separate agencies and at different scales. For example, housing data were available to CPLP by address, but information on children with elevated blood lead levels was aggregated to the zip code to protect privacy. Conversely, air quality in California is monitored regionally, but research showed that health effects varied over very small distances from transportation hubs. Thus, a major early effort in each case was to produce an overview synthesizing relevant health and environmental information at similar scales (Matsuoka et al. 2011; Gilley, Gangl, and Skoog 2011; Boyce and Hood 2002).

Each initiative also used external information from government reports, academic research, and case studies of other communities. This information helped build a common understanding of the environmental health problem, but local data was also essential to building credible arguments for local decision makers. The initiatives faced challenges in trying to connect environmental health determinants to local health outcomes because of the multifactorial relationships involved. Environmental contributions to health are difficult to demonstrate at a local level. This complicated the initiatives' efforts to develop a community consensus that addressing environmental factors would be a productive, ethical, and effective step toward reducing health disparities. Nonetheless, each group was successful in combining national research findings with available local data to support their systems change agendas.

All three initiatives devoted significant resources to synthesizing and sharing information in policy-relevant, audience-appropriate ways. Materials translating environmental health knowledge to varied audiences were key products of all three initiatives. These included policy briefs, storytelling videos, public service announcements, and researchers' testimony at public hearings.

Although each of the initiatives accessed, generated, and integrated multiple kinds of information in different ways, they all prioritized accessing and sharing credible information. This may reflect the fact that, as Wondolleck and Yaffee (2000, 244) point out, "Participants in these processes are investing considerable time and energy in trying to solve problems and resolve disputes. They can achieve their own ends and receive benefits from the effort they have invested only if the process is ultimately deemed acceptable to other participants and agency decision makers, as well as to those who would challenge the process's agreements. Hence, each participant has a considerable incentive to make sure that the group's decisions are credible and legitimate." Despite their limited resources, each initiative recognized that scientific credibility was a key source of their power to affect change.

Another common theme was that the process of building knowledge was a core part of the effort. As Ascher, Steelman, and Healy (2010, 210) note, "Knowledge generation, transmission, and use (can be) socially integrative." In other words, the very process of collaboratively developing a better understanding of the problem can strengthen partnerships. Each initiative's focus on knowledge sharing suggests this was a key unifying function of the partnership. Thus, leveraging credible multidisciplinary knowledge was both a key strategy of and important contributor to the effectiveness of the groups.

Financial Resources

All three initiatives began with members who had flexibility in their jobs or the capacity to volunteer that allowed them to convene partners, but did not have core funding to support an environmental health initiative. Each initiative eventually obtained financial resources from a variety of sources over time for staff, communications, and projects. The way each effort obtained financial resources, who controlled them, and how the resources were used to support collaboration differed greatly.

The Rochester CPLP started as an all-volunteer effort in 1999. Small private donations allowed it to hire a part-time staff to write grants to sustain the organization's capacity. Over time, CPLP received additional funding to coordinate the work of the committees, produce outreach materials, and support communications campaigns. These grants came from a variety of sources, including local foundations, government agencies, health insurers, in-kind donations of communications services, and the United Way.

Tracking Healthy Duluth's financial support is more complicated. The initiative was started as an unfunded effort by city parks and recreation staff. When Fit City Duluth was established as an independent not-for-profit group, it had no financial support and was staffed by an AmeriCorps volunteer. Fit City soon received the Pioneering Healthy Communities grant for core staff and activities. The Healthy Duluth Area Coalition (HDAC) obtained private foundation and government grant funding to hire an executive director. HDAC staff were supported through funding from the State Health Improvement Partnership (SHIP) and private foundations. Other projects like HIAs and brownfield plans were funded by grants.

THE Impact Project was primarily financed by private foundation grants that supported joint activities, member organizations' staff time, and administrative costs related to the project. These resources allowed the group to develop communications materials, produce reports, support community-based science, participate in policy processes, and translate scientific information to the news media. Even after dedicated funding ended, the project's members continued to meet monthly. Ongoing support from the National Institute for Environmental Health Sciences (NIEHS) and from the Moving Forward Network helped sustain THE Impact Project.

Thus, all three initiatives began as voluntary efforts but eventually leveraged financial resources to support core staff and activities. Obtaining funds to sustain collaboration was challenging. One strategy was to seek funding for projects related to their goals (i.e., producing materials, hosting meetings, providing training, conducting surveys, outreach initiatives) that in effect subsidized their convening functions. Another commonality was diversified financial support: none of them relied on one single sustained source of funding over time.

The initiatives' control of financial resources varied. CPLP's funds were managed by core staff in accordance with grant work plans and under the direction of its executive board. With the exception of foundation grants that provided support for HDAC, most of the funding for Healthy Duluth efforts was project-based and controlled by the organization that initiated the specific project. THE Impact Project developed grant proposals jointly and divided funds equally among the partners to implement the work plans. Thus, each initiative obtained financial resources to support convening functions that in turn leveraged human and knowledge resources.

Organizing Collaboration: Group Structuring and
Decision-Making Processes

Collaborative initiatives' structures and decision-making processes contribute to the stability, sustainability, and success of the efforts. The three local environmental health initiatives had diverse organizational structures, but each collaborative had an element of consensus decision-making, information sharing, and coordination of related decisions made by individual partners. Their structures and processes evolved over time.

The Coalition to Prevent Lead Poisoning relied on the fiscal and physical infrastructure of several different nongovernmental organizations at different times. The organization also changed its structure significantly over the years. After the lead law passed in 2005, active membership dwindled, the number of working committees was reduced to two, and CPLP relaxed its bylaws to allow for more informal decision-making. As of 2017, it had no dedicated staff, but the group continued to be active through regular meetings, communications services subsidized by a local public relations firm, and staff support contributed by long-standing members.

In Duluth, there was not a single convening body, but rather an increasingly well-connected network of professionals who collaborated on projects to promote healthy built environments. The HDAC did not have formal membership or decision-making rules, but rather served as a coordinating forum and provided input on the plans, projects, and funding proposals developed by staff and partners. Stakeholders asserted that because of the community's small size this informal network allowed them to identify opportunities to work together in pursuit of common goals.

THE Impact Project operated on a model of equal decision-making and resource sharing. The University of Southern California administered grants, meeting sites rotated between the partner groups' offices, and decisions were made by consensus. THE Impact Project had just six organizational members: four community partner organizations and two academic institutions, although the members worked regularly with additional groups involved in goods movement.

Every collaborative effort must balance between including diverse perspectives to inform consensus solutions and limiting partners to those with common interests. These initiatives were formed to advocate for environmental health equity by changing the actions of government and private-sector actors. They tried to build broad support but did not expect to develop a universal consensus around their solutions. Instead, they supported their members' advocacy for systems change. Each made efforts to understand and integrate the perspectives, knowledge, and constraints of the government or private-sector actors that their solutions targeted, but these affected organizations were not part of their decision-making structures.

All three initiatives had rather informal, loosely structured organizations. Much of the literature on collaborative organizations focuses on the importance of clear leadership, decision rules, and committed participation (Collective Impact Forum 2018). However, these three cases showed that progress is possible even when these conditions are not met. Only the CPLP had formal bylaws, and these were only in place during several years at its height of activity leading up to passage of the lead law. Healthy Duluth was comprised of loosely coordinated efforts of a number of separate agencies and organizations convened by different groups over time. THE Impact Project partners agreed to develop work plans by consensus to support their collaborative efforts and continued meeting after their funded work ended. Each group adapted its organizational and decision-making structures for collaboration as problem definitions, resources, and community needs shifted over time.

All three collaborative structures were able to balance their roles as partners with decision makers and as advocates for policy change. As noted, Healthy Duluth and CPLP engaged government agency staff as partners in non-decision-making roles, but they also advocated for changes in the policies and practices of these agencies. THE Impact Project members served as appointed members of government advisory committees, educated elected officials and agency staff about the health effects of goods movement, and testified as advocates at public hearings. This "inside-outside strategy" was evidenced in all three cases (Matsuoka 2014).

Impacts of Collaboration

These initiatives focused on changing local policies, systems, and environments to further health equity. Their strategies for impacting local decision processes were very different, however. Therefore, it is not surprising that their outputs and impacts varied as well. Nonetheless, participants and outsiders widely viewed each of these cases as a success.

As noted in chapter 3, defining "success" of a collaborative effort is complicated. On first blush, indicators that the initiative was successful might include answers to questions like: Did the initiative accomplish its initial goal? Did participants as well as outsiders view it as successful? Was there a concrete outcome—a new policy, process, or improvements in the environment—that can be traced to these efforts? The answers to these questions may not reflect the full value of the effort. For example, changed external conditions, unanticipated barriers, or new information may have altered the effort's goals over time. Different stakeholders may have different views about its success. Any assessment of accomplishments must consider what is likely to have happened absent the initiative. Finally, the initiative may have had unintended consequences that should also be considered in evaluating impacts. The conceptual framework presented in chapter 3 captures some of the complexities of assessing the impacts of collaborative efforts and provides a starting point for describing the impacts of these efforts in terms of their outputs, social outcomes, and systems-change impacts. Each initiative generated a wide range of products that supported its systems-change efforts. These initiatives also had social impacts that magnified their policies, systems, and environments influence. In each case, stakeholders noted unanticipated positive outcomes or "ripple effects" of their work, including sparking similar local efforts in other sectors and serving as a model for other communities.

Outputs

Each initiative produced a wide range of outputs in support of its overall goal. These outputs helped to develop, promote, and implement solutions to the identified health inequities.

The CPLP developed, promoted, and campaigned for the passage of a local lead law targeting rental housing. Its outreach work built support for the legislation. Once the law was passed, CPLP refocused on maintaining intergovernmental coordination, monitoring implementation of the law, and community education about lead poisoning. CPLP's outputs contributed to other primary prevention activities in the community, like the school district's lead policy, enhanced county inspections, and neighborhood-based outreach efforts.

Healthy Duluth's promotion of health equity in the built environment employed a variety of strategies and approaches. Most of the early projects involved conducting assessments, supporting neighborhood coalitions, and creating development plans. Partners later engaged in more direct actions, including commenting on street redesign projects, implementing community gardens, and organizing community events.

THE Impact Project engaged in decisions on a range of issues throughout the region. Its outputs supported the goal of ensuring that all decisions related to goods movement consider community environmental health impacts. A first step was to raise awareness of the comprehensive, cumulative, and inequitable impacts on vulnerable populations. Accordingly, project staff worked closely with the media and developed their own communication tools. The outputs included an array of storytelling videos, "Ports 101" training sessions, education materials, and policy briefs related to topics including trucking, railyards, warehouses, and port expansion. Because of the large geographic area, it was essential to build the capacity of local communities to advocate for themselves. This was the rationale for outputs such as the A-Teams, workshops, and trainings for community partners.

The varied outputs of the three initiatives all aimed to create the conditions for change in systems to promote environmental health. These outputs also reflected the initiatives' recognition of the two-way relationship between environmental and economic equity. For example, CPLP aimed to find an approach to primary prevention that would not damage the low-income rental housing market or cause major rent increases. It also produced a workforce development guide to advance training of unemployed community members in lead hazard control work. Healthy Duluth shifted its focus from "active living" to "transportation equity" with a focus on improving low-income residents' ability to access employment and nutritious food. The efforts supported job creation through the Deep Winter Greenhouse project and emphasized the cost savings of growing food in community gardens. THE Impact Project's "Driving Harm" policy brief addressed the challenges facing independent contractors who had to pay for pollution controls on their own trucks and recommended that trucking companies instead hire drivers as employees (THE Impact Project, 2012b). Later efforts emphasized creation of green jobs in neighborhoods affected by transportation industries. Thus, these initiatives' outputs focused on reducing environmental health inequities in ways that also improved (or at least did not detract from) other social determinants of health, particularly poverty.

Social Outcomes

The Local Environmental Health Initiative Framework delineates social outcomes as a distinct type of impact. Researchers and participants in coalitions frequently note that the trust, relationships, skills, and networks developed through the course of collaboration have positive impacts beyond the observable "outputs" of these efforts. These social outcomes can result in ripple effects in other sectors, decision forums, or time periods. Strong social outcomes were evidenced in all three initiatives. CPLP developed a network of lead-savvy community leaders and government staff who continued to collaborate, anticipate challenges, and take advantage of opportunities to further lead poisoning prevention efforts. In addition to continuing the lead work, many of the partners who worked together on CPLP later partnered on healthy homes, childhood obesity, and built environment collaborations. Healthy Duluth cultivated a tightly networked group of professionals in a range of organizations who "speak the language" of health equity. This network continued to focus on promoting health equity as new opportunities arose.

THE Impact Project increased the skills and knowledge of all its partners. Community partners learned about environmental health research, which bolstered their ability to participate in future goods movement decisions and enhanced their credibility. Academic partners gained experience in partnering with community organizations, interacting with the media, and engaging in a policy processes. The partners continued to interact on ongoing goods movement issues and through the national Moving Forward Network.

Participants in all three cases stated that the experience of collaboration had indirect effects on their ongoing work in the community. In all three cases, partners went on to work together on other community issues. However, participants also acknowledged that since the majority of these social outcomes were based on individual rather than institutional relationships, these impacts may attenuate with staff turnover over time. Although the initiatives did not aim to create permanent organizations, each made efforts to sustain convening functions that may refresh social outcomes over time.

Impacts on Policies, Systems, and Environments

It is difficult to comprehensively capture the impacts of collaborative initiatives on policies, systems, and environments. Uptake of outputs (e.g., participation in events, website hits, materials distributed) and stakeholders' reflections on social outcomes are intermediate indicators that the initiative's contributions will foster changes in policies, systems, and environments over time. To capture the potential for longer-term impacts, it is also important to document changes in policy, environmental health conditions, or external systems that may be attributed to the initiative's work. Impacts on decision processes and policies may be direct or indirect, long term and multilevel. In some cases, it may be possible identify trends in environmental determinants and health outcomes that can be attributed to the initiative's impacts on local systems change. Finally, many of the initiatives had effects outside of their local areas. Capturing such "external" impacts reflects the two-way interactions between local initiatives and broader efforts to improve environmental health. Table 7.3 provides an overview of some of the PSE impacts.

Decision Processes and Policies   CPLP's efforts contributed to several policy changes. The City of Rochester's 2006 lead law was the flagship outcome, but there were also changes in the practices of county health and human services departments, Rochester Housing Authority inspections, and the maintenance of school buildings. As well, CPLP established new processes for coordination that continue to affect how local governments plan, implement, and adapt their lead poisoning prevention efforts. Healthy Duluth's efforts supporting active living and better access to healthy food contributed to land use and brownfield redevelopment plans that reflected environmental health equity concerns. Adoption of health and fairness as aims for the comprehensive plan and discussions about passing a city resolution for a "Health in All Policies" approach suggest that decision processes in Duluth have been changed in durable ways. THE Impact Project concentrated on elevating health considerations in all decisions related to goods movement. To do so, the project partners first needed to increase the transparency of public decisions and expand opportunities for participation. In addition to promoting these procedural changes, partners and other stakeholders participated in multiple policy processes, including an environmental review of the I-710 and the Southern California International Gateway railyard proposed by Burlington Northern Santa Fe Railway. While

Table 7.3
Impacts on policies, systems and environments

	Coalition to Prevent Lead Poisoning	Healthy Duluth	THE Impact Project
Decision Processes and Policies	Passed local lead law; supported RCSD school lead policy; enhanced Rochester Housing Authority inspections.	Complete streets policy recommendation; health and fairness integrated into comprehensive plan.	Increased transparency and participation in goods movement decisions; enhanced consideration of health in EIR process; supported local "green" ordinances.
Environmental Health	City inspections show reduction in lead hazards in rental housing; rate of childhood lead poisoning declining faster than elsewhere.	New trails, gardens, and parks; Grocery Bus; complete streets; healthier brownfield developments; designing data system to capture health impacts.	Contributed to diesel emissions reductions through CAP; other impacts on health and environmental conditions difficult to measure due to scope and scale of issue.
External Impacts	Served as model for lead policy efforts in other cities; informed statewide lead policy network.	Highlighted as model for HIA and brownfields work; informed MN Brownfields health indicator tool.	Engaged in state and national EJ and policy analyses; initiated Moving Forward Network.

it is not yet clear to what extent the partners influenced the final decisions, their efforts increased the awareness of community health considerations and influenced decision processes. THE Impact Project partners also contributed to policy changes like local land use plans and truck-routing agreements to better protect communities' environmental health.

Indicators of Environmental Health Equity Each of the initiatives used data on health disparities to motivate, focus, and argue for the significance of its efforts. However, health outcomes are influenced by so many factors that it is difficult to attribute them to any single policy, educational effort, or funding stream aimed at improving the environment. Even the prevalence of childhood lead poisoning, which is directly caused by lead exposure, can be influenced by changes in housing markets, individual behaviors, consumer products, and population shifts (e.g., the increase in immigrant children from countries with high lead risk). For this reason, the efforts focused on impacting environmental determinants as well as measuring health outcomes.

For example, Rochester inspected more than 140,000 units in the first ten years of implementing the lead law. The unexpectedly high passing rate indicated that property owners were proactively making rental units lead safe. These efforts certainly contributed to the 82 percent decline in cases of children with elevated blood lead (EBL) levels from 2002 to 2012 (Kennedy et al. 2014). Although EBL cases are declining everywhere, the reduction in Rochester happened at a rate 2.4 times that in other upstate areas that lacked community lead coalitions. It is impossible to say whether CPLP's overall efforts—or the lead law in particular—caused these outcomes, but the data from other communities and reflections of a broad range of observers suggest that it made a significant contribution. Healthy Duluth influenced plans that have already resulted in a number of projects to improve environmental health equity in Duluth, including new trail segments, bike-friendly road improvements, community gardens, and the "Grocery Bus." Bridging Health Duluth is designing a community health tracking system that hopes to capture the cumulative effects of such efforts on health disparities over time. As already noted, THE Impact Project influenced a range of decision processes, policies, and plans that in turn have affected environmental conditions. For example, the Clean Air Action Plan significantly decreased diesel emissions from trucks at the ports. However, because of the complexity of goods movement decisions and multiple drivers of air quality, it is difficult to directly attribute any specific improvements in environmental conditions to THE Impact Project's efforts. Tracking any associated health effects is even more complex, because of the many non-air quality contributors to asthma, heart disease, and cancer. Thus, although in each of these cases there is some evidence of environmental improvement, it is important to remember that issues like air quality, housing markets, and economic development are significantly impacted by forces outside of local control, so lack of observed short-term improvements in environmental conditions does not necessarily mean the initiative failed to make a positive contribution. This is even more true of observed health effects, which often have multiple causes and long latency.

External Impacts   All three initiatives interacted with and were informed by efforts in other communities, national interest groups, and state or federal government agencies. These connections helped disseminate their experiences to other communities. The Rochester lead law has been widely recognized as a cost-effective approach to reduce hazards in high-risk private rental housing. Since it passed, over two dozen cities have reached out to Rochester to learn from its experiences, and some have passed their own lead laws. There is much to be learned from the CPLP experience in terms of building a coalition of diverse stakeholders, characterizing the local challenges and resources for reducing lead hazards in housing, designing an appropriate system of prevention, and coordinating efforts to monitor and adapt the program over time. CPLP and city staff frequently interact with other cities about how to adapt Rochester's approach to their local context. However, they always caution that while the coalition-building process is widely applicable, Rochester's specific policy solution may not be appropriate for other cities.

Several of Duluth's innovative efforts have been shared with wider audiences. For example, Minnesota Brownfields piloted a brownfield health indicator tool in Duluth that was published for statewide use in 2017. Former funders including the Pew Charitable Trusts and the Center for Prevention at Blue Cross Blue Shield of Minnesota have highlighted Duluth-based environmental health equity projects on their websites. Healthy Duluth stakeholders have also been invited to speak at numerous state and national conferences.

THE Impact Project discovered there was national interest in its efforts among attendees at the first Moving Forward conference. Recognizing the need to share lessons learned between groups in different regions led to formation of the Moving Forward Network (MFN). Additionally, the Moving Forward conferences showed the potential for local groups to come together to pursue a national policy agenda that would benefit all port-adjacent communities, giving rise to MFN's "zero campaign" on emissions. This unanticipated outcome of THE Impact Project may help to significantly reduce the future health impacts of ports around the country. Over the years, THE Impact Project members have been recognized by national awards, news articles, and academic publications praising it as a model community-university partnership.

Each of the initiatives learned from and informed other communities. Although it is not possible to attribute specific changes in other cities, state agencies, or federal policy to these interactions, there is clearly potential for these local initiatives to inform environmental health equity efforts in other communities.

Summary of Impacts   While it is difficult to prove that these initiatives directly reduced health disparities in the short term, there are many indicators that they influenced systems in ways that will reduce environmental health inequities over time. Rochester is the only case in which there is public health data that strongly suggest the community's efforts to reduce housing-based lead hazards have contributed directly to positive health outcomes. Both CPLP and Healthy Duluth can point to environmental changes attributed to their efforts. Because of the scope, scale, and timeline of goods movement decisions, it is difficult to connect specific environmental health impacts to THE Impact Project's activities, but the policies and processes the partners affected are likely to contribute to wide-ranging long-term improvements in the long term.

All the initiatives influenced processes and systems in ways that are likely to reduce environmental health inequities over time. In Duluth, the integration of health considerations into planning processes has already shaped the flow of resources into low-income neighborhoods. Adoption of health and fairness as goals for city decisions and the network of professionals committed to furthering health equity bodes well for implementation of these plans. THE Impact Project's success in increasing opportunities for participation by a broad range stakeholders, enhancing the engagement capacity of community partners, and elevating attention to health in decisions related to goods movement is likely to strengthen environmental health protections. However, it may never be possible to directly connect improvements in environmental health equity to the partnership. Acknowledging such challenges of evaluating collaborative efforts can help set appropriate expectations, develop intermediate indicators of progress, and help participants and funders appreciate the indirect, long-term, and often invisible nature of these initiatives' contributions toward environmental health equity.

Summary

These three cases differ by issue area, geography, demographics, scope, and scale—yet their collaborative approaches had several common features. First, each initiative addressed a problem in which the environmental determinant was managed by a well-established set of rules and regulations. Despite this existing management system, in each case the community identified a disproportionate health burden on a local population. Framing these problems as unacceptable inequities was necessary for launching a collaborative search for new solutions. The groups' ability to make systems changes supports the observation that "information, resources, and political support are often more readily available when multiple parties work together to collaboratively solve complex problems" (Wondolleck and Yaffee 2000, 245). Thus, their successes both depended on and contributed to boundary spanning, partnering, and collaboration.

In each case, the collaborative effort involved multiple sectors, but each had a unique constellation of government, health care, community, environmental, and academic partners. At least one member of each initiative had a directive to collaborate with community partners around environmental health issues. In Rochester and Southern California, these included NIEHS-funded Community Outreach and Engagement Cores; in Duluth, the guidelines for the local health department's State Health Improvement Partnership (SHIP) and the city's brownfield planning grants from the U.S. Environmental Protection Agency encouraged community collaboration. These organizations helped convene others who had the incentive, flexibility, and resources to participate and then leveraged these resources to expand community engagement.

Because these were informal collaboratives initiated by the community, there was no mandate for specific organizations or individuals to partner. Therefore, understanding the partners' barriers, incentives, and goals for their voluntary participation is essential to understanding the success of these initiatives. In each case, stakeholders perceived the initiative as an opportunity to make progress on an issue of concern by partnering with new groups. Each collaborative found ways to work around participants' professional constraints—for example, by focusing on building capacity, analysis, and sharing knowledge. This allowed professionals and academics to participate in the initiative, while also supporting the advocacy efforts of community partners, volunteers, and nongovernmental groups. Enabling participation from diverse sectors helped the initiatives access multidisciplinary knowledge and perspectives.

The organizational diversity of each initiative suggests that there is no one "right" structure for a successful local environmental health initiative.

Rather, the structure must be appropriate to the goals, needs, and capacity of members, and it may change over time. Each initiative used a different strategy to achieve systems change. CPLP focused on promoting a new local policy. Healthy Duluth developed a common vision among partners who then proceeded to integrate health into the practices of non-health agencies. THE Impact Project increased its members' environmental health literacy and capacity to advocate for awareness of health in public decisions. Many of their impacts were indirect, process-based, long-term, and even invisible to outsiders. Specific goals and approaches were not clear at the outset but rather emerged from the collaborative over time. This suggests that a developmental approach to evaluating these types of initiatives is most appropriate (Patton 2010).

These initiatives produced a wide range of outputs, social outcomes, and changes in policies, systems, or environments. In each case, the local environmental health initiative secured funding streams and influenced decision processes. There may be future shifts in the environmental, legal, technical, or economic context that require the collaborative energy of a local environmental health initiative adapt to these changes. Fortunately, the social impacts of these initiatives have increased the capacity of communities to address future needs. Finally, each contributed to change beyond the local community in unanticipated ways. This suggests an underappreciated potential for local-to-local learning to promote environmental health equity beyond the community scale.

Given this diversity of these collaborative efforts, it is clear that there are many paths to success. It also suggests that one initiative's approach is unlikely to have the same impact in another community. Although these initiatives' specific strategies, structures, and approaches may not be readily replicable, there is still much to learn from them about supporting progress toward environmental health equity in other communities. Certain community conditions may facilitate collaboration to address local environmental health and justice issues. These conditions—and how to foster them—are further discussed in chapter 8.

8 The Promise of Local Environmental Health Initiatives

> One of the most powerful ways to influence the behavior of a system is through its purpose or goal.
>
> —Donella Meadows, *Thinking in Systems* (2008, 138)

This book examines three local initiatives to promote urban environmental health equity by changing policies, systems, and environments. The initiatives developed to address diverse environmental health problems: lead hazards in rental housing in Rochester, New York; the built environment in Duluth, Minnesota; and goods movement around the ports of Los Angeles and Long Beach, California. In each case, stakeholders confronted a long-standing environmental health inequity. All three built collaborative efforts across disciplinary barriers and leveraged multiple sources of knowledge. They also built their partners' capacity and influenced how local decisions are made in ways that are likely to foster future reductions in health disparities. This chapter highlights the common themes across all the cases, reflects on the potential to disseminate lessons learned in other communities, and suggests how similar efforts might be supported elsewhere in the future.

Origins of the Local Initiatives

In each of these cases, an individual who was not an environmental public health professional played a significant formative role. These initiators called attention to the problem from an outsider's perspective, transcending existing management systems. Professionals in relevant organizations then

helped to characterize the nature of the problem, identify gaps in existing policies, and communicate relevant information. Community members
contributed their perspectives on their lived experience of the problem,
either directly or through community based organizations. The multifaceted understanding that emerged from this collaboration helped reframe
the problem and develop systems-change solutions.

In Rochester, elementary school principal Ralph Spezio made the connection between lead and his students' learning challenges. Through his efforts
to learn how to protect the children in his school from lead exposure, he
connected with the local health department, pediatricians, public interest
lawyers, researchers, and many others who helped characterize the nature
of this entrenched problem in Rochester. His focus on children's education
and well-being set the stage for a coalition that looked beyond existing
health department programs to respond to lead poisoning cases and identified the drivers of housing-based lead hazards facing low-income children.
The Coalition to Prevent Lead Poisoning (CPLP) went on to promote lead-
safe housing by promoting a local lead law and supporting actions.

Although many local government professionals contributed to the launch
of Duluth's health equity efforts, a concerned community member played
a key role in establishing durable collaboration. Mimi Stender's personal
passion to promote healthy living in Duluth motivated her to create Fit City
Duluth as a policy, systems, and environmental change-focused organization. With strong support from organizations including the YMCA and the
Local Initiatives Support Corporation (LISC) and an active board, Fit City
provided a hub where community, government, and private stakeholders
could work together to promote system changes. Both Fit City Duluth and
its successor organization, the Healthy Duluth Area Coalition, leveraged
government and private support for a wide range of local initiatives. The
training and technical assistance provided to Duluth stakeholders through
national initiatives like Pioneering Healthy Communities, Safe Routes to
School, and health impact assessments helped build local capacity to promote healthy food access and active living. At the same time, the city's planning and economic development efforts increased the community's focus
on health equity with support from the Minnesota Department of Health,
the U.S. Environmental Protection Agency, and Minnesota Brownfields,
among others. Together, these efforts influenced public decision processes
like neighborhood planning, complete streets design, community gardens,

transportation plans, and brownfield redevelopment efforts to benefit low-income neighborhoods.

At the 2001 town hall meeting on environmental health in Southern California, longtime environmental justice activist Jesse Marquez told the assembled group of community members, academics, and journalists that his community was suffering from air pollution from the ports. Marquez was one of several local community leaders who later joined with academic partners to form THE Impact Project. This initiative elevated the consideration of health in goods movement decisions by building on the complementary skills of academics and community groups—all of whom were outsiders to the government institutions responsible for regional goods movement decisions. The resulting effort had significant system-wide impacts on how community concerns and health information were considered in subsequent goods movement decisions in the region and beyond.

These genesis stories suggest that successful local environmental health initiatives may arise outside of the institutions officially responsible for managing environment and public health. When these community stakeholders teamed up with experts and agencies, they were able to collaboratively identify new strategies and solutions. Thus, although these efforts were not initiated by environmental or health agencies, governmental actors were important to the initiatives' sustainability, effectiveness, and impacts.

Sustaining Dynamics

Accounts of environmental justice initiatives often emphasize the role of crisis in initiating action. However, that was not the driving dynamic in these three cases. In fact, the trends surrounding each environmental hazard of concern were generally improving. Lead poisoning was on the decline in Rochester, Duluth was redeveloping, and regional air quality in Southern California had improved markedly. Thus, these initiatives called attention to environmental health inequities against the backdrop of overall improvement. Environmental injustices typically arise because of the lack of political power of affected populations. These collaborations derived persuasive power from highlighting health inequities.

These efforts to reframe a long-standing environmental issue in terms of health disparities brought together diverse stakeholders. Each initiative built on local resources including engaged university partners, active community groups, collaborative local government staff, or dedicated host organizations. In each case a significant role was played by a local entity that was mission-driven to promote environmental health partnerships. This commitment provided a base of support for collaboration. As already noted, each of these efforts was initiated outside existing management systems, but was later fostered by a local organization with a mission to promote collaboration, the ability to work across disciplines, and the capacity to leverage outside resources.

There are many other communities with lead problems, pollution from ports, and challenging built environments that have not given rise to systems-change initiatives. Why did collaboration occur in these cases? Looking back on their experiences, the stakeholders in each case reflected that the "stars aligned" in unexpected ways that allowed them to overcome the inertia of existing management systems. But the case descriptions also suggest that local organizations "helped the stars align" by seeking to promote partnerships, access multidisciplinary knowledge, and tap resources to support the effort. This suggests that absent increased support for these convening functions, such initiatives are not likely to proliferate.

Unfortunately, communities with the greatest needs are least likely to have the capacity to initiate efforts like those described in this book. Counterintuitively, environmental health equity may be a less powerful concept in the most vulnerable communities, where an intense focus on poverty, jobs, and economic development can supersede concerns about health and environment. Accordingly, Cummings (2018, 345) warns that "social movement efforts to build progressive cities may create islands of greater equality amid a larger sea of inequality—causing the gap between the politics of progressive big cities and the politics of everywhere else to grow wider, reinforcing polarization." Conscious efforts can be made in every sector to support proliferation of effective local environmental health initiatives in less economically well-endowed communities.

Common Themes of Local Environmental Health Initiatives

The three cases presented in this book represent very different issues, geographies, communities, and institutions. However, their experiences revealed several common themes that may be relevant to other local environmental health initiatives.

- *Health equity is a powerful idea in many environmental management issues.* In all three cases, a focus on combating health inequities brought energy, resources, and new partners to focus on a long-standing environmental problem. Although stakeholders may not have articulated the problem explicitly as "health equity" or "environmental justice," they motivated action by highlighting unfair access to environmental benefits or distribution of harms associated with health disparities.

- *Collaboration is a process, not an organization.* None of these initiatives formed a separate fiscal entity, but rather coordinated efforts between existing organizations. Each aimed to "put itself out of business" by changing systems and building capacity so that it was no longer needed. Creating opportunities for collaboration was more important than maintaining a new, standalone organization. Participants in all three cases emphasized that the opportunity to learn, plan, and develop solutions together allowed them to be successful despite lack of a formal organization.

- *Many types of organizations can be effective conveners if they are predisposed to partnering.* Each initiative included at least one organization that had coalition building as part of its mission. Rochester's lead coalition was hosted by several organizations that were committed to coordinating community partnerships, including the Rochester Primary Care Network, the Finger Lakes Health Systems Agency, and United Way. An academic environmental health outreach program whose goal was to support community partnerships played a key role in both CPLP and THE Impact Project. In Duluth, the state health department directed local health departments to develop community coalitions and promote systems change. Even though many of the core organizations were prohibited from direct policy advocacy, their commitment to partnering, informing, and developing public support helped sustain these efforts.

- *Boundary spanners are created, not born.* In each case, individuals stepped outside their institutional silos to address the problem in a new way. Many professionals welcomed the opportunity to work beyond their agency structures and program limitations. Several of the key actors in each case were longtime employees of key organizations and were given permission by their home agency to participate. For many, this was their first experience collaborating with different sectors. They became enthusiastic about partnering to solve long-standing community problems their home organization could not address alone.

- *Research can be helpful, but translation is essential.* In two cases (CPLP and THE Impact Project), a local university hosted an environmental health science center funded by the National Institute for Environmental Health Sciences (NIEHS) whose mission included translating research to address local environmental health concerns. These centers also provided access to leading researchers in lead and air pollution, respectively. In Duluth, public health agency partners provided analysis of health data while the city and consultants contributed environmental expertise. As a result, all three initiatives had the capacity to credibly synthesize, communicate, and apply environmental health information to local problems.

- *Locals are listening.* Although these cases were locally initiated, they were informed by national efforts. All three initiatives tapped into national resources through grants, training programs, pilot project funding, publications, or conferences. These interactions also benefited the national groups by providing evidence of successful dissemination of their ideas and serving as a model for other communities.

- *There are tradeoffs between measuring success in terms of environmental determinants versus health outcomes.* Each initiative highlighted data showing health disparities associated with an environmental concern. However, they all generally refrained from promising immediate health improvements as a result of the policy changes they promoted. Instead, they relied on existing environmental health research to argue that addressing environmental determinants would eventually contribute to health improvements. Tapping into concerns about human health to focus attention on environmental interventions required developing a consensus around causality and a community commitment to take actions with indirect, long-term, or unmeasurable effects on public health.

Although these insights relate to environmental health initiatives, they may also inform collaborations in other issue areas. Similar dynamics may exist around local initiatives to promote education, transportation, or criminal justice equity. Analysis of additional case studies could inform efforts to better support local environmental health initiatives in the future.

Supporting Local Environmental Health Initiatives

Most communities experiencing environmental health disparities do not give rise to local collaborative initiatives like those described in this book. This suggests that local initiatives will not spontaneously emerge under current conditions, but rather need to be intentionally encouraged. These case studies suggest several ways to better promote, support, and sustain such efforts.

Although increasing funding opportunities would likely encourage additional collaborative work, many other barriers remain, including institutional structures, individual incentives, and cultural constraints to partnering. Corburn (2005, 215) calls the "jazz of practice" an essential component of environmental justice collaborations, in which "professionals are expected to situate themselves in this struggle and make this a centerpiece of their work. By being playful, improvisational, and open to new 'players,' the jazz of practice encourages professionals to remake existing models of environmental-health decision making." However, many professionals face barriers to such "improvisation," including grant funding restrictions, limited budgets, hierarchical management systems, and simply having too much to do. As Steelman (2010, 196) notes, "Individuals working under conditions of weak structures and challenges to legitimacy will face daunting hurdles. Under these conditions, work first needs to take place within the structures and culture before innovation stands a reasonable chance of longer-term implementation." In other words, many of the key players needed for a successful local environmental health initiative may lack the capacity, training, guidance, or incentive to partner with community groups. Institutions may need to work consciously to change their cultures and structures in ways that facilitate their staff members' participation in innovative collaborative efforts. Community groups, academia, government agencies, and funders can all create conditions in their institutions that are more conducive to collaboration. Each sector may use different approaches to do so, as described below.

Community Groups

Community groups face numerous barriers to participating in local environmental health initiatives. The greatest challenge is usually time. Most community groups have limited core support, so participating in partnership meetings takes staff away from funded projects and essential activities. THE Impact Project addressed this challenge by building funding for partner groups' staff into its grants. However, before obtaining funding, the participants contributed significant time to develop the initiative. Under-resourced community groups must constantly make strategic decisions about whether participating in collaborative efforts is a wise investment of their limited staff time.

Environmental justice groups often build support and membership by organizing in opposition to established interests. Participating in collaborative initiatives with government or academic partners can thus threaten their independent identity and image in the community. As Corburn notes (2005, 216), communities can benefit from "shifting the discourse from protest and refusal to engagement with problem solving." However, they can also lose credibility among their base of support if the outcome of collaboration does not meet their members' needs. The expectations for community group roles in environmental health initiatives should recognize these dynamics as potential limits to their collaboration.

Finally, many small community groups have rapid staff, board, and membership turnover. This can undermine the social outcomes of collaborative initiatives: the development of individuals' capacity, networks, and relationships. Anticipating turnover, community groups can set up internal systems for maintaining institutional memory (i.e., rotating staff participation or regular reporting among staff) and communicating regularly with their constituents about their roles in collaborative initiatives and the value of such work. Community groups should seek funding opportunities that sustain their internal capacity for external collaboration, although these are notoriously difficult to find.

Academia

Both CPLP and THE Impact Project had strong involvement by academics. However, the universities involved both had a unique resource: an environmental health science center that was charged by its funder—the National Institute of Environmental Health Sciences—to use its research capacity to address community problems. In practice, this meant that the academic centers had Community Outreach and Engagement Core (COEC) staff that could convene meetings, initiate partnerships, write grants, and facilitate engagement by researchers. There are other models that similarly support community engagement, such as cooperative extension programs at land grant universities, but these are the exception rather than the rule among academic institutions. Most universities lack dedicated resources for outreach, engagement, and translation of research.

In fact, academics are often implicitly discouraged from engaging with community efforts because these activities detract from research, publication, and grant writing. Few universities take faculty members' community engagement activities into account in promotion and tenure decisions. Increasing funding opportunities for community-based participatory research can encourage academics' engagement but does not typically provide ongoing support for partnership building, collaborative problem-solving, applied analyses, and educational outreach. Additionally, academics may be discouraged from participating in politically controversial issues, particularly when they work at publicly funded institutions. For example, when Andrea Hricko wrote a letter to the Gateway Cities Council of Governments (GCCOG) in 2004 asking that minutes of meetings about the I-710 Major Corridor Study be made public, her dean received a letter of complaint from GCCOG questioning her efforts as "political" (Hricko 2016).

On the other hand, positive contributions to community efforts can be a source of goodwill and can enhance public relations. Such reputational benefits accrue to the institution as a whole, however, not the individual department, faculty, staff, and students involved. Recognizing this, some universities provide core support for engagement activities to encourage community engagement. A growing number of universities host "science shops," institutes focused on generating community solutions, and multidisciplinary problem-focused clinics (Trubek and Farnham 2000; Israel et al. 2006; Tryon and Ross 2012). Additional efforts to remove barriers, increase incentives, and provide support for academics to engage in local environmental health initiatives could make technical, strategic, and logistical support more widely available to community initiatives.

Government

Healthy Duluth and CPLP benefited from collaboration with government agencies. In Duluth, local health department staff was supported by the state health department's directive that they work with communities to promote systems change. The city's economic development staff became engaged through brownfield redevelopment grants that encouraged health assessments and the planning department partnered actively in several HIAs. Both the mayor of Rochester and the Monroe County public health director voiced strong support for CPLP's efforts to promote primary prevention. This endorsement provided city and county staff with flexibility, if not a mandate, to participate in CPLP. Later, both the city and county highlighted their support of CPLP in their lead hazard control grant applications to the U.S. Department of Housing and Urban Development (HUD), which gave extra points to applicants with strong community partnerships. Although THE Impact Project did not collaborate directly with agencies that govern goods movement decisions, its members participated in numerous advisory committees, hearings, and review processes alongside government staff and elected officials.

Thus, in all three cases, mandates, incentives, or opportunities established by higher levels of authority supported collaboration with government staff. When leaders or funders set clear expectations for participation, staff are more likely to collaborate. Nonetheless, even when given permission or encouragement, spending time in collaborative initiatives may seem like a luxury that overburdened government staff cannot afford. In the long run, government staff participation in partnerships can yield dividends in terms of leveraging community and private-sector support for agencies' goals. Matsuoka and colleagues (2011, 61) point out that "cities across the country face enormous economic and budgetary challenges. The result has been layoffs, furloughs, and elimination of environmental and regulatory enforcement programs. New partnerships with the nonprofit sector, when deeply rooted in the public sector, can provide local authorities more tools and resources to address health and environmental impacts." Integrating these kinds of collaborations into staff job descriptions, designating official positions on boards for government representatives, and requiring community engagement as part of program goals can help public servants prioritize partnering.

However, it is also important to acknowledge that direct participation by government agency staff can create conflict—or at least discomfort—if an initiative is targeting that agency for change. Recognizing this, the Rochester and Duluth initiatives did not include their government partners in decision-making roles. Efforts to facilitate government involvement in partnerships should be sensitive to this constraint. For example, government staff may be designated as "advisory" members to avoid appearing to endorse policy advocacy or positions critical of current agency practice.

These cases also show the importance of collaboration between sectors of government and how joining community partnerships can promote such interagency collaboration. As emphasized throughout this book, many environmental health problems fall between the purviews of institutions that focus on health and those responsible for environmental management. In all three cases, partnering with stakeholders *outside* government increased collaboration *between* government agencies. This was accomplished by providing a forum for collaboration that involved staff from multiple governmental agencies and publicly praising their joint efforts. As agency leaders explore the potential of collaborating with other government institutions to address ongoing issues of environmental health, they should recognize the role outside groups can play in promoting coordination with other governmental entities. As Koontz noted (2004, 184), "The interaction and shared deliberation inherent in collaboration may enhance relations both among and between nongovernment and government representatives by promoting trust, network development, and participatory democracy."

However, social scientists who have studied collaborations for ecosystem management have identified multiple institutional, structural, and social barriers to government agencies and staff members' ability to engage in effective collaborations (Koontz 2004; Wondolleck and Yaffee 2000). Civil service tends to reward strict implementation of agency programs and rules, which does not traditionally include forging partnerships and collaborating with new partners (Grenadier, Holtgrave, and Aldridge 2018). However, as agency goals and resources change, they may recognize the importance of collaboration with outside groups in systems change. Unfortunately, significant gaps in collaborative skills have been noted among the existing public health workforce (Trochim et al. 2006; McGinty, Castrucci, and Rios 2018). This suggests new training needs. For example, the San Francisco Health Department has developed a systematic training program to "foster a culture of learning, trust, and innovation, and to support our public health colleagues in promoting health equity" (San Francisco Department of Public Health 2018). This type of initiative recognizes that the incentives, structural barriers, and cultural norms facing government professionals need to be clearly recognized, and sometimes intentionally reoriented, in order to promote their successful participation in collaborative efforts (Wondolleck and Yaffee 2000; Steelman 2010).

A final way government agencies can support collaborative initiatives is as a funder. Changes in funding mechanisms that apply to all funders, including government agencies, may better support local environmental health initiatives.

Funders

All three initiatives faced challenges financing their collaborative efforts. Participants noted that it was particularly difficult to get financial support for the core functions of convening such as communicating with members, developing strategic plans, and supporting meetings. Accordingly, increased sources of financial support for local collaborations would likely spawn more environmental health initiatives. For example, the Duluth initiative benefited from national efforts to support local healthy built environment collaborations and health impact assessments. The fact that all these local groups leveraged external financial support suggests that additional national resources may foster more successful local initiatives.

Funders generally prefer to support efforts that are time-limited, well defined, and clearly measurable through objectively reported outcomes (Israel et al. 2006). However, collaborative environmental health initiatives are by definition emergent, unpredictable, and long term. It is difficult to evaluate their impacts, particularly their long-term contributions toward building capacity and changing relationships, their indirect effects, and their ability to shift priorities of existing systems. Nonetheless, these cases are rich with examples in which small amounts of funding for collaboration contributed to significant long-term changes in policies, systems, and environments. Therefore, it seems likely that expanding private, agency, and academic funding for collaborative initiatives could expand these kinds of efforts.

However, different *kinds* of funding are also needed. Funders increasingly acknowledge the value of community collaborations and aim to support them through longer-term funding of dedicated staff positions, nonrestricted funds, or increased overhead rates on grants to community groups. Funding of this kind is particularly important to provide community groups with flexibility in staff activities and the ability to invest time in building new partnerships, sustaining relationships, and developing institutional memory. Funders should explore additional mechanisms that provide core support for convening, flexibility to adapt as problems are reframed, developmental approaches to evaluation, and functions like monitoring, implementation, reporting, and dissemination to other communities.

The funding, cultural, and institutional constraints of many community groups, academics, and government institutions pose barriers to environmental health initiatives. Several of the initiatives presented in this book were often referred to by their participants as "stars aligning" moments, when their institutional goals, resources, and opportunities overcame such barriers in ways that allowed them to partner successfully. As described previously, community groups, academic institutions, government agencies, and funders all have roles to play in helping the stars align by changing their practices, processes, and programs to better incentivize collaborative efforts.

Developing Networks for Dissemination

Although each of these initiatives emerged from a unique local context, their experiences organizing for environmental health systems change may be informative for other communities. As noted previously, many cities have reached out to CPLP members to learn how Rochester developed and implemented its lead law. However, there is no established mechanism for active dissemination of these experiences through a national network; thus, there may be many other cities that could learn from the Rochester lead coalition but are not aware of its program. How can we help cities learn from each other's local environmental health initiatives? There are several options for promoting local-to-local learning to explore.

In some cases, there may be existing networks that could disseminate lessons from local initiatives into other communities. One past example of sharing a local initiative's learning with a wider audience through an existing national network is the Transportation Research Board (TRB) case study on THE Impact Project (National Academies of Sciences Transportation Research Board and Strategic Highway Research Program 2011). This report made THE Impact Project's collaborative experiences widely available to transportation planners nationwide. Several foundations have played important roles in sharing local community experiences, including the Robert Wood Johnson Foundation's case studies of local collaborations for active living and the Pew Charitable Trust Health Impact Project's online database of health impact assessments (Active Living by Design 2018; Pew Charitable Trusts 2018a). However, these resources are often limited to initiatives that are funded by the sponsoring foundation or program.

With growing interest in local approaches to promoting health equity and environmental justice, conferences and publications increasingly share lessons learned from local environmental health initiatives. In recent years, the American Public Health Association, the American Planning Association, and the National Association of County and City Health Officials have all featured local environmental health initiatives at their national conferences. Several peer-reviewed journals also regularly publish articles on community environmental health initiatives, both as research articles and in special sections designed to highlight community partnerships.

There are fewer opportunities for community groups to share perspectives nationwide. The Moving Forward Network initiated by THE Impact Project is a promising example of such a forum (Moving Forward Network 2018). Similarly, the Active Living by Design program promotes information exchange between communities about collaborative efforts (Active Living by Design 2018). It is important to note that both of these efforts are primarily funded by private foundations and that maintaining sustained funding for intercity networks of community groups may be challenging.

Thus, there are some issue-specific opportunities for local groups to share their stories and learn from others. However, local groups may have limited capacity to participate in these learning networks. Local initiatives seldom have the time or resources to tell their stories—never mind a venue to share them, identify which elements may be relevant to others, or even respond to questions from others. This suggests that funders of local environmental health initiatives should incorporate support for staff time and travel to participate in activities that make their experience accessible to and let them learn from others.

How these lessons are communicated, and the level of detail examined in each local case, is also important. Many traditional case study reports simply provide short summaries of accomplishments without reporting on the group's processes, struggles, and resources. Such cursory treatments may suggest that strategies, policies, or approaches can be simply transferred from one community to another. As shown by the lesson of Benton Harbor—the Michigan city that adopted but failed to implement a Rochester-like lead law—this is seldom the case. An essential part of dissemination involves unpacking the context and details of the collaborative process, the challenges of cross-sector data analysis, and the strategies for sustaining community engagement.

National organizations can play an important role in promoting local-to-local learning about collaborative environmental health initiatives. For example, the health impact assessment map from the Health Impact Project (Pew Charitable Trusts 2018a) makes HIAs from all over the country publicly available in a searchable database. The interactions each of the case studies had with national groups and other communities suggest that locals are receptive to learning from other efforts. However, their capacity to do so may be limited by the availability of information, time to do research, and skepticism that others' experiences will translate to their community.

A Message for Individuals

Government agencies, nonprofits, consultants, and researchers have produced numerous training materials, books, and guides on promoting successful collaboration. Although these resources can help people plan collaborative efforts by laying out key principles, process recommendations, and resource needs, they may paint an ideal picture of collaboration that can be hard to achieve in practice. There are often real barriers and risks to participants from all sectors. Collaboration can take time from other mission-essential (or career-enhancing) activities. Partnering with organizations that have aligned but not congruent interests can undermine credibility, and failure to achieve shared goals can erode crucial relationships.

The three case studies examined in this book suggest that changes are needed in every sector to support successful local environmental health initiatives. Even absent such systemic changes, individual community members, government employees, researchers, or other professionals can all play a role in promoting collaboration. Wondolleck and Yaffee (2000, 250) call collaboration "a kind of awkward dance that none of us knows the steps to." Similarly, the former surgeon general Joycelyn Elders once famously quipped, "Collaboration has been defined as an unnatural act between nonconsenting adults. We all say we want to collaborate, but what we really mean is that we want to continue doing things as we have always done them while others change to fit what we are doing" (Backer 2003).

These statements recognize that collaboration must be advanced by real people facing real political constraints, competing priorities, and resource limitations. Collaboration has become such a popular notion that people may fail to realistically consider their goals, barriers, and institutional interests—as well as those of their potential partners. This can lead to misunderstandings, conflict, and loss of trust. Wondolleck and Yaffee conclude their comprehensive analysis of successful collaboration for ecosystem management with a "message to individuals" considering partnering outside of their organization. To paraphrase their advice:

1. *Numerous opportunities exist*: build on the most immediate with small steps.

2. *There is no one right way to promote collaboration*: experiment, evaluate, and adapt.

3. *Collaboration does not always work*: don't take it personally, and don't lose sight of your own interests.

4. *Collaboration is not rocket science*: persistence, humility, honesty, sincerity, and listening carefully will get you a long way, *but also* ...

5. *Collaborative skills can be learned*: training in communication, group process, and facilitation—either as an individual or with the whole group—can improve effectiveness.

Thus, individuals should carefully consider their personal incentives, goals, and constraints before embarking on a collaborative effort, then ask the same questions of potential partners (Wondolleck and Yaffee 2000, 249).

A final point for individuals to remember: failure may not be failure. Well-conceived, focused, and amply supported collaborations often fail to achieve their initial objectives. Collaboration is not always the most productive or timely way to solve a problem of environmental health inequity. Even "failed" collaborations may provide an opportunity for the individuals involved to form relationships, gain knowledge, or incorporate new objectives in their future work. The potential for such "invisible successes" in the face of "visible failures" (Korfmacher 1998) is why the social outputs of collaborative efforts are emphasized in the Local Environmental Health Initiative Framework.

Poverty, Environment, and Health

Kjellstrom and others have noted that "poverty is not only a question of money, but it has ... other dimensions: lack of *opportunities* (for employment and access to productive resources), lack of *capabilities* (access to education, health, and other public services), lack of *security* (vulnerability to economic risks and violence), ... lack of *empowerment* (absence of voice, power, and participation), (and) lack of a *health-supporting physical living environment*. These five dimensions stem from inequality as the root causes of poverty" (2007, 86).

There is a positive feedback loop between environmental health inequities and poverty. Poorer people are more likely to be exposed to environmental hazards, live in neighborhoods with few health-supportive facilities, lack the resources to avoid hazards, or have limited resilience to environmental risks. Living in unhealthy environmental conditions can exacerbate economic challenges by limiting opportunities for education, transportation, and access to employment. Cumulative stress related to environmental hazards, poverty, and disordered neighborhoods contributes to health problems. These relationships between poverty and environmental health can be reinforced by discrimination, racism, and social stigma. Local environmental health initiatives cannot single-handedly end poverty, but they have the potential to mitigate the bidirectional connections between poverty and environmental injustice.

There are several ways that local environmental health initiatives can address the two-way relationship between environmental health and poverty. First, explicitly recognizing that poverty, racism, and historical marginalization of disadvantaged groups contribute to current environmental health inequities can help local environmental health initiatives argue for devoting additional resources to counteract observed disparities. Second, these initiatives can create opportunities to reduce poverty through their activities. This may require reaching out to stakeholders involved in economic development, education, antiracism initiatives, and workforce development to find ways that environmental health initiatives can support their efforts. Conversely, environmental health initiatives must be mindful of causing unintended negative consequences for neighborhood well-being, such as contributing to gentrification and community displacement. Third, environmental injustice is experienced at the neighborhood, home, and individual level. Therefore, the knowledge, values, and preferences of affected communities must inform the process, strategies, and approaches from problem identification through promoting specific solutions. This requires interaction between multidisciplinary experts and communities, often using a variety of approaches. Finally, making progress on an environmental health problem can inspire ongoing efforts to address the root causes of poverty.

These three cases provide examples of how collaboration around locally identified problems can develop solutions that help address both poverty and environmental health inequities. In fact, their local focus makes them better poised to identify complementary opportunities and avoid unintended negative consequences than state or federal programs. Local environmental health initiatives alone cannot end economic inequity, but they have the potential to augment community development efforts. Struggling municipalities may consider environmental improvements to be of secondary importance to economic development efforts. However, these cases suggest that local environmental health initiatives have the potential to help combat broader social inequities.

Toward Health Equity in Local Environmental Policies

In each case, local stakeholders identified an ongoing issue of environmental injustice and successfully reframed it as an issue of health inequity. They harnessed the expertise of community groups, technical experts, and government agencies to understand the issue. They learned about how existing federal and state policy, economic forces, local historical factors, demographics, and culture shaped the local environmental health problem. This allowed them to understand key drivers of trends, identity opportunities for systems change, and formulate strategies.

Although many of these efforts engaged governmental actors, none of the collaboratives had official authority. Therefore, they needed to work with existing institutions to achieve systems change. In so doing, they developed networks and built the capacity of participants to engage in future policy processes. In most cases, they fostered broader community engagement in local issues beyond their initial scope. They elevated health equity as a goal for environmental management systems. By increasing community awareness of and support for environmental health equity, they increased the likelihood of sustained systems change and laid the foundation for future efforts.

None of these initiatives had visible outcomes like shutting down an industrial polluter, blocking a development, or banning a dangerous chemical. Rather, they shifted existing management systems toward addressing the upstream drivers of environmental health inequities. Thus, these types of efforts may be a promising approach to resolving long-standing issues of environmental injustice. This begs the question: How might we build on these experiences to more universally, systematically, and proactively address the gaps in existing environmental management systems to reduce health inequities through local action?

First, removing barriers and increasing incentives for local stakeholders to engage in collaboration could promote this kind of cross sector problem-solving. As described previously, there are many barriers to collaboration. Funding collaborative efforts is part of the solution, but changes in institutional incentives and cultures are also needed. Second, we could enhance opportunities to learn from and disseminate local environmental health initiatives. These three cases are just a small sample of ongoing local efforts throughout the country to address environmental health injustices. Helping communities learn from each other could promote more effective local initiatives. It is also essential to extract lessons about the failures of existing environmental and health management systems that gave rise to the locally identified problems. Some of these failures could be addressed through changes at the state or federal level. Third, these efforts support the idea that considering "Health in All Policies" can be a powerful political, practical, and analytic approach to addressing local environmental health inequities. Although the "Health in All Policies" concept is gaining traction at the federal and state levels, few localities have embraced the idea. Developing tools to facilitate consideration of health in all local policies may help other communities, researchers, agencies, and funders promote health equity in multiple sectors.

It is important to design collaborative structures that are appropriate to the problem at hand. Indeed, the collaborative efforts profiled in this book exhibited a wide range of approaches, from informal to structured collaboration. None aimed to build a sustained formal partnership, but rather promoted new relationships, practices, and priorities within existing institutions. Such questions of appropriate collaborative processes and structures merit careful consideration by future researchers and practitioners.

Integrating health equity goals into policies in multiple sectors requires new ways of engaging communities; forming partnerships between government, academia, and interest groups; harnessing multidisciplinary sources of knowledge; and developing funding streams that support these efforts. This book shows how collaboration at the local level can help existing management systems better address environmental drivers of health disparities. An explicit focus on environmental health and justice can drive systems for managing the environment to more efficiently, effectively, and equitably promote healthy communities.

Public Health as an Ecosystem

Decades ago, environmental advocates, researchers, and agencies recognized that siloed, single-agency approaches were insufficient to protect the health of ecosystems. Environmental disasters, public conflict, failure to meet environmental quality standards, and slow species recovery efforts were taken as evidence that environmental protection needed a new approach: cross-sector collaboration, more public engagement, and holistic ecosystem management. In response, a wide range of collaborative ecosystem management institutions were developed to better protect natural resources as integrated systems. The aim of ecosystem management was to promote ecological integrity, a more holistic goal than the single-sector approach of most prior environmental management systems (Grumbine 1994).

Similarly, escalating health care costs and growing health inequities demonstrate that our current approaches to protecting public health are failing. Growing appreciation for the importance of social determinants of health suggests that protecting public health requires collaboration between multiple agencies, diverse sources of knowledge, and robust community involvement. Public health professionals increasingly recognize engagement in community collaboration as an important growth area for health departments seeking to reduce health disparities through systems change (McGinty, Castrucci, and Rios 2018; Fraser, Castrucci, and Harper 2017; DeSalvo et al. 2016; Trochim 2006).

The need for a systems approach to public health is particularly clear with respect to environmental health. The separate management of environment and public health has contributed to many environmental health inequities. Each of the cases in this book shows how siloed management systems failed to prevent cumulative, comprehensive, and inequitable impacts on health. Broader consideration of health equity in multiple decision-making arenas is needed to address environmental contributors to health disparities. These cases also suggest that adopting environmental health equity as a goal may facilitate new solutions to long-standing environmental problems.

The field of ecosystem management was built on the promising initial experiences of informal collaborations such as voluntary watershed protection associations. Over time, collaboration was institutionalized to various degrees by state, federal, and nongovernmental organizations. The promise of the local environmental health initiatives portrayed in this book suggests that these approaches have the potential to reduce environmental health inequities. Further research is needed to explore how such efforts could be better supported, disseminated, and institutionalized to help reduce health disparities. Treating public health like an ecosystem with many interdependent parts, perspectives, and processes requires new bridges between existing institutional silos. Communities, academics, public health professionals, environmental managers, urban planners, and funders all have roles to play in building these bridges. Collaborative management of urban environments can speed progress toward the goal of achieving environmental health equity.

Methodological Appendix

Chapter 4: The Coalition to Prevent Lead Poisoning: Promoting Primary Prevention in Rochester, New York

I have been a participant-observer in the Rochester, New York childhood lead poisoning prevention work since 2001, serving as co-chair of the Coalition to Prevent Lead Poisoning's Government Relations Committee since 2007. During this time, I was involved in many of the coalition's activities, discussions, and events. These experiences informed development of this case study. My involvement with CPLP was part of my role in the Community Outreach and Engagement Core of the University of Rochester's Environmental Health Sciences Center, which is supported by the National Institute of Environmental Health Sciences grant P30 ES001247. For this chapter, I also drew from numerous articles, reports, news articles, and case studies written about CPLP and community lead poisoning prevention efforts in Rochester. In-depth interviews with longtime CPLP partners and observers including Mel Callan, Dr. Andrew Doniger, Bryan Hetherington, Dr. Richard Kennedy, Ralph Spezio, and Wade Norwood provided additional perspectives. I am grateful to these interviewees as well as to Macayla Barnes for her assistance documenting CPLP's history. Many other CPLP members and national partners provided helpful input and reviewed portions of this chapter, including Patricia Brantingham, Vicki Brown, Paul Hunt, David Jacobs, Gary Kirkmire, Donna Lawrence, Kathy Lewis, Elizabeth McDade, Rebecca Morley, Tom Neltner, Katelin Pellett, and Dr. Stanley Schaffer. Theresa Green and Paul Haan provided invaluable orientation to the Benton Harbor case.

Chapter 5: Healthy Duluth: Toward Equity in the Built Environment

This case study relied primarily on interviews and correspondence with over two dozen individuals who have been involved in a wide range of environmental health equity initiatives in Duluth, Minnesota, over the past ten years. These informants included current and past government staff, state and national organizations involved in Duluth-based projects, members of community groups, and staff of private institutions. I am deeply indebted to all of these people, including Cate Bosserman, Natalie Brown, Tony Cuneo, Deb DeLuca, Jim Gangl, James Gittemeier, Annie Harala, Robert Herling, Kayla Keigley, John Kelley, Pam Kramer, Kelly Muellman, Julie Myhre, Jennifer Pelletier, Ellen Pillsbury, Kristin Raab, and Jim Skoog. I especially thank Jean Ayers, Heidi Timm-Bijold, Josh Gorham, Lisa Luokkala, Jenny Peterson, and Mimi Stender for multiple iterations of feedback on drafts. Richard Bunten created the map of Duluth. I greatly appreciate these generous contributions to my synthesis of the Healthy Duluth efforts. In addition to these firsthand sources, I drew from government and community organization websites, project reports, grant applications, news articles, and published literature.

Chapter 6: THE Impact Project: Trade, Health, and Environment around Southern California's Ports

Much has been written about THE Impact Project as a nationally significant initiative to address health and environmental issues related to global trade. Lisa Cacari-Stone, Analilia P. Garcia, Meredith Minkler, Nina Wallerstein, and others have written several insightful pieces on THE Impact Project as an exemplar of community-based participatory research. Reports highlighting the project were also important resources, including "Trade, Health, Environment: Making the Case for Change" (Sausser et al. 2009), "Global Trade Impacts: Addressing the Health, Social and Environmental Consequences of Moving International Freight through Our Communities" (Matsuoka et al. 2011), and "Democratizing Planning" (Matsuoka 2014). As well, the project has been highlighted as a case study in numerous reports, manuals, and news articles. THE Impact Project's own website, policy briefs, communications materials, presentations, and videos were also invaluable. To complement these published materials, I conducted phone and in-person interviews with several project partners and others involved in goods movement in Southern California, including Ed Avol, Bob Gottlieb, Jonathan Heller, Angelo Logan, and Carla Truax. I am particularly grateful to Andrea Hricko for sharing presentations, reports, and personal reflections on her experiences as the director of the University of Southern California's Community Outreach and Engagement Core (USC COEC) over a span of more than fifteen years, as well as for providing extensive references, resources, and feedback on drafts of this chapter. Her work with THE Impact Project was initiated through the USC's Environmental Health Sciences Center, which is supported by National Institute of Environmental Health Sciences grant P30 ES007048. Finally, Gunter Oberdorster, Stefania Squizzato, and Jamie Winebrake provided helpful reviews of sections on air pollution, health effects, and U.S. policy.

Notes

1 Changing Local Systems to Promote Environmental Health and Justice

1. These engagement cores have had several names since first being established by then-NIEHS director Kenneth Olden in 1996 as "Community Outreach and Education Programs." For most of the time period discussed in this book (2005–2016), they were called Community Outreach and Engagement Cores before being renamed "Community Engagement Cores" in 2017 (O'Fallon et al. 2003). See also NIEHS (2018a), "Community Engagement Cores: Environmental Health Sciences Core Centers."

2 Standing Silos

1. The terms "population health" and "public health" are often used interchangeably in the popular media, but they have different meanings to many researchers and professionals (Kindig and Stoddart 2003). According to the Institute of Medicine, "Population health (also referred to in this report as the health of the population, or the public's health) is the focus of public health efforts. It refers to 'the health of a population as measured by health status indicators and as influenced by social, economic and physical environments, personal health practices, individual capacity and coping skills, human biology, early childhood development and health services'" (Institute of Medicine 2002).

2. The Federal Water Pollution Control Act Amendments of 1972 are commonly referred to as the Clean Water Act of 1972.

3. In states governed by "Home Rule," local governments have more control over land use than in states governed by "Dillon's Rule," which gives state government more power (Dannenberg, Frumkin, and Jackson 2011).

4. In 2016, California incorporated guidelines for promoting environmental justice into state law overseeing local planning (State of California 2016; Office of Environmental Health and Hazard Assessment 2018). The state directed that comprehensive

plans should "(A) Identify objectives and policies to reduce the unique or compounded health risks in disadvantaged communities by means that include, but are not limited to, the reduction of pollution exposure, including the improvement of air quality, and the promotion of public facilities, food access, safe and sanitary homes, and physical activity. (B) Identify objectives and policies to promote civil engagement in the public decision-making process. (C) Identify objectives and policies that prioritize improvements and programs that address the needs of disadvantaged communities" (State of California 2016).

3 Building Bridges

1. Most definitions of social determinants of health include environmental factors. In this context, the "environment" is all the characteristics of where we live, work, and play. Some public health professionals use the term "environment" to refer to both the social environment (e.g., family, community, etc.) and the physical environment as a function of place. This book focuses primarily on the physical resources, conditions, and exposures in people's neighborhoods and built environments. Thus, as used here, the term "social determinants of health" includes environmental determinants of health.

2. The Alma-Ata Declaration stated that primary health care "involves, in addition to the health sector, all related sectors and aspects of national and community development, in particular agriculture, animal husbandry, food, industry, education, housing, public works, communications and other sectors; and demands the coordinated efforts of all those sectors" (WHO 1978).

3. Ecosystem management is by definition a collaborative process. The term "collaborative environmental management" reflects that fact that some collaborative management institutions focus on subsets of activities or dynamics within ecosystems. Thus, while both "ecosystem management" and "collaborative environmental management" are used in this book, the latter term emphasizes the collaborative nature and diverse scope of these efforts.

4 The Coalition to Prevent Lead Poisoning

1. In 1986, Congress limited lead content in pipes and fixtures to 8 percent and in solder to 0.2 percent; lead in brass fixtures was also limited to 8 percent. As of 2014, lead in pipes and fixtures was further limited to 0.25 percent. Thus, fixtures and solder labeled "lead free" in the United States may still contain some lead (U.S. EPA 2018k).

2. Health departments usually report elevated blood lead level rates (EBLL) as the percentage of children tested for lead whose blood lead levels exceeded a certain concentration (in this case, 10 µg/dL). When reporting EBLL rates, it is important to note the "screening rate"—or the percentage of all children whose blood was actually tested. If the screening rate is low, or if the sample of children tested is not

representative of the whole population, the reported EBLL rate may not represent the actual percentage of children affected by lead. In places where only high-risk children are tested, the EBLL rate may greatly exceed the rate of EBLL in the entire population. Conversely, in communities where high-lead-risk children are not effectively identified and tested, the EBLL rate may underestimate the population rate. Complicating matters further, "screening" sometimes refers to asking the parent questions to determine whether the child is at risk for exposure to lead and should be tested; other times it refers to actual blood lead testing.

Testing rates in Rochester were among the highest in the state in 2000, with over 70 percent of children in Monroe County tested for lead before their second birthday (New York State Department of Health 2001). What the Coalition to Prevent Lead Poisoning (CPLP) reported as the "national lead poisoning rate" was based on National Health and Nutrition Examination Survey data (NHANES) (CDC 2018b). NHANES surveys and conducts medical exams of a sample of the population that is selected to create statistical estimates of the prevalence of health conditions in the entire population. The "national rate" of 2.2% used in CPLP's early communication materials was based on the 1999–2000 NHANES prevalence estimate for U.S. children ages 1–5 (Meyer et al. 2003). The statewide 1999 EBLL rate reported by the New York State Department of Health was 5.8 percent (Boyce and Hood 2002).

3. The Advertising Council of Rochester changed its name to Causewave Community Partners ("Causewave") in 2016 (www.causewave.org/who-we-are/), just prior to becoming CPLP's fiscal agent. Because of the ongoing relationship with CPLP under this new name, for clarity's sake it is referred to as Causewave Community Partners throughout this book, even in reference to its role during the time it was officially called The Advertising Council of Rochester.

4. The Finger Lakes Health Systems Agency (FLHSA), a regional community health planning organization, changed its name to Common Ground Health in 2017 (www.commongroundhealth.org/). Since this case focuses on the period during which the agency was known as FLHSA, that name is used throughout the book.

5. HUD estimated in 1990 that abatement could cost from $7,700 to $11,900 (for full removal) per unit (HUD 1990). Despite emerging evidence from HUD-funded control programs that actual costs might be significantly lower, Rochester housing agencies cited these higher estimates based on their experiences with "full rehabilitation" (National Center for Healthy Housing and University of Cincinnati Department of Environmental Health 2004; Boyce and Hood 2002).

5 Healthy Duluth

1. The primary funders of this HIA were the Health Impact Project, a collaboration of the Robert Wood Johnson Foundation and the Pew Charitable Trusts, the Kresge Foundation, and the Center for Prevention at Blue Cross and Blue Shield of Minnesota (PolicyLink 2011).

2. In 2016, the Center for Prevention at Blue Cross and Blue Shield of Minnesota committed $4 million over three years to reduce smoking and to support Health in All Policies projects aimed at reducing health disparities. This initiative included a grant to the Zeitgeist Center to "drive a regional health equity agenda by engaging health systems, local government, school districts and nonprofit organizations throughout the Duluth area" (Center for Prevention at Blue Cross and Blue Shield of Minnesota 2018b).

3. Considering multiracial individuals ("race alone or in combination with one or more other races," according to the Census), these minority populations increase to 3.5 percent (black or African American), 4.1 percent (American Indian and Alaska native), and 2.0 percent (Asian).

4. As described by Bunnell (2002, 344), the negotiated agreement to trench I-35 necessitated blasting large quantities of rock, which the city proposed using to extend the waterfront, creating space for the Lakewalk and a waterfront park. The cost savings realized from this local solution for disposal of the blasted rock helped subsidize planning, design, and construction of the Lakewalk.

5. To be inclusive and for simplicity's sake, "Healthy Duluth" is used here as an umbrella term for the built environment and health equity work undertaken in Duluth between 2009 and 2018 under various auspices and names, including Fit City, Healthy Duluth Area Coalition, the City of Duluth's health-focused planning efforts, and related elements of the Community Health Needs Assessment (Bridging Health Duluth) process. HDAC was the longest-running and broadest forum for coordinating this work. However, this discussion includes initiatives that predated or worked separately from HDAC, particularly those of the City of Duluth. These varied efforts built on, learned from, and supported each other.

6. This project was originally called the Western Port Area Neighborhoods plan and was later renamed the Irving Fairmount Brownfields Revitalization Plan; for clarity, the latter name is used here.

7. The Zeitgeist Center for Arts and Community was initiated with support from the Zeppa Family Foundation, which was established in 2005 with the goals of promoting a healthy environment, sustainability, social justice, and the arts in Duluth (Passi 2014). The Zeitgeist Center for Arts and Community is a community and grant-supported not-for-profit organization maintaining the original mission of the foundation. The Zeitgeist Center, located in downtown Duluth, operates the Zinema 2 movie theater, a black box theater, restaurant, gallery, meeting spaces, and staff offices, including those of the HDAC (Cuneo 2016; Zeitgeist Center for Arts and Community 2018).

8. The survey was initially developed in 1995 by St. Mary's Hospital (now part of Essentia Health), and the hospital system remained involved as a funder and contributor to survey design after it was taken over by Generations Health Care in 2005 (Peterson 2017).

9. Although the City of Duluth had a strong tradition of physical planning, according to Bunnell the planning department was essentially disbanded in 1999 because of the sitting mayor's view that excessive regulation was impeding economic development (2002, 374). A series of development conflicts and successful plans for downtown, the waterfront, and west Duluth in the late 1990s showed the need for and potential of effective planning. City leaders revitalized the planning department in preparation for the 2006 Comprehensive Plan update, the first since 1958.

10. In her first State of the City address in March 2016, Larson referenced the eleven-year life expectancy disparity between adjacent zip codes in Duluth, commenting that "our right to a good and healthy life should not be determined by our zip code, or our income, education, race, gender or religion. ... My vision is of a healthy—prosperous—sustainable—fair—and inclusive community" (Larson 2016).

11. The "half and half tax" refers to authorization for Duluth to impose a half percent tax on food, beverage and hotel/motel sales, also known as the "tourism tax"(City of Duluth 2018b). The 2014 state legislative action allowed the city to reinstate tourism taxes that had previously funded improvements to the stadium and aquarium but sunsetted in 2012 (Pioneer Press 2014). The city council resolution authorizing the 2014 tax stated it was "for the purpose of funding an $18 million bond issue for the purpose of capital improvements to public facilities to support tourism and recreational activities in that part of Duluth lying west of 34th Avenue West." In 2015, this was amended to include areas "west of 14th Avenue West," allowing inclusion of Lincoln Park, the Cross City Trail, and other improvements in neighborhoods closer to the center city (City of Duluth 2018c).

12. Because of the age of the city, much of the infrastructure (roads, water lines, utilities) is aging and in need of repair. With the construction of the downtown Fond-du-Luth casino in 1988, the City received an annual payment based on the casino's profits (Bunnell 2002) (p. 361). This revenue stream was used to establish a fund, the interest from which was used for street improvements. However, in 2009 the casino successfully argued in court that the agreement was invalid and stopped paying the city what had amounted to $6 million a year (Kraker 2014). This loss compounded the city's budget challenges for funding infrastructure improvements.

13. Apparently this is not a new phenomenon. Jerry Kimball, Duluth's chief physical planner from 1968 to 1995, allegedly moved from St. Paul to Duluth because of its proximity to Boundary Waters canoeing (Bunnell 2002). According to Kimball, "More recently, Cirrus aircraft relocated because the owner just happened to drive through Duluth and liked what he saw" (Bunnell 2002, 377).

6 THE Impact Project

1. As of 2018, this "Global Trade Impacts" report had been downloaded over 1,500 times.

2. Multifamily residences and parks are required to post a sign reading: "NOTICE: Air pollution studies show a strong link between the chronic exposure of populations to vehicle exhaust and particulate matter from major roads and freeways and elevated risk of adverse health impacts, particularly in sensitive populations such as young children and older adults. Areas located within 500 feet of the freeway are known to experience the greatest concentration of ultrafine particulate matter and other pollutants implicated in asthma and other health conditions" (City of Los Angeles 2015).

7 Local Environmental Health Initiatives

1. With the development of tract-level data systems like the City Health Dashboard (www.cityhealthdashboard.com) and the Centers for Disease Control and Prevention's Environmental Public Health Tracking system (ephtracking.cdc.gov), finding local health data may be easier in the future. Nonetheless, health privacy laws and the geographic scale of data collection remain barriers to merging environmental and health data, particularly for smaller communities.

References

ACCLPP (Advisory Committee on Childhood Lead Poisoning Prevention). 2012. *Low Level Lead Exposure Harms Children: A Renewed Call for Primary Prevention.* Atlanta, GA: Centers for Disease Control and Prevention. https://www.cdc.gov/nceh/lead /acclpp/final_document_030712.pdf.

Active Living by Design. 2018. "Robert Wood Johnson Foundation: Active Living by Design." http://activelivingbydesign.org/project/robert-wood-johnson-foundation -active-living-by-design/.

ACT Rochester. 2015. "Children in Poverty." Rochester Area Community Foundation. http://www.actrochester.org/children-youth/family-support/children-poverty.

Ahrens, Katherine A., Barbara A. Haley, Lauren M. Rossen, Patricia C. Lloyd, and Yutaka Aoki. 2016. "Housing Assistance and Blood Lead Levels: Children in the United States, 2005–2012." *American Journal of Public Health* 106 (11): 2049–2056.

Alanen, Arnold Robert. 2007. *Morgan Park: Duluth, U.S. Steel, and the Forging of a Company Town.* Minneapolis: University of Minnesota Press.

American Cancer Society. 2015. "Policies, Systems, and Environmental Change Resource Guide." https://smhs.gwu.edu/cancercontroltap/sites/cancercontroltap/files /PSE_Resource_Guide_FINAL_05.15.15.pdf.

American Planning Association. 2015. *Sustaining Places: Best Practices for Comprehensive Plans—PAS Report 578.* Chicago: APA Planning Advisory Service.

American Planning Association. 2016. *The State of Health Impact Assessment in Planning.* Chicago: American Planning Association.

Amitai, Yona, John W. Graef, Mary Jean Brown, Robert S. Gerstle, Nancy Kahn, and Paul E. Cochrane. 1987. "Hazards of 'Deleading' Homes of Children with Lead Poisoning." *American Journal of Diseases of Children* 141 (7): 758–760.

Andersen, Z. J., M. Hvidberg, S. S. Jensen, M. Ketzel, S. Loft, M. Sorensen, A. Tjonneland, K. Overvad, and O. Raaschou-Nielsen. 2011. "Chronic Obstructive Pulmonary Disease and Long-Term Exposure to Traffic-Related Air Pollution: A Cohort

Study." *American Journal of Respiratory and Critical Care Medicine* 183 (4): 455–461. doi: 10.1164/rccm.201006-0937OC.

Andrews, Richard N. L. 1976. *Environmental Policy and Administrative Change: Implementation of the National Environmental Policy Act*. Lanham, MD: Lexington Books.

Andrews, Richard N. L. 2006. *Managing the Environment, Managing Ourselves: A History of American Environmental Policy*. New Haven, CT: Yale University Press.

Araujo, J. A., B. Barajas, M. Kleinman, X. Wang, B. J. Bennett, K. W. Gong, M. Navab, J. Harkema, C. Sioutas, A. J. Lusis, and A. E. Nel. 2008. "Ambient Particulate Pollutants in the Ultrafine Range Promote Early Atherosclerosis and Systemic Oxidative Stress." *Circulation Research* 102 (5): 589–596. doi: 10.1161/CIRCRESAHA.107.164970.

Ascher, William, Toddi A. Steelman, and Robert G. Healy. 2010. *Knowledge and Environmental Policy: Re-imagining the Boundaries of Science and Politics*. Cambridge, MA: MIT Press.

Ashe, Marice, Dora Barilla, Eileen Barsi, and Stephanie Cihon. 2016. "A Systems Thinking Approach to the Social Determinants of Health." In *Stakeholder Health: Insights into New Systems of Health*, edited by Teresa Cutts and James R. Cochrane. Winston-Salem, NC: FaithHealth Innovations.

Association of State and Territorial Health Officials. 2018. "State and Local Health Department Governance Classification System." http://www.astho.org/Research/Data-and-Analysis/State-and-Local-Governance-Classification-Tree/.

Attfield, Michael D., Patricia L. Schleiff, Jay H. Lubin, Aaron Blair, Patricia A. Stewart, Roel Vermeulen, Joseph B. Coble, and Debra T. Silverman. 2012. "The Diesel Exhaust in Miners Study: A Cohort Mortality Study with Emphasis on Lung Cancer." *Journal of the National Cancer Institute* 104 (11): 869–883.

Avendano, Mauricio, and Ichiro Kawachi. 2014. "Why Do Americans Have Shorter Life Expectancy and Worse Health than Do People in Other High-Income Countries?" *Annual Review of Public Health* 35 (1): 307–325. doi: 10.1146/annurev-publhealth-032013-182411.

Avol, Edward. 2018. Professor of Clinical Preventive Medicine, University of Southern California, *personal communication*.

Ayers, Jeanne. 2017. Assistant Commissioner, Minnesota Department of Health, *personal communication*.

Babcock, Richard F. 1966. *The Zoning Game: Municipal Practices and Policies*. Madison, WI: University of Wisconsin Press.

Babisch, Wolfgang. 2006. "Transportation Noise and Cardiovascular Risk: Updated Review and Synthesis of Epidemiological Studies Indicate That the Evidence Has Increased." *Noise and Health* 8 (30): 1–29.

Backer, Thomas E. 2003. "Evaluating Community Collaborations: An Overview." In *Evaluating Community Collaborations*, edited by Thomas E. Backer. New York: Springer Publishing.

Barboza, Tony. 2016a. "L.A. City Council Adopts Rules to Ease Health Hazards in Polluted Neighborhoods." *Los Angeles Times*, April 13. http://www.latimes.com/local/lanow/la-me-pollution-protection-20160412-story.html.

Barboza, Tony. 2016b. "The Port That Fuels L.A.'s Economy and Fouls Its Air Gets a Pollution-Reduction Team." *Los Angeles Times*, July 13. http://www.latimes.com/local/lanow/la-me-ln-port-advisory-board-20160712-snap-story.html.

Basu, R., M. Harris, L. Sie, B. Malig, R. Broadwin, and R. Green. 2014. "Effects of Fine Particulate Matter and Its Constituents on Low Birth Weight among Full-Term Infants in California." *Environmental Research* 128: 42–51. doi: 10.1016/j.envres.2013.10.008.

Bates, Kristin Ann, and Richelle S. Swan. 2010. *Through the Eye of Katrina*. Durham, NC: Carolina Academic Press.

Beaulac, Julie, Elizabeth Kristjansson, and Steven Cummins. 2009. "A Systematic Review of Food Deserts, 1966–2007." *Preventing Chronic Disease* 6 (3): 1–10.

Beier, E. E., J. R. Maher, T. J. Sheu, D. A. Cory-Slechta, A. J. Berger, M. J. Zuscik, and J. E. Puzas. 2013. "Heavy Metal Lead Exposure, Osteoporotic-like Phenotype in an Animal Model, and Depression of Wnt Signaling." *Environmental Health Perspectives* 121 (1): 97–104.

Bell, Michelle L., Devra L. Davis, and Tony Fletcher. 2003. "A Retrospective Assessment of Mortality from the London Smog Episode of 1952: The Role of Influenza and Pollution." *Environmental Health Perspectives* 112 (1): 6–8. doi: 10.1289/ehp.6539.

Bellinger, David C. 2016. "Lead Contamination in Flint—An Abject Failure to Protect Public Health." *New England Journal of Medicine* 374 (12): 1101–1103. doi: 10.1056/NEJMp1601013.

Benbrahim-Tallaa, Lamia, Robert A. Baan, Yann Grosse, Béatrice Lauby-Secretan, Fatiha El Ghissassi, Véronique Bouvard, Neela Guha, Dana Loomis, and Kurt Straif. 2012. "Carcinogenicity of Diesel-Engine and Gasoline-Engine Exhausts and Some Nitroarenes." *The Lancet Oncology* 13 (7): 663–664. doi: 10.1016/s1470-2045(12)70280-2.

Berke, Philip, and Edward John Kaiser. 2006. *Urban Land Use Planning*. Champaign, IL: University of Illinois Press.

Bernstein, J. A., N. Alexis, C. Barnes, I. L. Bernstein, J. A. Bernstein, A. Nel, D. Peden, D. Diaz-Sanchez, S. M. Tarlo, and P. B. Williams. 2004. "Health Effects of Air Pollution." *Journal of Allergy and Clinical Immunology* 114 (5): 1116–1123. doi: 10.1016/j.jaci.2004.08.030.

Berwick, Donald M., Thomas W. Nolan, and John Whittington. 2008. "The Triple Aim: Care, Health, and Cost." *Health Affairs* 27 (3): 759–769. doi: 10.1377/hlthaff.27.3.759.

Bhatia, R., K. Gilhuly, C. Harris, J. Heller, J. Lucky, and L. Farhang. 2011. *A Health Impact Assessment Toolkit: A Handbook to Conducting HIA*. 3rd ed. Oakland, CA: Human Impact Partners.

Bhatia, Rajiv, and Aaron Wernham. 2008. "Integrating Human Health into Environmental Impact Assessment: An Unrealized Opportunity for Environmental Health and Justice." *Environmental Health Perspectives* 116 (8): 991–1000. doi: 10.1289/ehp.11132.

Blackwell, Angela Glover. 2009. "Active Living Research and the Movement for Healthy Communities." *American Journal of Preventive Medicine* 36 (2): S50–S52.

Bogado, Aura. 2015. "Polluting Industries Took Over This California City. Now, Residents Are Taking It Back." *Grist*, November 5. https://grist.org/cities/polluting -industries-took-over-this-california-city-now-residents-are-taking-it-back/.

Boothe, Vickie L., and Derek G. Shendell. 2008. "Potential Health Effects Associated with Residential Proximity to Freeways and Primary Roads: Review of Scientific Literature, 1999–2006." *Journal of Environmental Health* 70 (8): 33–41.

Boschken, Herman L. 2009. "Spanning Policymaking Silos in Urban Development and Environmental Management: When Global Cities Are Coastal Cities Too." Presented at meeting of the American Political Science Association, Toronto, September.

Bouman, Evert A., Elizabeth Lindstad, Agathe I. Rialland, and Anders H. Strømman. 2017. "State-of-the-Art Technologies, Measures, and Potential for Reducing GHG Emissions from Shipping—A Review." *Transportation Research Part D: Transport and Environment* 52: 408–421. doi: https://doi.org/10.1016/j.trd.2017.03.022.

Bourcier, E., D. Charbonneau, C. Cahill, and A. Dannenberg. 2014. *Do Health Impact Assessments Make a Difference? A National Evaluation of HIAs in the United States: Supplement*. Seattle: Center for Community Health and Evaluation.

Boyce, Sarah, and Kim Hood. 2002. *Lead Poisoning among Young Children in Monroe County, NY: A Needs Assessment, Projection Model, and Next Steps*. Rochester, NY: Center for Governmental Research.

Boyce, Sarah, Rochelle Ruffer, and Maria Ayoob. 2008. *An Evaluation of Rochester's Lead Law: 2006–2008*. Rochester, NY: Center for Governmental Research.

Braveman, Paula. 2014. "What Are Health Disparities and Health Equity? We Need to Be Clear." *Public Health Reports* 129 (Suppl. 2): 5–8.

Braveman, Paula, Elaine Arkin, Tracy Orleans, Dwayne Proctor, and Alonzo Plough. 2017. *What Is Health Equity? And What Difference Does a Definition Make?* Princeton, NJ: Robert Wood Johnson Foundation.

Brennan Ramirez, Laura K., Elizabeth Anne Baker, and Marilyn Metzler. 2008. *Promoting Health Equity: A Resource to Help Communities Address Social Determinants of Health*. Atlanta, GA: Centers for Disease Control and Prevention.

Brewer, Garry D., and Peter DeLeon. 1983. *The Foundations of Policy Analysis*. Homewood, IL: Dorsey Press.

Breysse, Jill, Jack Anderson, Sherry Dixon, Warren Galke, and Jonathan Wilson. 2007. "Immediate and One-Year Post-Intervention Effectiveness of Maryland's Lead Law Treatments." *Environmental Research* 105 (2): 267–275.

Bridge to Health Survey. 2018. "About Bridge to Health Survey." http://bridgetohealth survey.org/index.php/about.

Bridging Health Duluth. 2016. "Working Together for a Healthy Duluth: 2016 Community Health Needs Assessment," City of Duluth, MN. http://www.slhduluth.com /documents/2016DuluthCHNA-web.pdf.

Brink, Susan. 2017. "What Country Spends the Most (and Least) on Health Care per Person?" *National Public Radio*, April 20. https://www.npr.org/sections/goatsandsoda /2017/04/20/524774195/what-country-spends-the-most-and-least-on-health-care -per-person.

Brown, David, Beth Weinberger, Celia Lewis, and Heather Bonaparte. 2014. "Understanding Exposure from Natural Gas Drilling Puts Current Air Standards to the Test." *Reviews on Environmental Health* 29 (4): 277–292.

Brown, M. J. 2002. "Costs and Benefits of Enforcing Housing Policies to Prevent Childhood Lead Poisoning." *Medical Decision Making: An International Journal of the Society for Medical Decision Making* 22 (6): 482–492.

Brown, Mary Jean, Jane Gardner, James D. Sargent, Katherine Swartz, Howard Hu, and Ralph Timperi. 2001. "The Effectiveness of Housing Policies in Reducing Children's Lead Exposure." *American Journal of Public Health* 91 (4): 621.

Brown, Mary Jean, and Patrick J. Meehan. 2004. "Health Effects of Blood Lead Levels Lower than 10 mg/dl in Children." *American Journal of Public Health* 94 (1): 8–9. doi: 10.2105/AJPH.94.1.8-a.

Browne, Geoffrey R., and Ian D. Rutherfurd. 2017. "The Case for 'Environment in All Policies': Lessons from the 'Health in All Policies' Approach in Public Health." *Environmental Health Perspectives* 125 (2): 149–154. doi: 10.1289/EHP294.

Bryant, Bunyan. 1995. *Environmental Justice: Issues, Policies, Solutions*. Washington, DC: Island Press.

Bryant, Bunyan I., and Paul Mohai. 1992. *Race and the Incidence of Environmental Hazards: A Time for Discourse*. Boulder, CO: Westview Press.

Bullard, Robert D. 2008. *Dumping in Dixie: Race, Class, and Environmental Quality.* Boulder, CO: Westview Press. First published 1990.

Bunnell, Gene. 2002. *Making Places Special: Stories of Real Places Made Better by Planning.* Chicago: American Planning Association.

Bureau of Labor Statistics. 2018. "Census of Fatal Occupational Injuries (CFOI)—Current and Revised Data (2016)." https://www.bls.gov/iif/oshcfoi1.htm#2016.

Bush Foundation. 2018. "Bush Foundation: Investing in Great Ideas and the People Who Power Them." https://www.bushfoundation.org/.

Butler, Lindsey J., Madeleine K. Scammell, and Eugene B. Benson. 2016. "The Flint, Michigan, Water Crisis: A Case Study in Regulatory Failure and Environmental Injustice." *Environmental Justice* 9 (4): 93–97. doi: 10.1089/env.2016.0014.

Butterfield, Patricia G. 2017. "Thinking Upstream: A 25-Year Retrospective and Conceptual Model Aimed at Reducing Health Inequities." *Advances in Nursing Science* 40 (1): 2–11.

Cacari-Stone, Lisa, Nina Wallerstein, Analilia P. Garcia, and Meredith Minkler. 2014. "The Promise of Community-Based Participatory Research for Health Equity: A Conceptual Model for Bridging Evidence with Policy." *American Journal of Public Health* 104 (9): 1615–1623.

California Air Resources Board. 2018. "Overview: Diesel Exhaust and Health." https://www.arb.ca.gov/research/diesel/diesel-health.htm.

Callan, Mel. 2018. Nurse Practitioner, Highland Family Medicine, Rochester, NY, *personal communication.*

Campbell, J. R., and P. Auinger. 2007. "The Association between Blood Lead Levels and Osteoporosis among Adults—Results from the Third National Health and Nutrition Examination Survey (NHANES III)." *Environmental Health Perspectives* 115 (7): 1018–1022.

Canfield, R. L., C. R. Henderson, Jr., D. A. Cory-Slechta, C. Cox, T. A. Jusko, and B. P. Lanphear. 2003. "Intellectual Impairment in Children with Blood Lead Concentrations below 10 Microg per Deciliter." *New England Journal of Medicine* 348 (16): 1517–1526. doi: 10.1056/NEJMoa022848.

Carlson, Susan A., Janet E. Fulton, Michael Pratt, Zhou Yang, and E. Kathleen Adams. 2015. "Inadequate Physical Activity and Health Care Expenditures in the United States." *Progress in Cardiovascular Diseases* 57 (4): 315–323.

Carruth, Russellyn S., and Bernard D. Goldstein. 2014. *Environmental Health Law: An Introduction.* San Francisco: Jossey-Bass.

Causewave Community Partners. 2018. "Partners in Community Change." http://www.causewave.org/#community-change.

Center for Prevention at Blue Cross and Blue Shield of Minnesota. 2015a. "Center for Prevention Minnesota." Blue Cross and Blue Shield of Minnesota. http://www .centerforpreventionmn.com/.

Center for Prevention at Blue Cross and Blue Shield of Minnesota. 2015b. "Our Approach." Blue Cross and Blue Shield of Minnesota. http://www.centerforpreven tionmn.com/our-approach.

Center for Prevention at Blue Cross and Blue Shield of Minnesota. 2018a. "A. H. Zeppa Family Foundation." https://www.centerforpreventionmn.com/what-we-do /our-current-initiatives/health-equity-in-prevention/a-h-zeppa-family-foundation.

Center for Prevention at Blue Cross and Blue Shield of Minnesota. 2018b. "Zeitgeist Center for the Arts and Community." https://www.centerforpreventionmn.com /what-we-do/our-current-initiatives/health-in-all-policies/zeitgeist-center-for-the -arts-and-community.

CDC (Centers for Disease Control and Prevention). 2004a. "150th Anniversary of John Snow and the Pump Handle." *Morbidity and Mortality Weekly Report (MMWR)* 53 (34): 783.

CDC (Centers for Disease Control and Prevention). 2004b. "Preventing Lead Exposure in Young Children. https://www.cdc.gov/nceh/lead/publications/primarypre ventiondocument.pdf.

CDC (Centers for Disease Control and Prevention). 2011. "CDC's Healthy Communities Program Funded Communities." https://www.cdc.gov/nccdphp/dch/programs /healthycommunitiesprogram/communities/pdf/phclist.pdf.

CDC (Centers for Disease Control and Prevention). 2012. "CDC Response to Advisory Committee on Childhood Lead Poisoning Prevention Recommendations." https://www.cdc.gov/nceh/lead/acclpp/cdc_response_lead_exposure_recs.pdf.

CDC (Centers for Disease Control and Prevention). 2013. "U.S. Totals Blood Lead Surveillance Report 1997–2012."

CDC (Centers for Disease Control and Prevention). 2014a. "Environmental Public Health Performance Standards (version 2.0)," Division of Emergency and Environmental Health Services National Center for Environmental Health. https://www.cdc .gov/nceh/ehs/envphps/docs/EnvPHPSv2.pdf.

CDC (Centers for Disease Control and Prevention). 2014b. "Definitions." https:// www.cdc.gov/nchhstp/socialdeterminants/definitions.html.

CDC (Centers for Disease Control and Prevention). 2014c. "QuickStats: Infant Mortality Rates, by Race and Hispanic Ethnicity of Mother—United States, 2000, 2005, and 2010." *Morbidity and Mortality Weekly Report (MMWR)* 63 (1): 25.

CDC (Centers for Disease Control and Prevention). 2015a. "Health in All Policies Resource Center." https://www.cdc.gov/policy/hiap/resources/.

CDC (Centers for Disease Control and Prevention). 2015b. "Healthy People 2020." https://www.cdc.gov/nchs/healthy_people/hp2020.htm.

CDC (Centers for Disease Control and Prevention). 2016a. "10 Essential Environmental Public Health Services." https://www.cdc.gov/nceh/ehs/10-essential-services /index.html.

CDC (Centers for Disease Control and Prevention). 2016b. "Deaths and Mortality." https://www.cdc.gov/nchs/fastats/deaths.htm.

CDC (Centers for Disease Control and Prevention). 2017a. "Adult Obesity Facts," last modified August 29. https://www.cdc.gov/obesity/data/adult.html.

CDC (Centers for Disease Control and Prevention). 2017b. "Communities Putting Prevention to Work (2010–2012)," last modified March 7. https://www.cdc.gov /nccdphp/dch/programs/communitiesputtingpreventiontowork/index.htm.

CDC (Centers for Disease Control and Prevention). 2017c. "Healthy Communities Program (2008–2012)," last modified March 7. https://www.cdc.gov/nccdphp/dch /programs/healthycommunitiesprogram/index.htm.

CDC (Centers for Disease Control and Prevention). 2017d. "Healthy Food Environments," last modified March 14. https://www.cdc.gov/obesity/strategies/healthy -food-env.html.

CDC (Centers for Disease Control and Prevention). 2017e. "Chronic Disease Overview." https://www.cdc.gov/chronicdisease/overview/.

CDC (Centers for Disease Control and Prevention). 2017f. "Leading Causes of Death." https://www.cdc.gov/nchs/fastats/leading-causes-of-death.htm.

CDC (Centers for Disease Control and Prevention). 2018a. "What is Safe Routes to School?" https://www.cdc.gov/policy/hst/hi5/saferoutes/index.html.

CDC (Centers for Disease Control and Prevention). 2018b. "National Health and Nutrition Examination Survey." https://www.cdc.gov/nchs/nhanes/about_nhanes .htm.

CDC (Centers for Disease Control and Prevention). 2018c. "One Health." https:// www.cdc.gov/onehealth/index.html.

CDC (Centers for Disease Control and Prevention). 2018d. "Health Impact Assessment." https://www.cdc.gov/healthyplaces/hia.htm.

CDC (Centers for Disease Control and Prevention). 2018e. "Infant Mortality Rates by State." https://www.cdc.gov/nchs/pressroom/sosmap/infant_mortality_rates /infant_mortality.htm.

CGR. 2015. "CGR at 100: A Remarkable Story." https://www.cgr.org/cmsb/uploads /cgr100years.pdf.

Chachere, Matthew. 2018. *Lead Paint Laws and Regulations in New York City*. New York: Northern Manhattan Improvement Corporation. https://www.nmic.org /nyccelp/documents/lead-training-manual.pdf.

Chadwick, Edwin. 1842. *Report on the Sanitary Condition of the Labouring Population of Great Britain: Supplementary Report on the Results of Special Inquiry into the Practice of Interment in Towns*. Vol. 1. London: HM Stationery Office.

ChangeLab Solutions. 2013. "Preemption and Public Health Advocacy: A Frequent Concern with Far-Reaching Consequences." Fact Sheet. http://www .changelabsolutions.org/sites/default/files/Preemption_PublicHealthAdvocacy_FS_ FINAL_20130911.pdf.

ChangeLab Solutions. 2014. "A Guide to Proactive Rental Inspection Programs." http://www.changelabsolutions.org/sites/default/files/Proactive-Rental-Inspection -Programs_Guide_FINAL_20140204.pdf.

ChangeLab Solutions. 2018a. "Healthier Food Environments." http://www.changelab solutions.org/landing-page/healthier-food-environments.

ChangeLab Solutions. 2018b. "PSE 101: Building Healthier Communities." http:// www.changelabsolutions.org/publications/pse-101.

Chen, Alice, Emily Oster, and Heidi Williams. 2016. "Why Is Infant Mortality Higher in the United States than in Europe?" *American Economic Journal: Economic Policy* 8 (2): 89–124.

Chepesiuk, R. 2009. "Missing the Dark: Health Effects of Light Pollution." *Environmental Health Perspectives* 117 (1):A-20–27.

Chetty, Raj, Michael Stepner, Sarah Abraham, Shelby Lin, Benjamin Scuderi, Nicholas Turner, Augustin Bergeron, and David Cutler. 2016. "The Association between Income and Life Expectancy in the United States, 2001–2014." *JAMA* 315 (16): 1750–1766. doi: 10.1001/jama.2016.4226.

Chirls, Stuart. 2018. "BNSF, LA Port Look to Re-start Intermodal Transfer Project." *Railway Age*, August 31. https://www.railwayage.com/intermodal/bnsf-la-port-look -to-re-start-intermodal-transfer-project/.

Chisolm, J. Julian, Jr. 2001a. "Evolution of the Management and Prevention of Childhood Lead Poisoning: Dependence of Advances in Public Health on Technological Advances in the Determination of Lead and Related Biochemical Indicators of Its Toxicity." *Environmental Research* 86 (2): 111.

Chisolm, J. Julian, Jr. 2001b. "The Road to Primary Prevention of Lead Toxicity in Children." *Pediatrics* 107 (3): 581–583.

Cho, Y., S. H. Ryu, B. R. Lee, K. H. Kim, E. Lee, and J. Choi. 2015. "Effects of Artificial Light at Night on Human Health: A Literature Review of Observational and

Experimental Studies Applied to Exposure Assessment." *Chronobiology International* 32 (9): 1294–310. doi: 10.3109/07420528.2015.1073158.

City of Duluth. 2006. "Comprehensive Plan Historic Development Patterns." http://www.duluthmn.gov/community-planning/guiding-documents/comprehensive-plan/.

City of Duluth. 2011. "Duluth, Minnesota Trail and Bikeway Plan." http://www.duluthmn.gov/media/116291/Duluth_Bike_Report_Edited_October_2011.pdf.

City of Duluth. 2014a. "FY 2015 EPA Brownfields Area-Wide Planning Program: City of Duluth Western Port Area Neighborhood—St. Louis River Corridor." Workplan for CERCLA Section 104(k)(6) Cooperative Agreement.

City of Duluth. 2014b. "FY 2015 US EPA Brownfield Area-Wide Planning Grant Application for the Western Port Area Neighborhoods, City of Duluth, Minnesota."

City of Duluth. 2016a. "St. Louis River Corridor Initiative—Connecting People to the River." http://www.duluthmn.gov/media/541995/final-slrc-brochure.pdf.

City of Duluth. 2016b. "St. Louis River Corridor Initiative—Connecting People to the River 2016, update presentation." http://www.duluthmn.gov/media/506076/St-Louis-River-Corridor-Presentation-June-2016-.pdf.

City of Duluth. 2018a. "The Official Website." www.duluthmn.gov.

City of Duluth. 2018b. "Tourism Taxes." http://duluthmn.gov/finance/tourism-taxes/.

City of Duluth. 2018c. "Western Waterfront Renewal and Restoration." http://duluthmn.gov/st-louis-river-corridor/western-waterfront-renewal-restoration/.

City of Los Angeles. 2015. "Clean Up Green Up Proposed Ordinance," Ordinance 184245; 184246. L.A. City Planning Commission. https://cityclerk.lacity.org/lacityclerkconnect/index.cfm?fa=ccfi.viewrecord&cfnumber=15-1026.

City of Rochester. 2005. Municipal Code, pt. 2, chap. 90: Property Code, art. III, Lead-Based Paint Poisoning Prevention, §§90–50 to 90–69.

City of Rochester. 2018. "Lead Paint—Essential Links and Documents." http://www.cityofrochester.gov/lead/.

City of Rochester. 2019. "Certificate of Occupancy." http://www.cityofrochester.gov/article.aspx?id=8589935004.

Clark, E. Ray, and Larry W. Canter. 1997. *Environmental Policy and NEPA: Past, Present, and Future.* Boca Raton, FL: CRC Press. (See https://www.crcpress.com/Environmental-Policy-and-NEPA-Past-Present-and-Future/Clark-Canter/p/book/9781574440720.).

Clean Up Green Up. 2018. "Welcome to Clean Up Green Up." https://cleanupgreenup.wordpress.com/.

Clougherty, Jane E., Jonathan I. Levy, Laura D. Kubzansky, P. Barry Ryan, Shakira Franco Suglia, Marina Jacobson Canner, and Rosalind J. Wright. 2007. "Synergistic Effects of Traffic-Related Air Pollution and Exposure to Violence on Urban Asthma Etiology." *Environmental Health Perspectives* 115 (8): 1140.

Coalition for Environmental Health and Justice. 2009. "I-710 Corridor Project Fact Sheet." http://eycej.org/wp-content/uploads/2012/09/FS_I-710-11.2.09.pdf.

Cole, Claire, and Adam Winsler. 2010. "Protecting Children from Exposure to Lead: Old Problem, New Data, and New Policy Needs." *Social Policy Report/Society for Research in Child Development* 24 (1): 1–30.

Cole, Luke W., and Sheila R. Foster. 2001. *From the Ground Up: Environmental Racism and the Rise of the Environmental Justice Movement*. New York: NYU Press.

Colgrove, James. 2011. *Epidemic City: The Politics of Public Health in New York*. New York: Russell Sage Foundation.

Collective Impact Forum. 2018. "What Is Collective Impact?" https://www.collective impactforum.org/what-collective-impact.

Commission on Social Determinants of Health and World Health Organization. 2008. *Closing the Gap in a Generation: Health Equity through Action on the Social Determinants of Health: Commission on Social Determinants of Health, Final Report*. Geneva: World Health Organization. https://www.who.int/social_determinants/final_report /csdh_finalreport_2008.pdf.

Community Action Duluth. 2018. "Seeds of Success: Green Jobs in Urban Farming." https://www.communityactionduluth.org/seeds-of-success-and-duluth-stream-corps /seeds-of-success/.

Community Prevention Services Task Force. 2018. "The Community Guide. Physical Activity: Built Environment Approaches Combining Transportation System Interventions with Land Use and Environmental Design." https://www.thecommunityguide .org/findings/physical-activity-built-environment-approaches.

Cooperative Extension Service. 2018. "Elements of a Comprehensive Plan." http:// articles.extension.org/pages/26490/elements-of-a-comprehensive-plan.

Corbett, J. J., J. J. Winebrake, E. H. Green, P. Kasibhatla, V. Eyring, and A. Lauer. 2007. "Mortality from Ship Emissions: A Global Assessment." *Environmental Science & Technology* 41 (24): 8512–8518.

Corburn, Jason. 2002. "Combining Community-Based Research and Local Knowledge to Confront Asthma and Subsistence-Fishing Hazards in Greenpoint/Williamsburg, Brooklyn, New York." *Environmental Health Perspectives* 110 (suppl. 2): 241–248.

Corburn, Jason. 2005. *Street Science: Community Knowledge and Environmental Health Justice, Urban and Industrial Environments.* Cambridge, MA: MIT Press.

Corburn, Jason. 2009. *Toward the Healthy City: People, Places, and the Politics of Urban Planning.* Cambridge, MA: MIT Press.

Council on Environmental Quality. 2014. "NEPA and CEQA: Integrating Federal and State Environmental Reviews." Office of the President of the United States and the California Governor's Office of Planning and Research. https://ceq.doe.gov/docs /ceq-publications/NEPA_CEQA_Handbook_Feb_2014.pdf.

Council on Environmental Quality. 2018. "States and Local Jurisdictions with NEPA-like Environmental Planning Requirements." https://ceq.doe.gov/laws-regulations /states.html.

County of Los Angeles. 2018. "Part 9: Rural Outdoor Lighting District." https://library .municode.com/ca/los_angeles_county/codes/code_of_ordinances?nodeId=16274.

CPLP (Coalition to Prevent Lead Poisoning). 2006. "About the Coalition." http:// theleadcoalition.org/wp-content/uploads/2019/01/About-CPLP-History.pdf.

Cradock, Angie L., Philip J. Troped, Billy Fields, Steven J. Melly, Shannon V. Simms, Franz Gimmler, and Marianne Fowler. 2009. "Factors Associated with Federal Transportation Funding for Local Pedestrian and Bicycle Programming and Facilities." *Journal of Public Health Policy* 30 (1): S38–S72.

Crouse, D. L., M. S. Goldberg, N. A. Ross, H. Chen, and F. Labreche. 2010. "Postmenopausal Breast Cancer Is Associated with Exposure to Traffic-Related Air Pollution in Montreal, Canada: A Case-Control Study." *Environmental Health Perspectives* 118 (11): 1578–83. doi: 10.1289/ehp.1002221.

Crowe, Timothy D. 2000. *Crime Prevention through Environmental Design: Applications of Architectural Design and Space Management Concepts.* Boston: Butterworth-Heinemann.

Cummings, Scott L. 2018. *Blue and Green: The Drive for Justice at America's Port.* Cambridge, MA: MIT Press.

Cuneo, Tony. 2016. Executive Director, Zeitgeist Center for Arts and Community, Duluth, MN, *personal communication.*

Cunningham Group Architecture. 2014. "Sixth Avenue East Corridor Redevelopment Strategy, Draft," October. http://www.duluthmn.gov/media/258437/130840Rpt _BookNov5.pdf.

Dahlgren, Göran, and Margaret Whitehead. 1991. *Policies and Strategies to Promote Social Equity in Health.* Stockholm: Institute for Future Studies.

Dallmann, Timothy R., and Robert A. Harley. 2010. "Evaluation of Mobile Source Emission Trends in the United States." *Journal of Geophysical Research: Atmospheres* 115 (D14).

Dannenberg, Andrew L., Howard Frumkin, and Richard Jackson. 2011. *Making Healthy Places: Designing and Building for Health, Well-Being, and Sustainability*. Washington, DC: Island Press.

Dannenberg, Andrew L., Rajiv Bhatia, Brian L. Cole, Sarah K. Heaton, Jason D. Feldman, and Candace D. Rutt. 2008. "Use of Health Impact Assessment in the U.S.: 27 Case Studies, 1999–2007." *American Journal of Preventive Medicine* 34 (3): 241–256.

Davis, Devra L. 2003. *When Smoke Ran Like Water: Tales of Environmental Deception and the Battle against Pollution*. New York: Basic Books.

Delreux, Tom, and Sander Happaerts. 2016. *Environmental Policy and Politics in the European Union*. New York: Palgrave Macmillan.

DeSalvo, Karen B., Patrick W. O'Carroll, Denise Koo, John M. Auerbach, and Judith A. Monroe. 2016. "Public Health 3.0: Time for an Upgrade." *American Journal of Public Health* 106 (4): 621.

DeSalvo, Karen B., Y. Claire Wang, Andrea Harris, John Auerbach, Denise Koo, and Patrick O'Carroll. 2017. "Public Health 3.0: A Call to Action for Public Health to Meet the Challenges of the 21st Century." *Preventing Chronic Disease* 14.

Dissell, Rachel, and Brie Zeltner. 2015a. "Toxic Neglect: Curing Cleveland's Legacy of Lead Poisoning." *The Plain Dealer*, October 20. https://www.cleveland.com /healthfit/index.ssf/2015/10/toxic_neglect_curing_cleveland.html.

Dissell, Rachel, and Brie Zeltner. 2015b. "Without Enforcement, Laws to Tackle Lead Poisoning of Little Use: Toxic Neglect." *The Plain Dealer*, October 21. https://www .cleveland.com/healthfit/index.ssf/2015/10/without_enforcement_laws_to_ta.html.

Dissell, Rachel, and Brie Zeltner. 2019. "Cleveland Coalition Says City Will Be 'Lead Safe' within the Next Decade." *The Plain Dealer*, January 22. https://www.cleveland .com/metro/2019/01/cleveland-officials-say-city-will-be-lead-safe-by-2028.html.

Dixon, Sherry L., David E. Jacobs, Jonathan W. Wilson, Judith Y. Akoto, Rick Nevin, and C. Scott Clark. 2012. "Window Replacement and Residential Lead Paint Hazard Control 12 Years Later." *Environmental Research* 113: 14–20.

Dixon, S. L., J. W. Wilson, C. Scott Clark, W. A. Galke, P. A. Succop, and M. Chen. 2005. "Effectiveness of Lead-Hazard Control Interventions on Dust Lead Loadings: Findings from the Evaluation of the HUD Lead-Based Paint Hazard Control Grant Program." *Environmental Research* 98 (3): 303–314.

Doniger, Andrew. 2017. Former Director, Monroe County Department of Public Health, Rochester, NY, *personal communication*.

Drmacich, Dan. 2011. "Guest Essay: The Disturbing Truths about Urban Education." *Daily Messenger*, April 8. http://www.mpnnow.com/article/20110408/NEWS /304089863?start=2.

Duffy, John. 1990. *The Sanitarians*. Champaign, IL: University of Illinois Press.

Duluth Area Chamber of Commerce. 2017. "History and Area Information." https://duluthchamber.com/local-living/history-area-information/.

Duluth Economic Development Authority. 2018a. "Brownfield Redevelopment." http://www.dulutheda.org/do-business-here/key-industries/brownfield-redevelopment.

Duluth Economic Development Authority. 2018b. "Fast Duluth Facts." http://www.dulutheda.org/choose-duluth/why-duluth/living-in-duluth/fast-duluth-facts.

Duluth News Tribune. 2007. "Duluth To Be Named 'Governor's Fit City.'" *Duluth News Tribune*, March 20. http://www.duluthnewstribune.com/content/duluth-be-named-governors-fit-city.

Duluth News Tribune. 2014. "Fit City Duluth Picked for CDC Forum." *Duluth News Tribune*, May 30. http://www.duluthnewstribune.com/content/fit-city-duluth-picked-cdc-forum.

Duluth-Superior Metropolitan Interstate Council. 2018. "Guiding the Future of Twin Ports Transportation." http://dsmic.org/.

Eccleston, Charles H. 2008. *NEPA and Environmental Planning: Tools, Techniques, and Approaches for Practitioners*. Boca Raton, FL: CRC Press.

Eder, Waltraud, Markus J. Ege, and Erika von Mutius. 2006. "Current Concepts: The Asthma Epidemic." *New England Journal of Medicine* 355 (21): 2226–2269.

Ehlinger, Edward P. 2015. "We Need a Triple Aim for Health Equity." *Minnesota Medicine* 98 (10): 28–29.

ENVIRON International Corporation. 2012. "Air Quality and Health Risk Assessments Technical Study for the I-710 Corridor Environmental Impact Report/Environmental Impact Statement." http://media.metro.net/projects_studies/I710/images/tech_study/AQ_HRA_ENVIRON_Final_020312.pdf.

Ettinger, Adrienne S., Monica L. Leonard, and Jacquelyn Mason. 2019. CDC's Lead Poisoning Prevention Program: A Long-standing Responsibility and Commitment to Protect Children From Lead Exposure. JPHMP. doi: 10.1097/PHH.0000000000000868. https://www.ncbi.nlm.nih.gov/pmc/articles/PMC6320665/.

Evans, G. W. 2006. "Child Development and the Physical Environment." *Annual Reviews in Psychology* 57: 423–451. doi: 10.1146/annurev.psych.57.102904.190057.

EYCEJ (East Yard Communities for Environmental Justice). 2009. "Why a Comprehensive Health Analysis in the I-710 EIR/EIS? A Brief on Health Impact Assessments." http://eycej.org/wp-content/uploads/2012/09/PB_HIA-710_v2.pdf.

EYCEJ (East Yard Communities for Environmental Justice). 2010. "Cumulative Impacts: Recommendation for Buffer Zones to Address Environmental Burdens & Incompatible

Land-Uses." http://eycej.org/wp-content/uploads/2012/09/PB_Cumulative-Impacts_v2b.pdf.

EYCEJ (East Yard Communities for Environmental Justice). 2017. "I-710 Corridor: Community Alternative 7." http://eycej.org/campaigns/i-710/.

EYCEJ (East Yard Communities for Environmental Justice). 2018a. "Collaboratives and Coalitions." http://eycej.org/about/collaboratives-and-coalitions/.

EYCEJ (East Yard Communities for Environmental Justice). 2018b. "Green Zones in Commerce, CA." http://eycej.org/campaigns/green-zones-in-commerce-ca/.

Farhang, L., R. Bhatia, C. C. Scully, J. Corburn, M. Gaydos, and S. Malekafzali. 2008. "Creating Tools for Healthy Development: Case Study of San Francisco's Eastern Neighborhoods Community Health Impact Assessment." *Journal of Public Health Management and Practice* 14 (3): 255–265. doi: 10.1097/01.PHH.0000316484.72759.7b.

Federal Interagency Working Group on Environmental Justice and NEPA Committee. 2016. "Promising Practices for EJ Methodologies in NEPA Reviews," EPA 300B16001, March.

Fox, Maggie. 2016. "United States Comes in Last Again on Health, Compared to Other Countries." *NBC News*, November 16. https://www.nbcnews.com/health/health-care/united-states-comes-last-again-health-compared-other-countries-n684851.

Franko, E. M., J. M. Palome, M. J. Brown, C. M. Kennedy, and L. V. Moore. 2009. "Children with Elevated Blood Lead Levels Related to Home Renovation, Repair, and Painting Activities—New York State, 2006–2007." *Morbidity and Mortality Weekly Report (MMWR)* 58 (3): 55–58.

Fraser, Michael, Brian Castrucci, and Elizabeth Harper. 2017. "Public Health Leadership and Management in the Era of Public Health 3.0." *Journal of Public Health Management and Practice* 23 (1): 90–92. doi: 10.1097/phh.0000000000000527.

French, Bryan. 2014a. "Cooking, Gardening, and Food Preservation Classes in Lincoln Park." http://www.zeitgeistarts1.com/HealthDul/healthy-eating/cooking-gardening-and-food-preservation-classes-in-lincoln-park/.

French, Bryan. 2014b. "Duluth's 'Front Door' Is Up for Redesign." http://www.zeitgeistarts1.com/HealthDul/active-living/duluths-front-door-is-up-for-redesign/.

French, Bryan. 2014c. "Lincoln Park Fair Food Access Update." http://www.zeitgeistarts1.com/HealthDul/healthy-eating/lincoln-park-fair-food-access-update/.

French, Bryan. 2014d. "May Is Bus/Bike/Walk Month." http://www.zeitgeistarts1.com/HealthDul/active-living/may-is-bus-bike-walk-month/.

French, Bryan. 2015a. "A Different Kind of Food Truck." http://www.zeitgeistarts1.com/HealthDul/healthy-eating/a-different-kind-of-food-truck/.

French, Bryan. 2015b. "Parklet Applications Are Open!" http://www.zeitgeistarts1
.com/HealthDul/active-living/parklet-applications-are-open/.

Freudenberg, N., and M. Golub. 1987. "Health Education, Public Policy, and Disease
Prevention: A Case History of the New York City Coalition to End Lead Poisoning."
Health Education Quarterly 14 (4): 387–401.

Freudenberg, Nicholas. 2004. "Community Capacity for Environmental Health Promotion: Determinants and Implications for Practice." *Health Education & Behavior* 31
(4): 472–490.

Freudenberg, Nicholas, Manuel Pastor, and Barbara Israel. 2011. "Strengthening
Community Capacity to Participate in Making Decisions to Reduce Disproportionate Environmental Exposures." *American Journal of Public Health* 101 (S1): S123–S130.

Frieden, Thomas R. 2010. "A Framework for Public Health Action: The Health
Impact Pyramid." *American Journal of Public Health* 100 (4): 590–595.

Fulton, Janet E., David M. Buchner, Susan A. Carlson, Deborah Borbely, Kenneth M.
Rose, Ann E. O'Connor, Janelle P. Gunn, and Ruth Petersen. 2018. "CDC's Active
People, Healthy Nation[SM]: Creating an Active America, Together." *Journal of Physical
Activity and Health* 15 (7): 1–5.

Galloway, Ian. 2014. "Using Pay-for-Success to Increase Investment in the Nonmedical Determinants of Health." *Health Affairs* 33 (11): 1897–1904. doi: 10.1377/
hlthaff.2014.0741.

Gallucci, Maria. 2018. "At Last, the Shipping Industry Begins Cleaning Up Its
Dirty Fuels." *Yale Environment 360*, June 28. https://e360.yale.edu/features/at-last-the
-shipping-industry-begins-cleaning-up-its-dirty-fuels.

Gangl, Jim. 2016. Public Health Analyst and Emergency Preparedness Coordinator, St. Louis County Public Health and Human Services, Duluth, MN, *personal
communication.*

Garcia, Analilia P., Nina Wallerstein, Andrea Hricko, Jesse N. Marquez, Angelo Logan,
Elina Green Nasser, and Meredith Minkler. 2013. "THE (Trade, Health, Environ-
ment) Impact Project: A Community-Based Participatory Research Environmental
Justice Case Study." *Environmental Justice* 6 (1): 17–26. doi: 10.1089/env.2012.0016.

Garshick, E., F. Laden, J. E. Hart, M. E. Davis, E. A. Eisen, and T. J. Smith. 2012.
"Lung Cancer and Elemental Carbon Exposure in Trucking Industry Workers." *Environmental Health Perspectives* 120 (9): 1301–6. doi: 10.1289/ehp.1204989.

Gateway Cities Council of Governments. 2006. "Proposal for Major Corridor Study
and RSTIS Peer Review," October. http://www.gatewaycog.org/media/userfiles
/subsite_9/files/rl/RSTISPeerReview91-605October20062.pdf.

Gateway Cities Council of Governments. 2018. "I-710 Corridor." http://www.gatewaycog.org/gateway/who-we-are/committees/i710-corridor/?cat=I-710+Corridor.

Gauderman, James, Edward Avol, Frank Gilliland, Hita Vora, Duncan Thomas, Kiros Berhane, Rob McConnell, Nino Kuenzli, Fred Lurmann, Edward Rappaport, Helene Margolis, David Bates, and John Peters. 2004. "The Effect of Air Pollution on Lung Development from 10 to 18 Years of Age." *New England Journal of Medicine* 351 (11): 1057–1067.

Gauderman, W. James, Edward Avol, Fred Lurmann, Nino Kuenzli, Frank Gilliland, John Peters, and Rob McConnell. 2005. "Childhood Asthma and Exposure to Traffic and Nitrogen Dioxide." *Epidemiology* 16 (6): 737–743. doi: 10.1097/01.ede.0000181308.51440.75.

Gauderman, W. James, Hita Vora, Rob McConnell, Kiros Berhane, Frank Gilliland, Duncan Thomas, Fred Lurmann, Edward Avol, Nino Kunzli, Michael Jerrett, and John Peters. 2007. "Effect of Exposure to Traffic on Lung Development from 10 to 18 Years of Age: A Cohort Study." *The Lancet* 369 (9561): 571–577. doi: 10.1016/s0140-6736(07)60037-3.

Georgetown Law. 2012. "Moving Ahead for Progress in the 21st Century Act (MAP-21): Short Summary." Georgetown Climate Center.

Gibson, J. Lockhart. 1904. "A Plea for Painted Railings and Painted Walls of Rooms as the Source of Lead Poisoning amongst Queensland Children." *Australian Medical Gazette* 23: 149–153.

Gibson, J. L., W. Love, D. Hardie, P. Bancroft, and A. J. Turner. 1892. "Notes on Lead-Poisoning as Observed among Children in Brisbane." Proceedings of the Third Intercolonial Medical Congress, Sydney, Australia.

Gillespie, Cathleen D., Charles Wigington, and Yuling Hong. 2013. "Coronary Heart Disease and Stroke Deaths—United States, 2009." *Morbidity and Mortality Weekly Report (MMWR) Supplement* 62 (3): 157–160.

Gilley, Jane, Jim Gangl, and Jim Skoog. 2011. *St. Louis County Health Status Report.* Duluth, MN: St. Louis County Public Health and Human Services Department.

Gittemeier, James. 2018. Principal Planner, Duluth-Superior Metropolitan Interstate Council, Duluth, MN, *personal communication.*

Go Duluth MN. 2018. "The Duluth Lakewalk." http://www.goduluthmn.com/best-duluth-attractions/lakewalk/.

Gorham, Josh. 2016a. "Inequity Is Public Health Issue No. 1." *Duluth Budgeteer*, April 9. http://www.duluthnewstribune.com/opinion/columns/4005975-inequity-public-health-issue-no-1.

Gorham, Josh. 2016b. Public Health Nurse, St. Louis County Public Health and Human Services Department, Duluth, MN, *personal communication.*

Gould, E. 2009. "Childhood Lead Poisoning: Conservative Estimates of the Social and Economic Benefits of Lead Hazard Control." *Environmental Health Perspectives* 117 (7): 1162–1167. doi: 10.1289/ehp.0800408.

Gray, Alastair McIntosh. 1982. "Inequalities in Health. The Black Report: A Summary and Comment." *International Journal of Health Services* 12 (3): 349–380.

Greater Downtown Council. 2017. "Duluth's Roots Run Deep and Strong." https://www.downtownduluth.com/about/history.php.

Greco, Susan L., Andrew M. Wilson, Steven R. Hanna, and Jonathan I. Levy. 2007. "Factors Influencing Mobile Source Particulate Matter Emissions-to-Exposure Relationships in the Boston Urban Area." *Environmental Science Technology* 41 (22): 7675–7682.

Green L.A. Port Working Group. 2018. "Stop the SCIG! Railroads Belong at the Port Not in Our Communities." http://www.lb4health.org/contact/.

Green, Rochelle S., Brian Malig, Gayle C. Windham, Laura Fenster, Bart Ostro, and Shanna Swan. 2009. "Residential Exposure to Traffic and Spontaneous Abortion." *Environmental Health Perspectives* 117 (12): 1939.

Grenadier, Andrea, Peter Holtgrave, and Chris Aldridge. 2018. "Fostering Agency through Local Public Health." *Journal of Public Health Management and Practice* 24 (5): 499–501. doi: 10.1097/phh.0000000000000864.

Grimm, Kirsten A., Latetia V. Moore, and Kelley S. Scanlon. 2013. "Access to Healthier Food Retailers—United States, 2011." *CDC Health Disparities and Inequalities Report—United States, 2013* 62 (3): 20.

Grumbine, R. Edward. 1994. "What Is Ecosystem Management?" *Conservation Biology* 8 (1): 27–38.

Guston, David H. 2001. "Boundary Organizations in Environmental Policy and Science: An Introduction." *Science, Technology & Human Values* 26 (4): 399.

Haley, V. B., and T. O. Talbot. 2004. "Geographic Analysis of Blood Lead Levels in New York State Children Born 1994–1997." *Environmental Health Perspectives* 112 (15): 1577–1582.

Hand, Ron, Ph.D. Pingkuan Di, P. E., P. E. Anthony Servin, P. E. Larry Hunsaker, and Carolyn Suer. 2004. "Roseville Rail Yard Study." California Environmental Protection Agency, Air Resources Board. https://www.arb.ca.gov/diesel/documents/rrstudy/rrstudy101404.pdf.

Hanley, M. 2007. "A Matter of Racial Justice: The Alarming Disparities of Lead-Poisoning Rates in New York State." *Empire Justice Center Legal Services Journal* (April): 19–21.

Harala, Annie. 2016. Northeast Minnesota Regional Coordinator, Healthy Northland, Statewide Health Improvement Program, *personal communication.*

Harris, Kamala. 2012. "Environmental Justice at the Local and Regional Level: Legal Background." https://oag.ca.gov/sites/all/files/agweb/pdfs/environment/ej_fact_sheet.pdf.

Harris-Roxas, Ben, Francesca Viliani, Alan Bond, Ben Cave, Mark Divall, Peter Furu, Patrick Harris, Matthew Soeberg, Aaron Wernham, and Mirko Winkler. 2012. "Health Impact Assessment: The State of the Art." *Impact Assessment and Project Appraisal* 30 (1): 43–52. doi: 10.1080/14615517.2012.666035.

Harvard School of Public Health. 2018. "Obesity Prevention Source." https://www.hsph.harvard.edu/obesity-prevention-source/obesity-prevention/food-environment/.

Hasheminassab, Sina, Nancy Daher, Bart D. Ostro, and Constantinos Sioutas. 2014. "Long-Term Source Apportionment of Ambient Fine Particulate Matter (PM2.5) in the Los Angeles Basin: A Focus on Emissions Reduction from Vehicular Sources." *Environmental Pollution* 193: 54–64.

Headwaters Foundation for Justice. 2011. "Mission and Vision." https://headwatersfoundation.org/about-us/mission-vision.

Healthy Duluth Area Coalition. 2018. "Coalition Members." http://www.zeitgeistarts1.com/HealthDul/about-us/coalition-members/.

Healthy Northland Statewide Health Improvement Program. 2018. "About Us." http://healthynorthland.org/about-us/.

Healthy People. 2013. "Conclusion and Future Directions: CDC Health Disparities and Inequalities Report—United States, 2013." *CDC Health Disparities and Inequalities Report—United States, 2013* 62 (3):184.

Healthy Places by Design. 2018. "Our History." https://healthyplacesbydesign.org/our-history/.

Heller, Jonathan. 2016. Executive Director, Human Impact Partners, Oakland, CA, *personal communication.*

Herling, Robert. 2016. Senior Planner, Duluth-Superior Metropolitan Interstate Council, Duluth, MN, *personal communication.*

HERO. 2018. "HERO Scorecard." https://hero-health.org/hero-scorecard/.

Hetherington, Bryan. 2016. Chief Counsel, Empire Justice Center, Rochester, NY, *personal communication.*

Hetherington, Bryan, and Patricia Brantingham. 2004. "Recent Lead Summit Revealed Community's Will to Aid Children." *Democrat and Chronicle*, June 29.

Hofer, Helene Biandudi. 2012. "New Report: RCSD Graduates Lowest Rate of Black Males in U.S." *WXXI News*, September 20. http://wxxinews.org/post/new-report-rcsd-graduates-lowest-rate-black-males-us.

Hofrichter, Richard. 2002. *Toxic Struggles: The Theory and Practice of Environmental Justice.* Salt Lake City: University of Utah Press.

Honeycutt, Sally, Jennifer Leeman, William J. McCarthy, Roshan Bastani, Lori Carter-Edwards, and Heather Clark. 2015. "Evaluating Policy, Systems, and Environmental Change Interventions: Lessons Learned from CDC's Prevention Research Centers." *Preventing Chronic Disease* 12: E174. doi: 10.5888/pcd12.150281.

Hoy, Suellen. 1995. *Chasing Dirt: The American Pursuit of Cleanliness.* Oxford: Oxford University Press.

Hricko, Andrea. 2008. "Global Trade Comes Home: Community Impacts of Goods Movement." *Environmental Health Perspectives* 116 (2): A78.

Hricko, Andrea. 2016. Former Director, Community Outreach and Engagement Core, University of Southern California Environmental Health Sciences Center, *personal communication.*

Hricko, A., G. Rowland, S. Eckel, A. Logan, M. Taher, and J. Wilson. 2014. "Global Trade, Local Impacts: Lessons from California on Health Impacts and Environmental Justice Concerns for Residents Living near Freight Rail Yards." *International Journal of Environmental Research and Public Health* 11 (2): 1914–41. doi: 10.3390/ijerph110201914.

HUD (U.S. Department of Housing and Urban Development). 1990. "Comprehensive and Workable Plan for the Abatement of Lead-Based Paint in Privately Owned Housing." https://www.huduser.gov/portal/publications/affhsg/comp_work_plan_1990.html.

HUD (U.S. Department of Housing and Urban Development). 2011. "American Healthy Homes Survey: Lead and Arsenic Findings." Office of Healthy Homes and Lead Hazard Control. https://www.hud.gov/sites/documents/AHHS_REPORT.PDF.

HUD (U.S. Department of Housing and Urban Development). 2012. "Chapter 11: Interim Controls." In *Guidelines for the Evaluation and Control of Lead-Based Paint Hazards in Housing.* 2nd ed. Washington, DC: HUD Office of Healthy Homes and Lead Hazard Control. http://portal.hud.gov/hudportal/HUD?src=/program_offices/healthy_homes/lbp/hudguidelines.

HUD (U.S. Department of Housing and Urban Development). 2017. "Revised Dust-Lead Action Levels for Risk Assessment and Clearance, Clearance of Porch Floors." https://www.hud.gov/sites/documents/LEADDUSTCLEARANCE.PDF.

HUD (U.S. Department of Housing and Urban Development). 2018a. "The Lead-Safe Housing Rule." https://www.hud.gov/program_offices/healthy_homes/enforcement /lshr.

HUD (U.S. Department of Housing and Urban Development). 2018b. "Noise Abatement and Control." https://www.hudexchange.info/programs/environmental -review/noise-abatement-and-control/.

HUD (U.S. Department of Housing and Urban Development). 2018c. The University of Rochester Medical Center Partners to Eliminate Lead Poisoning. Office of Policy Development and Research. https://www.huduser.gov/portal/casestudies/study -061118.html.

Human Impact Partners. 2011. "I-710 Corridor Project Health Impact Assessment." https://humanimpact.org/wp-content/uploads/2017/09/HIA-I710-Air-Quality-Plan .pdf.

Human Impact Partners. 2013. "Frequently Asked Questions about Integrating Health Impact Assessment into Environmental Impact Assessment." https://humanimpact .org/wp-content/uploads/2013/11/FAQs-about-HIA-and-EIA.pdf.

Iannantuono, Adele, and John Eyles. 2000. "Environmental Health Policy: Analytic "Framing" of the Great Lakes Picture." *Environmental Management* 26 (4): 385–392.

IARC (International Agency for Research on Cancer). 2012. "IARC: Diesel Engine Exhaust Carcinogenic." *Journal of the National Cancer Institute* 104(11): 855–868.

Institute of Medicine. 1988. *The Future of Public Health*. Washington, DC: The National Academies Press.

Institute of Medicine. 2002. *The Future of the Public's Health in the 21st Century*. Washington, DC: National Academies of Science.

International Code Council. 2015. 2015 *International Property Maintenance Code*. 4th printing. Washington, DC: ICC.

International Labour Organization. 2018. "Convention C013—White Lead (Painting) Convention, 1921 (No. 13)." http://www.ilo.org/dyn/normlex/en/f?p=NORML EXPUB:12100:0::NO::P12100_INSTRUMENT_ID:312158.

International Maritime Organization. 2018. "Sulphur 2020—Cutting Sulphur Oxide Emissions." http://www.imo.org/en/mediacentre/hottopics/pages/sulphur-2020.aspx.

Israel, Barbara A., James Krieger, David Vlahov, Sandra Ciske, Mary Foley, Princess Fortin, J. Ricardo Guzman et al. 2006. "Challenges and Facilitating Factors in Sustaining Community-Based Participatory Research Partnerships: Lessons Learned from the Detroit, New York City and Seattle Urban Research Centers." *Journal of Urban Health* 83: 1022–1040.

I-710 Major Corridor Study Tier 2 Community Advisory Committee. 2004. "Major Opportunity/Strategy Recommendations and Conditions." http://www.gatewaycog .org/media/userfiles/subsite_9/files/rl/RL-I710/I-710Tier2CommunityAdvisoryCom mitteeFinalReport-2004.pdf.

Jacobs, David E. 1995. "Lead-Based Paint as a Major Source of Childhood Lead Poisoning: A Review of the Evidence." In *Lead in Paint, Soil, and Dust: Health Risks, Exposure Studies, Control Measures, Measurement Methods, and Quality Assurance*, edited by Michael E. Beard and S. D. Allen Iske, 175–187. Philadelphia: ASTM International.

Jacobs, D. E., R. P. Clickner, J. Y. Zhou, S. M. Viet, D. A. Marker, J. W. Rogers, D. C. Zeldin, P. Broene, and W. Friedman. 2002. "The Prevalence of Lead-Based Paint Hazards in U.S. Housing." *Environmental Health Perspectives* 110 (10): A599–606.

Jacquemin, B., V. Siroux, M. Sanchez, A. E. Carsin, T. Schikowski, M. Adam, V. Bellisario et al. 2015. "Ambient Air Pollution and Adult Asthma Incidence in Six European Cohorts (ESCAPE)." *Environmental Health Perspectives* 123 (6): 613–21. doi: 10.1289/ehp.1408206.

John, DeWitt. 1994. *Civic Environmentalism: Alternatives to Regulation in States and Communities*. Washington, DC: CQ Press.

Johnson, Nicole Blair, Locola D. Hayes, Kathryn Brown, Elizabeth C. Hoo, and Kathleen A. Ethier. 2014. "CDC National Health Report: Leading Causes of Morbidity and Mortality and Associated Behavioral Risk and Protective Factors—United States, 2005–2013." *Morbidity and Mortality Weekly Report (MMWR)* 63 (4): 3–27.

Jurewicz, Joanna, Kinga Polanska, and Wojciech Hanke. 2013. "Chemical Exposure Early in Life and the Neurodevelopment of Children—An Overview of Current Epidemiological Evidence." *Annals of Agricultural and Environmental Medicine* 20 (3): 465–486.

Keehan, Sean P., Devin A. Stone, John A. Poisal, Gigi A. Cuckler, Andrea M. Sisko, Sheila D. Smith, Andrew J. Madison, Christian J. Wolfe, and Joseph M. Lizonitz. 2017. "National Health Expenditure Projections, 2016–25: Price Increases, Aging Push Sector to 20 Percent of Economy." *Health Affairs* 36 (3): 553–563. doi: 10.1377/ hlthaff.2016.1627.

Keigley, Kayla. 2016. Former Program Manager, Essentia Health, Duluth, MN, *personal communication*.

Kelley, John. 2016. Planner II, Community Planning, City of Duluth, MN, *personal communication*.

Kennedy, Byron S., Andrew S. Doniger, Susan Painting, Lee Houston, Michael Slaunwhite, Frank Mirabella, John Felsen, Paul Hunt, Dawn Hyde, and Earl Stich. 2014. "Declines in Elevated Blood Lead Levels among Children, 1997– 2011." *American Journal of Preventive Medicine* 46 (3): 259–264.

Kennedy, Richard. 2018. Family Medicine Physician, Jordan Health Center, Rochester, NY, *personal communication.*

Kent, Jennifer, and Susan Thompson. 2012. "Health and the Built Environment: Exploring Foundations for a New Interdisciplinary Profession." *Journal of Environmental and Public Health* 2012: 958175. doi: 10.1155/2012/958175.

Khan, Laura Kettel, Kathleen Sobush, Dana Keener, Kenneth Goodman, Amy Lowry, Jakub Kakietek, and Susan Zaro. 2009. "Recommended Community Strategies and Measurements to Prevent Obesity in the United States." *Morbidity and Mortality Weekly Report (MMWR) Recommendations and Reports* 58 (7): 1–29.

Kim, Eugene, and Philip K. Hopke. 2008. "Source Characterization of Ambient Fine Particles at Multiple Sites in the Seattle Area." *Atmospheric Environment* 42 (24): 6047–6056.

Kim, Eugene, Katarzyna Turkiewicz, Sylvia A. Zulawnick, and Karen L. Magliano. 2010. "Sources of Fine Particles in the South Coast Area, California." *Atmospheric Environment* 44 (26):3095–3100.

Kindig, David, and Greg Stoddart. 2003. "What Is Population Health?" *American Journal of Public Health* 93 (3): 380–383.

Kirkmire, Gary. 2018. Director of Buildings and Zoning, City of Rochester, NY, *personal communication.*

Kjellstrom, Tord, Sharon Friel, Jane Dixon, Carlos Corvalan, Eva Rehfuess, Diarmid Campbell-Lendrum, Fiona Gore, and Jamie Bartram. 2007. "Urban Environmental Health Hazards and Health Equity." *Journal of Urban Health* 84 (1): 86–97.

Kneese, A. V., and C. L. Schultze. 1975. *Pollution, Prices, and Public.* Washington, DC: Brookings Institution.

Kochanek, Kenneth D., Elizabeth Arias, and Robert N. Anderson. 2015. "Leading Causes of Death Contributing to Decrease in Life Expectancy Gap between Black and White Populations: United States, 1999–2013." Centers for Disease Control and Prevention NCHS Data Brief No. 218, November.

Kochtitzky, Chris S., H. Frumkin, R. Rodriguez, A. L. Dannenberg, J. Rayman, K. Rose, R. Gillig, and T. Kanter. 2006. "Urban Planning and Public Health at CDC." *Morbidity and Mortality Weekly Report (MMWR) Supplement* 55 (2): 34–38.

Koontz, Tomas M. 2006. "Collaboration for Sustainability? A Framework for Analyzing Government Impacts in Collaborative-Environmental Management." *Sustainability: Science, Practice, and Policy* 2 (1): 15–24.

Koontz, Tomas M., T. A. Steelman, J. Carmin, K. S. Korfmacher, C. Moseley, and C. W. Thomas 2004. *Collaborative Environmental Management: What Roles for Government?* Washington, DC: Resources for the Future.

Koontz, Tomas M., and Craig W. Thomas. 2006. "What Do We Know and Need to Know about the Environmental Outcomes of Collaborative Management?" *Public Administration Review* 66 (1): 111–121.

Korfmacher, Katrina S. 1998. "Invisible Successes, Visible Failures: Paradoxes of Ecosystem Management in the Albemarle–Pamlico Estuarine Study." *Coastal Management* 26 (3). doi.org/10.1080/08920759809362352.

Korfmacher, Katrina S. 2008. "Collaborating for Primary Prevention: Rochester's New Lead Law." *Journal of Public Health Management and Practice* 14 (4): 400–406. doi: 10.1097/01.PHH.0000324570.95404.84.

Korfmacher, Katrina S. 2010. "Boundary Networks and Rochester's 'Smart' Lead Law: The Use of Multidisciplinary Information in a Collaborative Policy Process." *NEW SOLUTIONS: A Journal of Environmental and Occupational Health Policy* 20 (3): 317–336.

Korfmacher, Katrina S. 2014. "Local Housing Policy Approaches to Preventing Childhood Lead Poisoning." http://phlr.org/product/local-housing-policy-approaches -preventing-childhood-lead-poisoning.

Korfmacher, Katrina S., Maria Ayoob, and Rebecca Morley. 2012. "Rochester's Lead Law: Evaluation of a Local Environmental Health Policy Innovation." *Environmental Health Perspectives* 120 (2): 309–315.

Korfmacher, Katrina S., and Michael L. Hanley. 2013. "Are Local Laws the Key to Ending Childhood Lead Poisoning?" *Journal of Health Politics, Policy, and Law* 38 (4): 757–813.

Korfmacher, Katrina S., and Kathleen D. Holt. 2018. "The Potential for Proactive Housing Inspections to Inform Public Health Interventions." *Journal of Public Health Management and Practice* 24 (5): 444–447. doi: 10.1097/phh.0000000000000757.

Korfmacher, Katrina S., Kristianna Grass Pettibone, Kathleen M. Gray, and Ogonnaya D. Newman. 2016. "Collaborating for Systems Change: A Social Science Framework for Academic Roles in Community Partnerships." *NEW SOLUTIONS: A Journal of Environmental and Occupational Health Policy* 26 (3): 429–457.

Korfmacher, Katrina S., and Kate Kuholski. 2007. "Do the Same Houses Poison Many Children? An Investigation of Lead Poisoning in Rochester, New York, 1993–2004." *Public Health Reports* 122 (4): 482–487.

Kota, Sri Harsha, Hongliang Zhang, Gang Chen, Gunnar W Schade, and Qi Ying. 2014. "Evaluation of On-Road Vehicle CO and NOx National Emission Inventories Using an Urban-Scale Source-Oriented Air Quality Model." *Atmospheric Environment* 85: 99–108.

Kraker, Dan. 2014. "Duluth's Roads Need Work, but City Needs Money First." *MPR News*, April 23. http://www.mprnews.org/story/2014/04/23/duluth-road-repairs.

Kramer, U., C. Herder, D. Sugiri, K. Strassburger, T. Schikowski, U. Ranft, and W. Rathmann. 2010. "Traffic-Related Air Pollution and Incident Type 2 Diabetes: Results from the SALIA Cohort Study." *Environmental Health Perspectives* 118 (9): 1273–9. doi: 10.1289/ehp.0901689.

Kunzli, N., R. McConnell, D. Bates, T. Bastain, A. Hricko, F. Lurmann, E. Avol, F. Gilliland, and J. Peters. 2003. "Breathless in Los Angeles: The Exhausting Search for Clean Air." *American Journal of Public Health* 93 (9): 1494–1499.

Laker, Barbara, Wendy Ruderman, and Dylan Purcell. 2016. "Philly's Shame: City Ignores Thousands of Poisoned Kids." *The Inquirer*, October 30. http://www.philly.com/philly/news/Philadelphia_ignores_thousands_of_kids_poisoned_by_lead_paint.html.

LA Metro (Los Angeles County Metropolitan Transportation Authority). 2011. "Project Alternatives Fact Sheet." http://media.metro.net/projects_studies/I710/images/i710_c_project_alternatives_fact_sheet.pdf.

LA Metro (Los Angeles County Metropolitan Transportation Authority). 2014. "Corridor Advisory Committee Meeting #39." I-710 Corridor Project EIR/EIS. http://media.metro.net/projects_studies/I710/images/cac_32014.pdf.

LA Metro (Los Angeles County Metropolitan Transportation Authority). 2015. "I-710 Corridor Project EIR/EIS: Alternative 5C." http://media.metro.net/projects_studies/I710/images/factsheet_I710_alternative5c_2015-10.pdf.

LA Metro (Los Angeles County Metropolitan Transportation Authority). 2018a. https://thesource.metro.net/2018/02/14/staff-recommends-alternative-5c-for-710-corridor-project.

LA Metro (Los Angeles County Metropolitan Transportation Authority). 2018b. "Community Participation Framework." http://media.metro.net/projects_studies/I710/images/710_fact_sheet_cpf.pdf.

LA Metro (Los Angeles County Metropolitan Transportation Authority). 2018c. "I-710 Corridor Project." https://www.metro.net/projects/i-710-corridor-project/.

LA Metro (Los Angeles County Metropolitan Transportation Authority). 2018d. "Overview." https://www.metro.net/about/agency/mission/.

Landon, P., P. Breysse, and Y. Chen. 2005. "Noise Exposures of Rail Workers at a North American Chemical Facility." *American Journal of Industrial Medicine* 47 (4): 364–9. doi: 10.1002/ajim.20152.

Landrigan, P. J., C. B. Schechter, J. M. Lipton, M. C. Fahs, and J. Schwartz. 2002. "Environmental Pollutants and Disease in American Children: Estimates of Morbidity, Mortality, and Costs for Lead Poisoning, Asthma, Cancer, and Developmental Disabilities." *Environmental Health Perspectives* 110 (7): 721–728.

Lanphear, B. P., R. S. Byrd, P. Auinger, and S. J. Schaffer. 1998. "Community Characteristics Associated with Elevated Blood Lead Levels in Children." *Pediatrics* 101 (2): 264–271.

Lanphear, B. P., K. Dietrich, P. Auinger, and C. Cox. 2000. "Cognitive Deficits Associated with Blood Lead Concentrations <10 microg/dL in U.S. Children and Adolescents." *Public Health Reports* 115 (6): 521–529.

Lanphear, B. P., M. Emond, D. E. Jacobs, M. Weitzman, M. Tanner, N. L. Winter, B. Yakir, and S. Eberly. 1995. "A Side-by-Side Comparison of Dust Collection Methods for Sampling Lead-Contaminated House Dust." *Environmental Research* 68 (2): 114–123. doi: 10.1006/enrs.1995.1015.

Lanphear, B. P., R. Hornung, and M. Ho. 2005. "Screening Housing to Prevent Lead Toxicity in Children." *Public Health Reports* 120 (3): 305–310.

Lanphear, B. P., R. Hornung, J. Khoury, K. Yolton, P. Baghurst, D. C. Bellinger, R. L. Canfield et al. 2005. "Low-Level Environmental Lead Exposure and Children's Intellectual Function: An International Pooled Analysis." *Environmental Health Perspectives* 113 (7): 894–899.

Larson, Emily. 2016. "State of the City—Forward Together," address to City of Duluth, MN, April 27.

Lee, I-Min, Eric J. Shiroma, Felipe Lobelo, Pekka Puska, Steven N. Blair, Peter T. Katzmarzyk, and Lancet Physical Activity Series Working Group. 2012. "Effect of Physical Inactivity on Major Non-Communicable Diseases Worldwide: An Analysis of Burden of Disease and Life Expectancy." *The Lancet* 380 (9838): 219–229.

Lee, Kai N. 1993. *Compass and Gyroscope: Integrating Science and Politics for the Environment.* Washington, DC: Island Press.

Leeman, Jennifer, Allison E. Myers, Kurt M. Ribisl, and Alice S. Ammerman. 2015. "Disseminating Policy and Environmental Change Interventions: Insights from Obesity Prevention and Tobacco Control." *International Journal of Behavioral Medicine* 22 (3): 301–311. doi: 10.1007/s12529-014-9427-1.

Lercher, P., G. W. Evans, M. Meis, and W. W. Kofler. 2002. "Ambient Neighbourhood Noise and Children's Mental Health." *Occupational Environmental Medicine* 59 (6): 380–386.

Lester, Julia. 2008. "I-710 Corridor Project Air Quality and Health Risk Assessment." http://media.metro.net/projects_studies/I710/images/710_AirQuality_HealthRiskAssessment1008.pdf.

Levi, Jeffrey. 2012. "Making the Healthy Choice the Easy Choice: Eliminating Health Disparities." *HuffPost*, January 23. http://www.huffingtonpost.com/jeffrey-levi/making-the-healthy-choice_b_1445342.html.

Levin, R., M. J. Brown, M. E. Kashtock, D. E. Jacobs, E. A. Whelan, J. Rodman, M. R. Schock, A. Padilla, and T. Sinks. 2008. "Lead Exposures in U.S. Children, 2008: Implications for Prevention." *Environmental Health Perspectives* 116 (10): 1285–1293.

Levitt, Jeremy I., and Matthew C. Whitaker. 2009. *Hurricane Katrina: America's Unnatural Disaster*. Lincoln: University of Nebraska Press.

Lewis, Jack. 1985. "Lead Poisoning: A Historical Perspective." *EPA Journal* 11 (4): 15.

Lewis, Kathy. 2018. Former Director of Community Partnerships, United Way of Greater Rochester, NY, *personal communication*.

Li, Ning, Steve Georas, Neil Alexis, Patricia Fritz, Tian Xia, Marc A Williams, Elliott Horner, and Andre Nel. 2016. "A Work Group Report on Ultrafine Particles (American Academy of Allergy, Asthma & Immunology): Why Ambient Ultrafine and Engineered Nanoparticles Should Receive Special Attention for Possible Adverse Health Outcomes in Human Subjects." *Journal of Allergy and Clinical Immunology* 138 (2): 386–396.

Li, W., S. Han, T. R. Gregg, F. W. Kemp, A. L. Davidow, D. B. Louria, A. Siegel, and J. D. Bogden. 2003. "Lead Exposure Potentiates Predatory Attack Behavior in the Cat." *Environmental Research* 92 (3): 197–206.

Lindstrom, Laura. 2017. "Rochester's Lead Law Spurs Success; Toledo Tries Similar Effort" *The Blade*, July 16. http://www.toledoblade.com/local/2017/07/16/Rochester -s-lead-law-spurs-success-Toledo-tries-similar-effort.html.

Listokin, David, and David B. Hattis. 2005. "Building Codes and Housing." *Cityscape: A Journal of Policy Development and Research* 8 (1): 21–67.

Liu, Cuiqing, Zhekang Ying, Jack Harkema, Qinghua Sun, and Sanjay Rajagopalan. 2013. "Epidemiological and Experimental Links between Air Pollution and Type 2 Diabetes." *Toxicologic Pathology* 41 (2): 361–373.

Logan, Angelo. 2016. Former Executive Director, East Yard Communities for Environmental Justice, Commerce, CA, *personal communication*.

Los Angeles Harbor Department. 2013. "Southern California International Gateway Project: Final Environmental Impact Report." https://www.portoflosangeles.org /pola/pdf/eir/scig/feir/01_introduction_scig_feir.pdf.

Los Angeles Harbor Department. 2018. "Southern California International Gateway Project Description." A1–A6. https://www.portoflosangeles.org/NOP/SCIG/NOP_ SCIG_PROJECT_DESCRIPTION2.pdf.

Luan, Hui, Jane Law, and Matthew Quick. 2015. "Identifying Food Deserts and Swamps Based on Relative Healthy Food Access: A Spatio-Temporal Bayesian Approach." *International Journal of Health Geographics* 14: 37. doi: 10.1186/s12942-015-0030-8.

Lundy, John. 2016. "Changes in Store for Grocery Express." *Duluth News Tribune*, July 25. http://www.duluthnewstribune.com/news/4081116-changes-store-grocery-express.

Lundy, John. 2017. "Grocery Express Routes Redesigned." *Duluth News Tribune*, March 3. http://www.duluthnewstribune.com/news/4229006-grocery-express-routes-redesigned.

Luokkala, Lisa. 2012. "Are You a Walker or Biker? We Want Your Input!" http://www.zeitgeistarts1.com/HealthDul/active-living/are-you-a-walker-or-biker-we-want-your-input/.

Luokkala, Lisa. 2013a. "Bike Friendly Duluth Stakeholder Meeting." http://www.zeitgeistarts1.com/HealthDul/active-living/bike-friendly-duluth-stakeholder-meeting/.

Luokkala, Lisa. 2013b. "The Hillside Counts!" http://www.zeitgeistarts1.com/HealthDul/active-living/the-hillside-counts/.

Luokkala, Lisa. 2013c. "Hiring for Position of Fair Food Access AmeriCorps." http://www.zeitgeistarts1.com/HealthDul/healthy-eating/hiring-for-position-of-fair-food-access-americorps/.

Luokkala, Lisa. 2016. Former Director, Healthy Duluth Area Coalition, *personal communication*.

Maantay, Juliana. 2001. "Zoning, Equity, and Public Health." *American Journal of Public Health* 91 (7): 1033.

Maantay, Juliana. 2002. "Zoning Law, Health, and Environmental Justice: What's the Connection?" *Journal of Law, Medicine & Ethics* 30 (4): 572–593. doi: 10.1111/j.1748-720X.2002.tb00427.x.

MacDorman, Marian F., T. J. Mathews, Ashna D. Mohangoo, and Jennifer Zeitlin. 2014. "International Comparisons of Infant Mortality and Related Factors: United States and Europe, 2010." *National Vital Statistics Reports* 63 (5).

MacKenzie, Susan H. 1996. *Integrated Resource Planning and Management: The Ecosystem Approach in the Great Lakes Basin*. Washington, DC: Island Press.

Mack, Thomas. 2004. *Cancers in the Urban Environment*. 1st ed. Oxford: Elsevier Academic Press.

Madamala, Kusuma, Katie Sellers, Leslie M. Beitsch, Jim Pearsol, and Paul E. Jarris. 2011. "Structure and Functions of State Public Health Agencies in 2007." *American Journal of Public Health* 101 (7): 1179–1186. doi: 10.2105/AJPH.2010.300011.

Mair, Julie Samia, and Michael Mair. 2003. "Violence Prevention and Control through Environmental Modifications." *Annual Review of Public Health* 24 (1): 209–225.

Mares, Rafael. 2003. "Enforcement of the Massachusetts Lead Law and Its Effect on Rental Prices and Abandonment." *Journal of Affordable Housing and Community Development Law* 12 (3): 343–365.

Markowitz, Gerald, and David Rosner. 2000. "'Cater to the Children': The Role of the Lead Industry in a Public Health Tragedy, 1900–1955." *American Journal of Public Health* 90 (1): 36–46.

Markowitz, Gerald, and David Rosner. 2013. *Deceit and Denial: The Deadly Politics of Industrial Pollution*. Oakland: University of California Press.

Marmot, M. G., and R. Bell. 2009. "Action on Health Disparities in the United States: Commission on Social Determinants of Health." *JAMA* 301 (11): 1169–1171. doi: 10.1001/jama.2009.363.

Marmot, Michael G., Martin J. Shipley, and Geoffrey Rose. 1984. "Inequalities in Death—Specific Explanations of a General Pattern?" *The Lancet* 323 (8384): 1003–1006.

Marmot, Michael G., Stephen Stansfeld, Chandra Patel, Fiona North, Jenny Head, Ian White, Eric Brunner, Amanda Feeney, and G. Davey Smith. 1991. "Health Inequalities among British Civil Servants: The Whitehall II Study." *The Lancet* 337 (8754): 1387–1393.

Massachusetts Department of Environmental Conservation. 2018. "MassDEP Environmental Justice." http://www.mass.gov/eea/agencies/massdep/service/justice/.

Mathews, T. J., Marian F. MacDorman, and Marie E. Thoma. 2015. "Infant Mortality Statistics from the 2013 Period Linked Birth/Infant Death Data Set." *National Vital Statistics Report* 64 (9): 1–28.

Matsuoka, Martha. 2008. "Clean and Safe Ports: Building a Movement, Region by Region." *Race, Poverty & the Environment* 15 (2): 26–28.

Matsuoka, Martha M. 2014. "Democratizing Planning: How Communities Are Raising Their Voices to Transform the I-710 Corridor Project." The California Endowment. http://www.calendow.org/wp-content/uploads/I-710-Case-Study-final_print1.pdf.

Matsuoka, Martha, Andrea Hricko, Robert Gottlieb, and Juan DeLara. 2011. "Global Trade Impacts: Addressing the Health, Social and Environmental Consequences of Moving International Freight through Our Communities." http://scholar.oxy.edu /uep_faculty/411.

May, Ashleigh L., David Freedman, Bettylou Sherry, and Heidi M. Blanck. 2013. "Obesity—United States, 1999–2010." *Morbidity and Mortality Weekly Report (MMWR) Supplement* 62 (3): 120–128.

Mays, Glen P., and Rachel A. Hogg. 2015. "Economic Shocks and Public Health Protections in U.S. Metropolitan Areas." *American Journal of Public Health* 105 (S2): S280–S287.

McCarthy, Gina. 2018. Former Administrator, U.S. Environmental Protection Agency, *personal communication.*

McConnell, R., T. Islam, K. Shankardass, M. Jerrett, F. Lurmann, F. Gilliland, J. Gauderman, E. Avol, N. Kunzli, L. Yao, J. Peters, and K. Berhane. 2010. "Childhood Incident Asthma and Traffic-Related Air Pollution at Home and School." *Environmental Health Perspectives* 118 (7): 1021–6. doi: 10.1289/ehp.0901232.

McDade, Elizabeth. 2018. "The Mission: End Childhood Lead Poisoning in Rochester." *Shelterforce: The Voice of Community Development,* Nov. 13. https://shelterforce.org/2018/11/13/the-mission-end-childhood-lead-poisoning-in-rochester/.

McDonnell, Patrick J., and Natalie Kitroeff. 2016. "$5.4-Billion Expansion of Panama Canal Could Reshape World Trade Routes." *Los Angeles Times,* June 24. http://www.latimes.com/world/mexico-americas/la-fg-panama-canal-20160624-snap-story.html.

McGarvey, Kathleen. 2010. "Home Work." *Rochester Review.* 76(2) http://www.rochester.edu/pr/Review/V72N6/0401_feature2.html.

McGinnis, J. Michael, Pamela Williams-Russo, and James R. Knickman. 2002. "The Case for More Active Policy Attention to Health Promotion." *Health Affairs* 21 (2): 78–93.

McGinty, Meghan D., Brian C. Castrucci, and Debra M. Rios. 2018. "Assessing the Knowledge, Skills, and Abilities of Public Health Professionals in Big City Governmental Health Departments." *Journal of Public Health Management and Practice* 24 (5): 465.

McGovern, Laura, George Miller, and Paul Hughes-Cromwick. 2014. "The Relative Contribution of Multiple Determinants to Health Outcomes." *Health Affairs Health Policy Brief,* August 21. doi: 10.1377/hpb20140821.404487.

McKnight Foundation. 2019. "Our Mission." https://www.mcknight.org/about/mission-values/.

MDH (Minnesota Department of Health). 2008. "Minnesota's 2008 Health Reform Law." http://www.health.state.mn.us/healthreform/about/.

MDH (Minnesota Department of Health). 2011. *Statewide Health Improvement Program Progress Brief: Results from the First Year.* St. Paul, MN: Minnesota Department of Health. http://www.health.state.mn.us/healthreform/ship/docs/SHIPbriefMARCH2011.pdf.

MDH (Minnesota Department of Health). 2013. "Statewide Health Improvement Program Progress Brief—Year 3," February 22. http://www.health.state.mn.us/divs/oshii/ship/docs/shiprpt2012.pdf.

MDH (Minnesota Department of Health). 2014. *Advancing Health Equity in Minnesota: Report to the Legislature.* St. Paul, MN: Minnesota Department of Health.

MDH (Minnesota Department of Health). 2017a. "SHIP Quick Facts." http://www .health.state.mn.us/divs/oshii/ship/facts.html.

MDH (Minnesota Department of Health). 2017b. "SHIP Strategies." http://www .health.state.mn.us/divs/oshii/ship/strategies.html.

MDH (Minnesota Department of Health). 2018. "Health Impact Assessment (HIA)." http://www.health.state.mn.us/divs/hia/hiainmn.html.

Meadows, Donella H. 2008. *Thinking in Systems: A Primer.* White River Junction, VT: Chelsea Green Publishing.

Melosi, Martin V. 1980. *Pollution and Reform in American Cities: 1870–1930.* Austin: University of Texas Press.

Melosi, Martin V. 2001. *Effluent America: Cities, Industry, Energy, and the Environment.* Pittsburgh, PA: University of Pittsburgh Press.

Meyer, Pamela A., Ana Penman-Aguilar, Vincent A. Campbell, Corinne Graffunder, Ann E. O'Connor, and Paula W. Yoon. 2013. "Conclusion and Future Directions: CDC Health Disparities and Inequalities Report—United States, 2013." *Morbidity and Mortality Weekly Report (MMWR) Supplement* 62 (3): 184.

Meyer, P. A., T. Pivetz, T. A. Dignam, D. M. Homa, J. Schoonover, and D. Brody. 2003. "Surveillance for Elevated Blood Lead Levels among Children—United States, 1997–2001." *Morbidity and Mortality Weekly Report (MMWR) Surveillance Summaries* 52 (10): 1–21.

Meyer, P. A., F. Staley, P. Staley, J. Curtis, C. Blanton, and M. J. Brown. 2005. "Improving Strategies to Prevent Childhood Lead Poisoning Using Local Data." *International Journal of Hygiene and Environmental Health* 208 (1–2): 15–20.

Mid-Michigan Regional HIA Program. 2018. "Mid-Michigan Mapping and Impact Assessment Toolkit." https://hiatoolkit.weebly.com/.

Mielke, Howard W., Christopher R. Gonzales, M. Kelley Smith, and Paul W. Mielke. 1999. "The Urban Environment and Children's Health: Soils as an Integrator of Lead, Zinc, and Cadmium in New Orleans, Louisiana, USA." *Environmental Research* 81 (2): 117–129.

Milazzo, Paul Charles. 2006. *Unlikely Environmentalists: Congress and Clean Water, 1945–1972.* Lawrence: University Press of Kansas.

Minkler, Meredith, Analilia P. Garcia, Victor Rubin, and Nina Wallerstein. 2012. "Community-Based Participatory Research: A Strategy for Building Healthy Communities and Promoting Health through Policy Change." http://www.policylink.org /sites/default/files/CBPR.pdf.

Minnesota Brownfields. 2018a. "About Minnesota Brownfields." http://mnbrown fields.org/.

Minnesota Brownfields. 2018b. "Brownfield Health Indicator Tool." http://mnbrown fields.org/home/available-resources/brownfield-health-indicator-tool/.

Minnesota Department of Health Climate and Health Program. 2014. "Gary-New Duluth Small Area Plan Health Impact Assessment." City of Duluth Planning Division. http://www.health.state.mn.us/divs/hia/docs/gnd_hia.pdf.

Minnesota Department of Health Climate and Health Program. 2015. "Lincoln Park/ Duluth Small Area Plan Health Impact Assessment." City of Duluth Planning Division. https://www.pewtrusts.org/-/media/assets/2018/08/lincoln-hia-final.pdf?la=en &hash=7EB53B192145B2D5E375820D3FF37DE111360F64.

Minnesota Pollution Control Agency. 2011. "Atlas Cement Plant #4 Duluth, St. Louis County, Minnesota." https://www.pca.state.mn.us/sites/default/files/Atlas _Cement_Plant4c-brwnfld2-22.pdf.

Minnesota Pollution Control Agency. 2016. "St. Louis River Area of Concern Resources." https://www.pca.state.mn.us/waste/st-louis-river-area-concern-resources.

Minnesota Pollution Control Agency. 2018. "Brownfields." https://www.pca.state .mn.us/waste/brownfields.

Modesta Avila Coalition. 2006. The Modesta Avila Coalition. https://www.arb.ca .gov/gmp/p2comments/set2/modesta_avila_coalition.pdf.

Mongelluzzo, Bill. 2016. "BNSF Uncertain It Will Pursue LA-Long Beach Terminal." JOC.com, April 8. https://www.joc.com/rail-intermodal/intermodal-shipping/bnsf -uncertain-about-moving-forward-scig_20160408.html.

Monroe County Department of Public Health. 2018. Blood Lead Screening Data, 2003-2016.https://www2.monroecounty.gov/files/health/Lead/2016%20FINAL%20 Screening%20Totals.pdf.

Morrissey, Wayne A., Jeffrey A. Zinn, and M. Lynne Corn. 1994. "Ecosystem Management: Federal Agency Activities." Congressional Research Service.

Moving Forward Network. 2018. "Moving Forward Network: Transforming Global Trade for Healthy Communities." http://www.movingforwardnetwork.com/.

Multnomah County. 2018. "Health Equity Initiative." https://multco.us/health/public -health-practice/health-equity-initiative.

Municipal Research and Services Center. 2016. "Light Nuisances—Ambient Light, Light Pollution, Glare," last modified January 8. http://mrsc.org/Home/Explore -Topics/Legal/Regulation/Nuisances-Regulation-and-Abatement/Light-Nuisances -Ambient-Light-Light-Pollution-Gl.aspx.

Murphy, Brett. 2017. "Rigged." USA Today, June 16, Investigative Report. https:// www.usatoday.com/pages/interactives/news/rigged-forced-into-debt-worked-past -exhaustion-left-with-nothing/.

Murray, Christopher J. L., Sandeep C. Kulkarni, Catherine Michaud, Niels Tomijima, Maria T. Bulzacchelli, Terrell J. Iandiorio, and Majid Ezzati. 2006. "Eight Americas: Investigating Mortality Disparities across Races, Counties, and Race-Counties in the United States." *PLoS Medicine* 3 (9): e260.

NACCHO (National Association of County and City Health Officials). 1999. "The Integration of Environmental Health and Public Health Practice, Resolution 99–13." http://www.precaution.org/lib/06/prn_naccho_integrate_enviro_and_public_health .19991107.htm.

NACCHO (National Association of County and City Health Officials). 2005. *Operational Definition of a Functional Local Health Department*. Washington, DC: NACCHO. https://www.naccho.org/uploads/downloadable-resources/Operational-Definition -of-a-Functional-Local-Health-Department.pdf.

NACCHO (National Association of County and City Health Officials). 2015. *Local Health Departments Protect the Public's Health*. Washington, DC: NACCHO.

NACCHO (National Association of County and City Health Officials). 2016. "NACCHO'S 2016 Profile Study: Environmental Health." http://nacchoprofilestudy.org /wp-content/uploads/2017/07/Environmental-Health-One-Pager_FINAL.pdf.

NACCHO (National Association of County and City Health Officials). 2017. *2016 National Profile of Local Health Departments*. Washington, DC: NACCHO.

National Academies of Sciences. 2015. *The Growing Gap in Life Expectancy by Income: Implications for Federal Programs and Policy Responses*. Washington, DC: The National Academies Press.

National Academies of Sciences Transportation Research Board and Strategic Highway Research Program. 2011. "Case Study California I-710: Engaged Community Supports Corridor Study Partnership." https://onlinepubs.trb.org/onlinepubs/shrp2 /SHRP2_CS_C01_California-I-710.pdf.

National Cancer Institute. 2008. "Cancer Health Disparities." National Institutes of Health, last modified March 11. https://www.cancer.gov/about-nci/organization /crchd/cancer-health-disparities-fact-sheet.

National Center for Healthy Housing. 2017. "Introducing Find It, Fix It, Fund It." http://nchh.org/build-the-movement/find-fix-fund/.

National Center for Healthy Housing. 2018a. "Hospital Community Benefits." https://nchh.org/tools-and-data/financing-and-funding/healthcare-financing /hospital-community-benefits/.

National Center for Healthy Housing. 2018b. "Policy: State and Local Lead Laws." http://www.nchh.org/Policy/StateandLocalPolicy/StateandLocalLeadLaws .aspx.

National Center for Healthy Housing and University of Cincinnati Department of Environmental Health. 2004. "Evaluation of the HUD Lead-Based Paint Hazard Control Grant Program Final Report." http://nchh.org/LinkClick.aspx ?fileticket=1jFfxfohcig%3d&tabid=273.

National Center for Safe Routes to School. 2018. "Safe Routes." http://www.saferoutes info.org/.

National Conference of State Legislatures. 2016. "States Shut Out Light Pollution," last modified May 23. http://www.ncsl.org/research/environment-and-natural-resources /states-shut-out-light-pollution.aspx.

National Environmental Health Association. 2018. "Definitions of Environmental Health." https://www.neha.org/about-neha/definitions-environmental-health.

National League of Cities. 2017. "City-Level Models to Advance Healthy Housing: Lessons from NLC's Mayors' Institute on Housing, Hazards, and Health." https://nlc .org/sites/default/files/users/user75/FINAL-Healthy%20Housing.pdf.

National Prevention Council. 2011. *National Prevention Strategy: America's Plan for Better Health and Wellness*. Washington, DC: US Department of Health and Human Services, Office of the Surgeon General. https://ntp.niehs.nih.gov/pubhealth/hat /noms/lead/index.html.

National Toxicology Program. 2012. "Health Effects of Low-Level Lead." NTP Monograph. Raleigh, NC: National Institutes of Health.

Natural Resources Defense Council. 2002a. "Appeals Court Stops China Shipping Terminal Construction," press release, October 30. https://www.nrdc.org/media/2002 /021030-1.

Natural Resources Defense Council Inc, v. City of Los Angeles. 2002b. Cal. Ct. App., 2nd Dist., Div. 4.

Navas-Acien, A., E. Guallar, E. K. Silbergeld, and S. J. Rothenberg. 2007. "Lead Exposure and Cardiovascular Disease—A Systematic Review." *Environmental Health Perspectives* 115 (3): 472–482. doi: 10.1289/ehp.9785.

Needleman, Herbert. 2009. "Low Level Lead Exposure: History and Discovery." *Annals of Epidemiology* 19 (4): 235–238.

NEJAC (National Environmental Justice Advisory Council). 2009. "Reducing Air Emissions Associated with Goods Movement: Working towards Environmental Justice." https://www.epa.gov/sites/production/files/2015-02/documents/2009-goods -movement.pdf.

Nelson, Arthur C., and Mitch Moody. 2003. *Paying for Prosperity: Impact Fees and Job Growth*. Washington DC: Brookings Institution.

Ness, Don. 2010. "Duluth Minnesota's Interest in the ATSDR Brownfield/Land Reuse Initiative Program," *personal communication.*

Ness, Don. 2012. Mayor, City of Duluth, MN, *personal communication.*

Ness, Don. 2014. "Re: Area-wide Planning Grant Application for the Western Port Area Neighborhoods, City of Duluth, MN," *personal communication.*

Newman, Nick, Camille Jones, Elena Page, Diana Ceballos, and Aalok Oza. 2015. "Investigation of Childhood Lead Poisoning from Parental Take-Home Exposure from an Electronic Scrap Recycling Facility—Ohio, 2012." *Morbidity and Mortality Weekly Report (MMWR)* 64 (27): 743.

New Ulm Minnesota. 2006. "Governor's Fit City." http://www.ci.new-ulm.mn.us /index.asp?SEC=7220A3BF-18EC-4FCB-ACF7-29EBA92DA595&Type=B_BASIC.

New York State Department of Environmental Conservation. 2018. "Environmental Justice: Office of Environmental Justice." http://www.dec.ny.gov/public/333.html.

New York State Department of Health. 2001. "Promoting Lead Free Children in New York State: A Report of Lead Exposure Status among New York Children, 2000–2001," https://www.health.ny.gov/environmental/lead/exposure/report/.

New York State Department of Health. 2019. "Lead Poisoning Prevention Programs and Plans of New York State." https://www.health.ny.gov/environmental /lead/programs_plans/index.htm.

NIEHS (National Institute of Environmental Health Sciences). 2012a. "2012–2017 Strategic Plan: Advancing Science, Improving Health: A Plan for Environmental Health Research." https://www.niehs.nih.gov/about/strategicplan/strategicplan2012_508.pdf.

NIEHS (National Institute of Environmental Health Sciences). 2012b. "Partnerships for Environmental Public Health Evaluation Metrics Manual: Workshop Materials for the Participants." https://www.niehs.nih.gov/research/supported/assets/docs/j_q /peph_mm_handouts_508.pdf.

NIEHS (National Institute of Environmental Health Sciences). 2013. "Partnerships for Environmental Public Health Evaluation Metrics Manual." NIH publication no. 12-7825. https://www.niehs.nih.gov/research/supported/assets/docs/a_c/complete_ peph_evaluation_metrics_manual_508.pdf.

NIEHS (National Institute of Environmental Health Sciences). 2018a. "Community Engagement Cores: Environmental Health Sciences Core Centers." https://www .niehs.nih.gov/research/supported/centers/core/coe/index.cfm.

NIEHS (National Institute of Environmental Health Sciences). 2018b. "Environmental Health Disparities and Environmental Justice." https://www.niehs.nih.gov /research/supported/translational/justice/index.cfm.

NIEHS (National Institute of Environmental Health Sciences). 2018c. "THE (Trade, Health, Environment) Impact Study." https://www.niehs.nih.gov/research/supported /translational/community/the-impact/index.cfm.

Northridge, Mary E., Elliot D. Sclar, and Padmini Biswas. 2003. "Sorting Out the Connections between the Built Environment and Health: A Conceptual Framework for Navigating Pathways and Planning Healthy Cities." *Journal of Urban Health* 80 (4): 556–568.

Norwood, Wade. 2007. Former City Councilman, City of Rochester, NY, *personal communication.*

Novotny, Patrick. 2000. *Where We Live, Work, and Play: The Environmental Justice Movement and the Struggle for a New Environmentalism.* Westport, CT: Greenwood Publishing Group.

NYCCELP (New York City Coalition to End Lead Poisoning). 2016. "New York City Coalition to End Lead Poisoning." http://www.nmic.org/nyccelp.htm.

Oakar, Catherine. 2017. "Making the Healthy Choice the Easy Choice: What the Record Shows." *Let's Move Blog*, January 23. https://letsmove.obamawhitehouse .archives.gov/blog/2017/01/01/making-healthy-choice-easy-choice-what-record -shows.

Oberdorster, G., Z. Sharp, V. Atudorei, A. Elder, R. Gelein, W. Kreyling, and C. Cox. 2004. "Translocation of Inhaled Ultrafine Particles to the Brain." *Inhalation Toxicology* 16 (6–7): 437–45. doi: 10.1080/08958370490439597.

Oberle, Mark W. 1969. "Lead Poisoning: A Preventable Childhood Disease of the Slums." *Science* 165 (3897): 991–992. doi: 10.1126/science.165.3897.991.

O'Fallon, Liam R. 2004. "Go for the GLO." *Environmental Health Perspectives* 112 (6): A349.

O'Fallon, Liam R., Geraldine M. Wolfle, David Brown, Allen Dearry, and Kenneth Olden. 2003. "Strategies for Setting a National Research Agenda That Is Responsive to Community Needs." *Environmental Health Perspectives* 111 (16): 1855.

Office of Disease Prevention and Health Promotion. 2018a. "Environmental Health, Healthy People 2020." https://www.healthypeople.gov/2020/topics-objectives/topic /environmental-health.

Office of Disease Prevention and Health Promotion. 2018b. "Healthy People 2020 Framework." https://www.healthypeople.gov/sites/default/files/HP2020Framework .pdf.

Office of Environmental Health and Hazard Assessment. 2018. "CalEnviroScreen 3.0." State of California. https://oehha.ca.gov/calenviroscreen/report/calenviroscreen-30.

Ogden, Cynthia L., Molly M. Lamb, Margaret D. Carroll, and Katherine M. Flegal. 2010. *Obesity and Socioeconomic Status in Adults: United States, 2005–2008*. Atlanta, GA: Centers for Disease Control and Prevention.

Olivieri, D., and E. Scoditti. 2005. "Impact of Environmental Factors on Lung Defences." *European Respiratory Review* 14 (95): 51–56. doi: 10.1183/09059180.05.00009502.

Oregon Health Authority. 2013. "Strategic Health Impact Assessment on Wind Energy Development in Oregon." https://www.oregon.gov/oha/ph/HealthyEnvironments /TrackingAssessment/HealthImpactAssessment/Documents/Wnd%20Energy%20 HIA/Wind%20HIA_Final.pdf.

Orleans, C. Tracy, Laura C. Leviton, Kathryn A. Thomas, Terry L. Bazzarre, Jamie B. Bussel, Dwayne Proctor, Celeste M. Torio, and Stephanie M. Weiss. 2009. "History of the Robert Wood Johnson Foundation's Active Living Research Program: Origins and Strategy." *American Journal of Preventive Medicine* 36 (2, Supplement): S1–S9. doi: https://doi.org/10.1016/j.amepre.2008.11.001.

Osborn, Chandra Y., Mary de Groot, and Julie A. Wagner. 2013. "Racial and Ethnic Disparities in Diabetes Complications in the Northeastern United States: The Role of Socioeconomic Status." *Journal of the National Medical Association* 105 (1): 51–58.

Osorio, Arturo E., Maria G. Corradini, and Jerome D. Williams. 2013. "Remediating Food Deserts, Food Swamps, and Food Brownfields: Helping the Poor Access Nutritious, Safe, and Affordable Food." *AMS Review* 3 (4): 217–231.

Ostrov, Barbara Feder. 2012. "Pollution, Health, and Activism at the Port of Los Angeles." *Center for Health Journalism Fellowships Blog*, December 8. https://www .centerforhealthjournalism.org/blogs/pollution-health-and-activism-port-los-angeles.

Pardee, Jessica Warner. 2005. *Surviving Katrina: The Experiences of Low-Income African American Women*. Boulder, CO: First Forum Press.

Parker, Molly. 2018. "HUD Is Failing to Protect Children from Lead Paint Poisoning, Audits Find." *The Southern Illinoisan*, June 22. https://www.propublica.org/article /hud-is-failing-to-protect-children-from-lead-paint-poisoning-audits-find.

Parkin, Charles. 2016. "Trial Court Sets Aside Approvals for BNSF's Controversial SCIG Railyard, A Victory for West Long Beach Residents," press release, March 30. http://www.longbeach.gov/Attorney/Press-Releases/Court-finds-Environmental -Review-Defective-for-BNSF-s-SCIG-Project/.

Parks, Troy. 2016. "Death by ZIP Code: Investigating the Root Causes of Health Inequity." *AMA Wire*, August 25.

Passi, Peter. 2014. "As Foundation Funds Dwindle, Zeitgeist Seeks Community Support." *Duluth News Tribune*, October 19. http://www.duluthnewstribune.com/content /foundation-funds-dwindle-zeitgeist-seeks-community-support.

Pastor, Manuel, Robert Doyle Bullard, James K. Boyce, Alice Fothergill, Rachel Morello-Frosch, and Beverly Wright. 2006. *In the Wake of the Storm: Environment, Disaster, and Race after Katrina*. New York: Russell Sage Foundation.

Patel, Kant, and Mark E. Rushefsky. 2005. *The Politics of Public Health in the United States*. Armonk, NY: M. E. Sharpe.

Patrick, Ruth, Faith Douglass, Drew M. Palavage, and Paul M. Stewart. 1992. *Surface Water Quality: Have the Laws Been Successful?* Princeton, NJ: Princeton University Press.

Patton, Michael Quinn. 2010. *Developmental Evaluation: Applying Complexity Concepts to Enhance Innovation and Use*. New York: Guilford Press.

Pauley, Stephen M. 2004. "Lighting for the Human Circadian Clock: Recent Research Indicates That Lighting Has Become a Public Health Issue." *Medical Hypotheses* 63 (4): 588–596.

Payne-Sturges, D. C., K. S. Korfmacher, D. A. Cory-Slechta, M. Jimenez, E. Symanski, J. L. Carr Shmool, O. Dotson-Newman, J. E. Clougherty, R. French, J. I. Levy, R. Laumbach, K. Rodgers, R. Bongiovanni, and M. K. Scammell. 2015. "Engaging Communities in Research on Cumulative Risk and Social Stress-Environment Interactions: Lessons Learned from EPA's STAR Program." *Environmental Justice* 8 (6): 203–212. doi: 10.1089/env.2015.0025.

Pearson, Stephanie. 2014. "Why Duluth Is the Best Town in America." *Outside Magazine*, August 12.

Peel, Jennifer L., Paige E. Tolbert, Mitchel Klein, Kristi Busico Metzger, W. Dana Flanders, Knox Todd, James A. Mulholland, P. Barry Ryan, and Howard Frumkin. 2005. "Ambient Air Pollution and Respiratory Emergency Department Visits." *Epidemiology* 16 (2): 164–174. doi: 10.1097/01.ede.0000152905.42113.db.

Peterson, Erin L., Susan A. Carlson, Thomas L. Schmid, David R. Brown, and Deborah A. Galuska. 2018. "Supporting Active Living through Community Plans: The Association of Planning Documents with Design Standards and Features." *American Journal of Health Promotion* (June): doi: 10.1177/0890117118779011.

Peterson, Jenny. 2017. Executive Director, Generations Health Care Initiatives, *personal communication*.

Peterson, Jon A. 2003. *The Birth of City Planning in the United States, 1840–1917*. Baltimore, MD: Johns Hopkins University Press.

Pettit, David. 2008. "China Shipping Redux." *Expert Blog*, December 23. https://www.nrdc.org/experts/david-pettit/china-shipping-redux.

Pew Charitable Trusts. 2017. *10 Policies to Prevent and Respond to Childhood Lead Exposure*. Health Impact Project. Washington, DC: Pew Charitable Trusts.

Pew Charitable Trusts. 2018a. "Health Impact Project." http://www.pewtrusts.org/en/projects/health-impact-project.

Pew Charitable Trusts. 2018b. "The HIA Process." http://www.pewtrusts.org/en/research-and-analysis/analysis/2014/08/28/the-hia-process.

Pine, Adam and John Bennett, John. 2011. "Food Access in Duluth's Lincoln Park/West End Neighborhood." University of Minnesota Extension. Duluth, MN. https://conservancy.umn.edu/handle/11299/171650.

Pingkuan Di. 2006. "Diesel Particulate Matter Exposure Assessment Study for the Ports of Los Angeles and Long Beach." California Air Resources Board.

Pioneer Press. 2014. "New Duluth Tourism Tax Would Promote City's Riverside, West Side," March 23. http://www.twincities.com/2014/03/23/new-duluth-tourism-tax-would-promote-citys-riverside-west-side/.

Plough, Alonzo L. 2015. "Building a Culture of Health: A Critical Role for Public Health Services and Systems Research." *American Journal of Public Health* 105 (S2): S150–S152. doi: 10.2105/ajph.2014.302410.

Polakovic, Gary. 2002. "Finally Tackling L.A.'s Worst Air Polluter." *Los Angeles Times*, February 10. http://articles.latimes.com/2002/feb/10/local/me-smog10.

PolicyLink. 2011. "Healthy Corridor for All: A Community Health Impact Assessment of Transit-Oriented Development Policy in Saint Paul, Minnesota." http://www.policylink.org/resources-tools/healthy-corridor-for-all.

Pope, C. A., 3rd, R. T. Burnett, G. D. Thurston, M. J. Thun, E. E. Calle, D. Krewski, and J. J. Godleski. 2004. "Cardiovascular Mortality and Long-Term Exposure to Particulate Air Pollution: Epidemiological Evidence of General Pathophysiological Pathways of Disease." *Circulation* 109 (1): 71–7. doi: 10.1161/01.CIR.0000108927.80044.7F.

Pope, C. Arden, III, and Douglas W Dockery. 2006. "Health Effects of Fine Particulate Air Pollution: Lines That Connect." *Journal of the Air and Waste Management Association* 56: 709–742.

Port of Long Beach. 2018a. "Environmental Documents." Long Beach Harbor Department. http://www.polb.com/environment/docs.asp.

Port of Long Beach. 2018b. "Yearly TEUs." Long Beach Harbor Department. http://www.polb.com/economics/stats/yearly_teus.asp.

Port of Long Beach and Port of Los Angeles. 2006a. "Clean Air Action Plan: About the Plan." http://www.cleanairactionplan.org/about-the-plan.

Port of Long Beach and Port of Los Angeles. 2006b. "Final 2006 San Pedro Bay Ports Clean Air Action Plan." https://www.portoflosangeles.org/CAAP/CAAP_Overview_Final.pdf.

Port of Long Beach and Port of Los Angeles. 2017. "San Pedro Bay Ports Clean Air Action Plan." http://www.cleanairactionplan.org/.

Port of Long Beach and Port of Los Angeles. 2018. "Clean Air Action Plan Strategies: Trucks." http://www.cleanairactionplan.org/strategies/trucks/.

Port of Los Angeles. 2007. "The Port of Los Angeles Inventory of Air Emissions." Los Angeles: Starcrest Consulting Group, LLC. https://www.portoflosangeles.org /environment/progress/resources/air-emissions-inventory-reports/.

Port of Los Angeles. 2013. "Final EIR—Southern California International Gateway (SCIG) Project." https://www.portoflosangeles.org/EIR/SCIG/FEIR/feir_scig.asp.

Port of Los Angeles. 2018a. "Historical TEU Statistics." https://www.portoflosangeles .org/maritime/stats.asp.

Port of Los Angeles. 2018b. "San Pedro Bay Ports Clean Air Action Plan (CAAP)." https://www.portoflosangeles.org/environment/caap.asp.

Presidential Documents. 1994. "Executive Order 12898 of February 11, 1994. Federal Actions to Address Environmental Justice in Minority Populations and Low-Income Populations." *Federal Register* 59 (32).

Prevention Institute. 2010. "Coalition to Prevent Childhood Lead Poisoning: Making Lead History in Western New York State." http://preventioninstitute.org /publications/coalition-prevent-childhood-lead-poisoning-making-lead-history -western-new-york-state.

Prüss-Ustün, A., J. Wolf, C. Corvalán, R. Bos, and M. Neira. 2016. *Preventing Disease through Healthy Environments: A Global Assessment of the Burden of Disease from Environmental Risks*. Geneva: World Health Organization.

Public Health Institute. 2018. "Working Together: Policy, Systems and Environmental Change for Community Health." http://www.phi.org/resources/?resource=working -together-policy-systems-environmental-change-for-community-health.

Public Health Law Center. 2015. *State and Local Public Health: An Overview of Regulatory Authority*. St. Paul, MN: William Mitchell College of Law.

Public Health Law Center. 2017. "Minnesota Tobacco Control." http://www .publichealthlawcenter.org/topics/tobacco-control/minnesota-tobacco-control.

Public Health Law Center. 2018. "Healthcare Can Lead the Way—Making the Healthy Choice the Easy Choice." http://www.publichealthlawcenter.org/sites /default/files/resources/MN.healthcare.Healthcare%20Can%20Lead%20the%20 Way.pdf.

Pueschel, S. M., and M. E. Fadden. 1975. "Childhood Lead Poisoning and Legislative Action." *Journal of Legal Medicine* 3 (10): 16.

Raab, Barbara. 2013. "'Almost Death by Zip Code': Study Suggests Link between Health and Wealth." *NBC News.* https://www.nbcnews.com/feature/in-plain-sight /almost-death-zip-code-study-suggests-link-between-health-wealth-v19397882.

Raab, Kristin. 2017. Health Impact Assessment (HIA) and Climate Change Program Director, Minnesota Department of Health, *personal communication.*

Rabin, Richard. 2008. "The Lead Industry and Lead Water Pipes: 'A MODEST CAMPAIGN.'" *American Journal of Public Health* 98 (9): 1584–1592. doi: 10.2105/ AJPH.2007.113555.

Ranft, U., T. Schikowski, D. Sugiri, J. Krutmann, and U. Kramer. 2009. "Long-Term Exposure to Traffic-Related Particulate Matter Impairs Cognitive Function in the Elderly." *Environmental Research* 109 (8): 1004–11. doi: 10.1016/j.envres.2009.08.003.

Renalls, Candace. 2014. "Kwik Trip Expansion in Twin Ports Area Is Underway." *Duluth News Tribune*, June 16. http://www.duluthnewstribune.com/news/traffic-and -construction/3280968-kwik-trip-expansion-twin-ports-area-underway.

Renalls, Candace. 2015. "More Kwik Trip Stores Coming to Region." *Duluth News Tribune*, Nov 2, 2015. http://www.duluthnewstribune.com/business/3873702-more -kwik-trip-stores-coming-region.

Reyes, N. L., L. Y. Wong, P. M. MacRoy, G. Curtis, P. A. Meyer, A. Evens, and M. J. Brown. 2006. "Identifying Housing That Poisons: A Critical Step in Eliminating Childhood Lead Poisoning." *Journal of Public Health Management and Practice* 12 (6): 563–569.

Richard, Chris. 2017. "How California's Greenhouse Gas Laws Can Better Serve Disadvantaged Communities." https://ensia.com/features/ca-environmental-justice/.

Robert Wood Johnson Foundation. 2012. "New Hospital Community Benefit Briefs: Reporting Requirements and Community Building." *Culture of Health Blog*, February 10. https://www.rwjf.org/en/culture-of-health/2012/10/new_hospital_communi .html.

Robert Wood Johnson Foundation. 2015. "Mapping Life Expectancy: Short Distances to Large Gaps in Health," last modified September 11. http://www.rwjf.org /en/library/articles-and-news/2015/09/city-maps.html.

Robert Wood Johnson Foundation. 2018a. "Healthy Communities." https://www .rwjf.org/en/our-focus-areas/focus-areas/healthy-communities.html.

Robert Wood Johnson Foundation. 2018b. "Healthy Eating Research." https://health yeatingresearch.org/.

Rochester City School District. 2007. Lead-Safe Schools Policy. In *7010*. http://www .theleadcoalition.org/wp-content/uploads/2017/03/RCSD_Lead_Safe_Schools_Policy .pdf.

Roeder, Amy. 2014. "Zip Code Better Predictor of Health than Genetic Code," *Harvard T. H. Chan School of Public Health*, August 4. https://www.hsph.harvard.edu /news/features/zip-code-better-predictor-of-health-than-genetic-code/.

Roosevelt, Margot. 2009. "A New Crop of Eco-Warriors Take to Their Own Streets." *Los Angeles Times*, September 24. http://www.latimes.com/local/la-me-air -pollution24-2009sep24-story.html.

Rosen, George. 2015. *A History of Public Health.* Baltimore, MD: Johns Hopkins University Press.

Rosenbaum, Arlene, Seth Hartley, and Chris Holder. 2011. "Analysis of Diesel Particulate Matter Health Risk Disparities in Selected U.S. Harbor Areas." *American Journal of Public Health* 101 (S1): S217–S223.

Rosner, D., G. Markowitz, and B. Lanphear. 2005. "J. Lockhart Gibson and the Discovery of the Impact of Lead Pigments on Children's Health: A Review of a Century of Knowledge." *Public Health Reports* 120 (3): 296–300.

Rosner, David, and Gerald Markowitz. 1985. "A 'Gift of God'?: The Public Health Controversy over Leaded Gasoline during the 1920s." *American Journal of Public Health* 75 (4): 344–352.

Rotman, Michael. 2017. "Cuyahoga River Fire." *Cleveland Historical.* https://cleveland historical.org/items/show/63#.WYM5YIQrLIU.

RTI International. 2015. *BenMAP: Environmental Benefits Mapping and Community Analysis Program—Community Edition: User's Manual Appendices.* Research Triangle Park, NC: RTI.

Rudolph, Linda, Karen Ben-Moshe, Julia Caplan, and Lianne Dillon. 2013. *Health in All Policies: A Guide for State and Local Governments.* Washington, DC: American Public Health Association.

Ryan, Don, Barry Levy, S. Pollack, and B. Walker, Jr. 1999. *Protecting Children from Lead Poisoning and Building Healthy Communities.* Washington, DC: American Public Health Association.

Rynbrandt, Linda J. 1999. *Caroline Bartlett Crane and Progressive Reform: Social Housekeeping as Sociology.* London: Taylor & Francis.

Sabatier, Paul A., Will Focht, Mark Lubell, Zev Trachtenberg, Arnold Vedlitz, and Marty Matlock. 2005. *Swimming Upstream: Collaborative Approaches to Watershed Management.* Cambridge, MA: MIT Press.

Saegert, Susan C., Susan Klitzman, Nicholas Freudenberg, Jana Cooperman-Mroczek, and Salwa Nassar. 2003. "Healthy Housing: A Structured Review of Published Evaluations of U.S. Interventions to Improve Health by Modifying Housing in the United States, 1990–2001." *American Journal of Public Health* 93 (9): 1471–1477.

Salinsky, Eileen. 2010. "Governmental Public Health: An Overview of State and Local Public Health Agencies." In *National Health Policy Forum.* Paper 244. Washington, DC: George Washington University.

Sallis, James F., Robert B. Cervero, William Ascher, Karla A. Henderson, M. Katherine Kraft, and Jacqueline Kerr. 2006. "An Ecological Approach to Creating Active Living Communities." *Annual Review of Public Health* 27: 297–322.

Salzman, James, and Barton Thompson Jr. 2014. *Environmental Law and Policy, 4th ed.* St. Paul, MN: West Academic.

San Francisco Department of Public Health. 2018. "The Center for Learning and Innovation: Catalyzing Innovation and Investing in People Who Are Advancing Public Health." https://www.sfdph.org/dph/comupg/tools/cli.asp.

Sanger-Katz, Anahad O'Connor and Margot. 2018. "California, of All Places, Has Banned Soda Taxes. How a New Industry Strategy Is Succeeding." *New York Times,* June 27. https://www.nytimes.com/2018/06/27/upshot/california-banning-soda -taxes-a-new-industry-strategy-is-stunning-some-lawmakers.html.

Sargent, J. D., A. Bailey, P. Simon, M. Blake, and M. A. Dalton. 1997. "Census Tract Analysis of Lead Exposure in Rhode Island Children." *Environmental Research* 74 (2): 159–168.

Sarnat, Jeremy A., and Fernando Holguin. 2007. "Asthma and Air Quality." *Current Opinion in Pulmonary Medicine* 13: 63–66.

Sausser, Ann, Robert Gottlieb, Angelo Logan, Penny Newman, Andrea Hricko, Jesse N. Marquez, and Elisa Nicholas. 2009. "Trade, Health, Environment: Making the Case for Change." In *Report on the History and Accomplishments of THE Impact Project.* https://envhealthcenters.usc.edu/wp-content/uploads/2019/02/THE-Impact-Project -Report-Making-the-Case-for-Change-2009.pdf.

SCAQMD (South Coast Air Quality Management District). 2012. "2012 Program Environmental Impact Report: Subchapter 3.7-Noise." http://www.aqmd.gov/docs /default-source/clean-air-plans/air-quality-management-plans/2012-air-quality -management-plan/final-2012-aqmp-(february-2013)/final-ceqa-eir/2012-program- environmental-impact-report-ch-3-7.pdf?sfvrsn=2.

SCAQMD (South Coast Air Quality Management District). 2017. "Final 2016 Air Quality Management Plan." http://www.aqmd.gov/docs/default-source/clean-air -plans/air-quality-management-plans/2016-air-quality-management-plan/final -2016-aqmp/final2016aqmp.pdf?sfvrsn=15.

SCAQMD (South Coast Air Quality Management District). 2018a. "About South Coast AQMD." http://www.aqmd.gov/nav/about.

SCAQMD (South Coast Air Quality Management District). 2018b. "Clean Port." https://www.aqmd.gov/nav/about/initiatives/clean-port.

SCAQMD (South Coast Air Quality Management District). 2018c. "Health Risk Assessment." http://www.aqmd.gov/home/rules-compliance/compliance/toxic-hot-spots-ab-2588/health-risk-assessment.

Schneider, Mary-Jane. 2016. *Introduction to Public Health*. Burlington, MA: Jones & Bartlett Learning.

Schoch, Deborah. 2003a. "710 Panel's Action Angers Residents: Confusion over Project Leaves Some Fearing Loss of Homes along the Busy Long Beach Freeway." *Los Angeles Times*, May 30. http://articles.latimes.com/2003/may/30/local/me-freeway30.

Schoch, Deborah. 2003b. "Hundreds Learn Plans to Expand 710 Freeway Threaten Their Homes." *Los Angeles Times*, April 13.

Schoch, Deborah. 2005. "Proposed Rail Yard Angers Residents of Nearby Long Beach Community: Foes Say Diesel-Spewing Trucks Carrying Cargo to the Site Would Worsen Air Pollution. Railway Promises a 'Green' Facility." *Los Angeles Times*, October 6. https://www.valleyair.org/recent_news/News_Clippings/2005/In%20the%20News%20--%20Oct.%206,%202005.pdf.

Senge, Peter M. 2013. *The Fifth Discipline: The Art and Practice of the Learning Organization*. New York: Crown Business.

Shapiro, Sidney A. 1992. "Lessons from a Public Policy Failure: EPA and Noise Abatement." *Ecology Law Quarterly* 19: 1.

Sharp, Brian. 2014. "Over 50% of Rochester's Kids Live in Poverty" *Democrat and Chronicle*, September 18. https://www.democratandchronicle.com/story/news/2014/09/18/rochesters-children-live-poverty/15856493/?from=global&sessionKey=&autologin=.

Shearer, Gail. 2010. "Prevention Provisions in the Affordable Care Act." *American Public Health Association Issue Brief*. October.

Shi, Liuhua, Antonella Zanobetti, Itai Kloog, Brent A. Coull, Petros Koutrakis, Steven J. Melly, and Joel D. Schwartz. 2016. "Low-Concentration PM2. 5 and Mortality: Estimating Acute and Chronic Effects in a Population-Based Study." *Environmental Health Perspectives* 124 (1): 46.

Silverman, Debra T., Claudine M. Samanic, Jay H. Lubin, Aaron E. Blair, Patricia A. Stewart, Roel Vermeulen, Joseph B. Coble, Nathaniel Rothman, Patricia L. Schleiff, and William D. Travis. 2012. "The Diesel Exhaust in Miners Study: A Nested Case–Control Study of Lung Cancer and Diesel Exhaust." *Journal of the National Cancer Institute* 104 (11): 855–868.

Sivulka, Juliann. 1999. "From Domestic to Municipal Housekeeper: The Influence of the Sanitary Reform Movement on Changing Women's Roles in America, 1860–1920." *Journal of American Culture* 22 (4): 1–7. doi: 10.1111/j.1542–734X.1999.2204_1.x.

Skihut. 2018. "Duluth Area Cycling Guide." https://bikeduluth.com/winter-riding/.

Skoog, Jim. 2016. Retired Public Health Educator, St. Louis County Public Health and Human Services, Duluth, MN, *personal communication*.

Smart Growth America. 2018. "What Are Complete Streets?" https://smartgrowth america.org/program/national-complete-streets-coalition/what-are-complete-streets/.

Smith, Rebecca, David Bensman, and Paul A. Marvy. 2010. "The Big Rig: Poverty, Pollution, and the Misclassification of Truck Drivers at America's Ports," https://s27147.pcdn.co/wp-content/uploads/2015/03/PovertyPollutionandMiscla ssification.pdf.

Snibbe, Kurt. 2010. "BNSF Turns Down Polluter Award." *The Press Enterprise*, August 21. https://www.pe.com/2010/08/21/bnsf-turns-down-polluter-award/?clear UserState=true.

Snow, John. 1855. *On the Mode of Communication of Cholera*. London: John Churchill.

Society of Practitioners of Health Impact Assessment. 2018. "SOPHIA." https:// hiasociety.org/.

Sorensen, M., M. Hvidberg, Z. J. Andersen, R. B. Nordsborg, K. G. Lillelund, J. Jakobsen, A. Tjonneland, K. Overvad, and O. Raaschou-Nielsen. 2011. "Road Traffic Noise and Stroke: A Prospective Cohort Study." *European Heart Journal* 32 (6): 737–744. doi: 10.1093/eurheartj/ehq466.

Southern California Association of Governments. 2018. "Programs: Transportation." http://www.scag.ca.gov/programs/Pages/Programs/Transportation.aspx.

Southern California Environmental Health Sciences Center. 2012. "Community Outreach: Programs." University of Southern California. http://hydra.usc.edu/scehsc /web/Resources/Policy%20Briefs/Ports%20issue%20brief.%20January%202012.pdf.

Southern California Environmental Health Sciences Center. 2018a. "About the Center." University of Southern California. https://scehsc.usc.edu/about_the_center .php.

Southern California Environmental Health Sciences Center. 2018b. "Children's Health Study." University of Southern California. http://hydra.usc.edu/scehsc/about -studies-childrens.html.

Southern California Environmental Health Sciences Center. 2018c. "Community Outreach." University of Southern California. https://scehsc.usc.edu/community_ outreach_home.php.

Southern California Environmental Health Sciences Center. 2018d. "Programs." University of Southern California. https://web.archive.org/web/20150906205628 /http://hydra.usc.edu/scehsc/community-programs.html.

Spanier, Adam J., Stephen Wilson, Mona Ho, Richard Hornung, and Bruce P. Lanphear. 2013. "The Contribution of Housing Renovation to Children's Blood Lead Levels: A Cohort Study." *Environmental Health* 12 (1): 72.

Spezio, Ralph. 2011. TEDxRochester. https://www.youtube.com/watch?v=mSw HSE6_ZoI.

Spezio, Ralph. 2017. Former Principal, Enrico Fermi Elementary School No. 17, Rochester, NY, *personal communication.*

Squires, David, and Chloe Anderson. 2015. *U.S. Health Care from a Global Perspective: Spending, Use of Services, Prices, and Health in 13 Countries.* Washington, DC: The Commonwealth Fund.

St. Louis County Health and Human Services. 2011. "Sixth Avenue East Duluth Health Impact Assessment." http://www.pewtrusts.org/~/media/assets/2011/06/20 /6thavenueeastfinalreport.pdf?la=en.

Stansfeld, S. A., B. Berglund, C. Clark, I. Lopez-Barrio, P. Fischer, E. Ohrstrom, M. M. Haines, J. Head, S. Hygge, I. van Kamp, and B. F. Berry. 2005. "Aircraft and Road Traffic Noise and Children's Cognition and Health: A Cross-National Study." *The Lancet* 365 (9475): 1942–1949. doi: 10.1016/s0140–6736(05)66660–3.

Starr, Paul. 2008. *The Social Transformation of American Medicine: The Rise of a Sovereign Profession and the Making of a Vast Industry.* New York: Basic Books.

State of California. 2016. "SB-1000 Land Use: General Plans: Safety and Environmental Justice." https://leginfo.legislature.ca.gov/faces/billNavClient.xhtml?bill_ id=201520160SB1000.

State of California Department of Justice. 2017a. "Environmental Justice and Healthy Communities." https://oag.ca.gov/environment/communities.

State of California Department of Justice. 2017b. "Health in All Policies Task Force." https://oag.ca.gov/environment/communities/policies.

State of Massachusetts. 2016. "The Massachusetts Lead Law." http://www.mass.gov /eohhs/gov/departments/dph/programs/environmental-health/exposure-topics /lead/lead/.

Steelman, Toddi A. 2010. *Implementing Innovation: Fostering Enduring Change in Environmental and Natural Resource Governance.* Washington, DC: Georgetown University Press.

Stefanak, M., J. Diorio, and L. Frisch. 2005. "Cost of Child Lead Poisoning to taxpayers in Mahoning County, Ohio." *Public Health Reports* 120 (3): 311–315.

Steinemann, Anne. 2000. "Rethinking Human Health Impact Assessment." *Environmental Impact Assessment Review* 20 (6): 627–645.

Stender, Mimi. 2016. Former Director, Fit City Duluth, *personal communication.*

Stradling, David, and Richard Stradling. 2008. "Perceptions of the Burning River: Deindustrialization and Cleveland's Cuyahoga River." *Environmental History* 13 (3): 515–535.

SUNY (The State University of New York). 2016. "Panama Canal Expansion: The Effect of Imports and Exports Diverted from California Seaports on the Port of New York and New Jersey," Buffalo, NY: University Transportation Research Center.

Sunyer, J., C. Spix, P. Quenel, A. Ponce-de-Leon, A. Ponka, T. Barumandzadeh, G. Touloumi, T. Bacharova, B. Wojtyniak, J. Vonk, L. Bisanti, J. Schwartz, and K. Katsouyanni. 1997. "Urban Air Pollution and Emergency Admissions for Asthma in Four European Cities: The APHEA Project." *Thorax* 52: 760–765.

Sylvia. 2016. "Victory for City of Los Angeles! Clean Up Green Up, A New City Ordinance," last modified April 13. http://www.cbecal.org/victory-at-city-hall-clean-up -green-up-is-a-new-city-ordinance/.

Task Force on Community Preventive Services. 2000. "Strategies for Reducing Exposure to Environmental Tobacco Smoke, Increasing Tobacco-use Cessation, and Reducing Initiation in Communities and Health-care Systems: A Report on Recommendations of the Task Force on Community Preventive Services." *Morbidity and Mortality Weekly Report (MMWR) Recommendations and Reports* 49 (RR-12): 1.

Tevlock, Dan. 2014. "Rochester Leads on Lead While Buffalo Dallies." *Investigative Post.* Nov. 12. http://www.investigativepost.org/2014/11/12/buffalo-lacks-leadership -lead-poisoning-problem/.

THE Impact Project. 2009. "Interim Grant Report Number 1 to the California Endowment." University of Southern California.

THE Impact Project. 2010a. "Interim Grant Report Number 3 to the California Endowment." University of Southern California.

THE Impact Project. 2010b. "Moving Forward Together," October. http://hydra.usc .edu:80/scehsc/web/Conference 2007/Conference2010.html.

THE Impact Project. 2011. "Year 2 Progress Report to the Kresge Foundation." University of Southern California.

THE Impact Project. 2012a. "Final Report to the Kresge Foundation." University of Southern California.

THE Impact Project. 2012b. Driving Harm: Health and Community Impacts of Living near Truck Corridors. THE Impact Project Policy Brief Series. https://envhealthcenters .usc.edu/wp-content/uploads/2016/11/Driving-Harm.pdf.

THE Impact Project. 2012c. Importing Harm: U.S. Ports' Impacts on Health and Communities. THE Impact Project Policy Brief Series. https://envhealthcenters.usc .edu/wp-content/uploads/2016/11/Impact-Project-Ports-issue-brief-2012-1.pdf.

THE Impact Project. 2012d. Storing Harm: the Health and Community Impacts of Goods Movement Warehousing and Logistics. THE Impact Project Policy Brief Series. https://envhealthcenters.usc.edu/wp-content/uploads/2016/11/Storing-Harm.pdf.

THE Impact Project. 2012e. Tracking Harm: Health and Environmental Impacts of Rail Yards. THE Impact Project Policy Brief Series. https://envhealthcenters.usc.edu /wp-content/uploads/2016/11/Tracking-Harm.pdf.

THE Impact Project. 2018. "THE Impact Project." https://vimeo.com/user5492393.

Times Editorial Board. 2016. "L.A. Needs Fewer Platitudes and More Action on Port Air Pollution." *Los Angeles Times*, February 5. http://www.latimes.com/opinion /editorials/la-ed-0205-port-pollution-20160205-story.html.

Timm-Bijold, Heidi. 2016. Business Resources Manager, City of Duluth, MN, *personal communication*.

Town of Irondequoit, New York. 2018. "Permit Process and Application Requirements." http://www.irondequoit.org/phocadownload/Forms/CommunityDevelopment /building%20permit%20application%20info%20sheet.pdf.

Transportation for America. 2017. "Map-21 Program Explainer: Transportation Alternatives." http://t4america.org/maps-tools/map-21/ta/.

Trochim, William M., Derek A. Cabrera, Bobby Milstein, Richard S. Gallagher, and Scott J. Leischow. 2006. "Practical Challenges of Systems Thinking and Modeling in Public Health." *American Journal of Public Health* 96 (3): 538–546.

Truax, Carla, Andrea Hricko, Robert Gottlieb, Jessica Tovar, Sylvia Betancourt, and Miranda Chien-Hale. 2013. Neighborhood Assessment Teams: Case Studies from Southern California and Instructions on Community Investigations of Traffic-Related Air Pollution. *THE (Trade, Health, and Environment) Impact Project.* https://www.oxy.edu/sites/default/files/assets/UEP/Speakers/Neighborhood%20 Assessment%20Teams%20-%20Case%20Studies%20from%20Southern%20Califor-nia%20on%20traffic%20related%20air%20pollution.pdf.

Trubek, Louise G., and Jennifer J. Farnham. 2000. "Social Justice Collaboratives: Multidisciplinary Practices for People." *Clinical Law Review* 7: 227.

Tryon, Elizabeth, and J. Ashleigh Ross. 2012. "A Community-University Exchange Project Modeled after Europe's Science Shops." *Journal of Higher Education Outreach and Engagement* 16 (2): 197–211.

United Nations Development Program. 2013. "Breaking Down the Silos: Integrating Environmental Sustainability in the Post-2015 Agenda." http://www.pnuma

.org/sociedad_civil/reunion2013/documentos/POST-2015/2013%20Integrating%20 Environmental%20Sustainability%20Post-2015.pdf.

Unnatural Causes. 2018. "Unnatural Causes: Is Inequality Making Us Sick?" http:// www.unnaturalcauses.org/.

U.S. Census. 2000. "Profile of General Demographic Characteristics: 2000 Census 2000 Summary File 1 (SF1) 100-Percent Data." http://factfinder.census.gov/faces /tableservices/jsf/pages/productview.xhtml?src=CF.

U.S. Census. 2016. "American FactFinder: Duluth, Minnesota." www.factfinder.census .gov.

U.S. Congress. 1970. Congressional Findings and Declaration of Purpose. In *42 U.S.C. The Public Health and Welfare, Chapter 85 Air Pollution Prevention and Control, Subchapter I.* Washington, DC: Government Publishing Office.

U.S. DOT (Department of Transportation). 2012. "Safe Routes to School." https:// www.fhwa.dot.gov/environment/safe_routes_to_school/.

U.S. DOT (Department of Transportation). 2017. *The Transportation Planning Process Briefing Book: 2017 Update.* Washington, DC: Federal Highway Administration.

U.S. DOT (Department of Transportation). 2018a. "Air Quality: Transportation Conformity." https://www.fhwa.dot.gov/environment/air_quality/index.cfm.

U.S. DOT (Department of Transportation). 2018b. "Use of Federal Funds for Bicycle and Pedestrian Efforts." https://www.transportation.gov/mission/health/use-federal -funds-bicycle-pedestrian-efforts.

U.S. EPA (Environmental Protection Agency). 2000. "Work Practice Standards for Conducting Lead-Based Paint Activities: Target Housing and Child-Occupied Facilities." *Code of Federal Regulations,* Title 40, §745.227.

U.S. EPA (Environmental Protection Agency). 2002. *Health Assessment Document for Diesel Engine Exhaust.* Washington, DC: National Center for Environmental Assessment.

U.S. EPA (Environmental Protection Agency). 2005. "Stormwater Phase II Final Rule: An Overview." https://www3.epa.gov/npdes/pubs/fact1-0.pdf.

U.S. EPA (Environmental Protection Agency). 2009a. "Environmental Justice Achievement Award Winners." http://www3.epa.gov/environmentaljustice/awards/.

U.S. EPA (Environmental Protection Agency). 2009b. "Integrated Science Assessment (ISA) for Particulate Matter." https://cfpub.epa.gov/ncea/risk/recordisplay.cfm ?deid=216546.

U.S. EPA (Environmental Protection Agency). 2009c. "Lead Dust Sampling Technician Field Guide."

U.S. EPA (Environmental Protection Agency). 2011. "National Environmental Justice Advisory Council," last modified October 11. https://www.epa.gov/environmentaljustice/national-environmental-justice-advisory-council.

U.S. EPA (Environmental Protection Agency). 2013a. "The Clean Air Act in a Nutshell: How It Works." https://www.epa.gov/sites/production/files/2015-05/documents/caa_nutshell.pdf.

U.S. EPA (Environmental Protection Agency). 2013b. "EPA Survey Finds More than Half of the Nation's River and Stream Miles in Poor Condition." https://yosemite.epa.gov/opa/admpress.nsf/0/C967210C37CFFB6885257B3A004CFAF6.

U.S. EPA (Environmental Protection Agency). 2014a. "EPA Region 2 Environmental Justice Action Plan." https://www.epa.gov/sites/production/files/2016-03/documents/region_2_environmental_justice_action_plan.pdf.

U.S. EPA (Environmental Protection Agency). 2014b. "FY 2014–2018 EPA Strategic Plan." https://www.epa.gov/planandbudget/archive#StrategicPlan.

U.S. EPA (Environmental Protection Agency). 2014c. "Renovation, Repair, and Painting Program." http://www2.epa.gov/lead/renovation-repair-and-painting-program.

U.S. EPA (Environmental Protection Agency). 2015. "Brownfields 2015 Area-Wide Planning Grant Fact Sheet, Duluth, MN." https://cfpub.epa.gov/bf_factsheets/gfs/index.cfm?xpg_id=8784&display_type=HTML.

U.S. EPA (Environmental Protection Agency). 2016a. "Environmental Justice: National Environmental Justice Advisory Council," last modified October 11. https://www.epa.gov/environmentaljustice/national-environmental-justice-advisory-council.

U.S. EPA (Environmental Protection Agency). 2016b. "NAAQS Table," last modified December 20. https://www.epa.gov/criteria-air-pollutants/naaqs-table.

U.S. EPA (Environmental Protection Agency). 2016c. "Scoping a Health Impact Assessment (HIA) for the Ports of Los Angeles and Long Beach," last modified February 21. https://archive.epa.gov/region9/nepa/web/html/index-23.html.

U.S. EPA (Environmental Protection Agency). 2016d. "SIP Status Reports," last modified October 12. https://www.epa.gov/air-quality-implementation-plans/sip-status-reports.

U.S. EPA (Environmental Protection Agency). 2016e. "Summary of Executive Order 12898—Federal Actions to Address Environmental Justice in Minority Populations and Low-Income Populations." https://www.epa.gov/laws-regulations/summary-executive-order-12898-federal-actions-address-environmental-justice.

U.S. EPA (Environmental Protection Agency). 2017a. "Criteria Air Pollutants," last modified October 17. https://www.epa.gov/criteria-air-pollutants.

U.S. EPA (Environmental Protection Agency). 2017b. "Environmental Justice and National Environmental Policy Act." https://www.epa.gov/environmentaljustice /environmental-justice-and-national-environmental-policy-act.

U.S. EPA (Environmental Protection Agency). 2017c. "Environmental Justice Grants, Funding, and Technical Assistance." https://www.epa.gov/environmentaljustice /environmental-justice-grants-funding-and-technical-assistance.

U.S. EPA (Environmental Protection Agency). 2017d. "Learn about Clean Diesel," last modified August 31. https://www.epa.gov/cleandiesel/learn-about -clean-diesel.

U.S. EPA (Environmental Protection Agency). 2017e. "MARPOL Annex VI," last modified April 19. https://www.epa.gov/enforcement/marpol-annex-vi.

U.S. EPA (Environmental Protection Agency). 2017f. "Overview of the Clean Air Act and Air Pollution," last modified April 28. http://www.epa.gov/clean-air-act -overview.

U.S. EPA (Environmental Protection Agency). 2018a. "Draft Environmental Justice Primer for Ports." https://www.epa.gov/ports-initiative/draft-environmental-justice -primer-ports.

U.S. EPA (Environmental Protection Agency). 2018b. "The Environmental Justice Collaborative Problem-Solving Cooperative Agreement Program." https://www.epa .gov/environmental-justice/environmental-justice-collaborative-problem-solving -cooperative-agreement-0.

U.S. EPA (Environmental Protection Agency). 2018c. "EPA History." https://www .epa.gov/history.

U.S. EPA (Environmental Protection Agency). 2018d. "International Standards to Reduce Emissions from Marine Diesel Engines and Their Fuels." https://www.epa .gov/regulations-emissions-vehicles-and-engines/international-standards-reduce -emissions-marine-diesel.

U.S. EPA (Environmental Protection Agency). 2018e. "Learn about Environmental Justice." https://www.epa.gov/environmentaljustice/learn-about-environmental -justice.

U.S. EPA (Environmental Protection Agency). 2018f. "National Environmental Policy Act." https://www.epa.gov/nepa.

U.S. EPA (Environmental Protection Agency). 2018g. "Overview of the Brownfields Program." https://www.epa.gov/brownfields/brownfield-overview-and-definition.

U.S. EPA (Environmental Protection Agency). 2018h. "Ports Initiative," last modified February 5. http://www.epa.gov/ports-initiative.

U.S. EPA (Environmental Protection Agency). 2018i. "Sources of Greenhouse Gas Emissions." https://www.epa.gov/ghgemissions/sources-greenhouse-gas-emissions.

U.S. EPA (Environmental Protection Agency). 2018j. "Table of Historical Ozone National Ambient Air Quality Standards (NAAQS)." https://www.epa.gov/ozone-pollution/table-historical-ozone-national-ambient-air-quality-standards-naaqs.

U.S. EPA (Environmental Protection Agency). 2018k. "Use of Lead Free Pipes, Fittings, Fixtures, Solder, and Flux for Drinking Water." https://www.epa.gov/dwstandardsregulations/use-lead-free-pipes-fittings-fixtures-solder-and-flux-drinking-water.

U.S. EPA (Environmental Protection Agency). 2018l. "Great Lakes Areas of Concern." https://www.epa.gov/great-lakes-aocs.

U.S. Forest Service. 2018. "The Art of Collaboration." https://www.fs.usda.gov/main/prc/tools-techniques/collaboration.

U.S. Supreme Court. 2013. "Notice of Court Decision Affecting the Port of Los Angeles Clean Truck Program." https://kentico.portoflosangeles.org/getmedia/bc0a9b28-109c-4edf-8395-14db04f19b41/CTP_Notice_of_Court_Decision_June_2013.

Utell, Mark J., and Mark W. Frampton. 2000. "Acute Health Effects of Ambient Air Pollution: The Ultrafine Particle Hypothesis." *Journal of Aerosol Medicine* 13 (4): 355–359.

Vallentyne, John, and Alfred Beeton. 1988. "The 'Ecosystem' Approach to Managing Human Uses and Abuses of Natural Resources in the Great Lakes Basin." *Environmental Conservation* 15 (1): 58–62.

Ver Ploeg, Michele. 2010. "Access to Affordable, Nutritious Food is Limited in 'Food Deserts.'" *U.S. Department of Agriculture Economic Research Service*, March 1. https://www.ers.usda.gov/amber-waves/2010/march/access-to-affordable-nutritious-food-is-limited-in-food-deserts/.

Viessman Jr., Warren. 1990. "Water Management: Challenge and Opportunity." *Journal of Water Resources Planning and Management* 116 (2): 155–169.

Wailoo, Keith, Jeffrey Dowd, and Karen M. O'Neill. 2010. *Katrina's Imprint: Race and Vulnerability in America*. New Brunswick, NJ: Rutgers University Press.

Walker, Bailus. 1989. "'The Future of Public Health': The Institute of Medicine's 1988 Report." *Journal of Public Health Policy* 10 (1): 19–31. doi: 10.2307/3342941.

Weikel, Dan. 2012. "Pollution Drop from Building Rail Yard near L.A. Harbor Disputed." *Los Angeles Times*, October 21. http://articles.latimes.com/2012/oct/21/local/la-me-rail-yard-20121020.

Weis, Robert. 2012. *Bakers and Basques: A Social History of Bread in Mexico*. Albuquerque: University of New Mexico Press.

Weiser, Benjamin, and J. David Goodman. 2018. "New York City Housing Authority, Accused of Endangering Residents, Agrees to Oversight." *New York Times*, June 11. https://www.nytimes.com/2018/06/11/nyregion/new-york-city-housing-authority -lead-paint.html.

Wernham, Aaron, and Steven M. Teutsch. 2015. "Health in All Policies for Big Cities." *Journal of Public Health Management and Practice* 21 (suppl. 1): S56–S65. doi: 10.1097/PHH.0000000000000130.

Weuve, Jennifer, Robin C. Puett, Joel Schwartz, Jeff D. Yanosky, Francine Laden, and Francine Grodstein. 2012. "Exposure to Particulate Air Pollution and Cognitive Decline in Older Women." *Archives of Internal Medicine* 172 (3): 219–227.

White, Chris, and Grace Edgar. 2010. "Inequalities in Healthy Life Expectancy by Social Class and Area Type: England, 2001–03." *Health Statistics Quarterly* 45 (1): 28–56.

WHO (World Health Organization). 1978. "Declaration of Alma-Ata International Conference on Primary Health Care, Alma-Ata, USSR, 6–12 September 1978." http://www.who.int/publications/almaata_declaration_en.pdf.

WHO (World Health Organization). 2009. *Global Health Risks: Mortality and Burden of Disease Attributable to Selected Major Risks*. Geneva: World Health Organization. http://www.who.int/healthinfo/global_burden_disease/GlobalHealthRisks_report_full.pdf.

WHO (World Health Organization). 2014. "Helsinki Statement on Health in All Policies." Eighth World Health Organization Conference on Health Promotion, Helsinki, Finland. http://apps.who.int/iris/bitstream/10665/112636/1/9789241506908_eng.pdf?ua=1.

WHO (World Health Organization). 2015. *Health in All Policies: Training Manual*. Geneva: World Health Organization. http://apps.who.int/iris/bitstream/10665/151788/1/9789241507981_eng.pdf?ua=1&ua=1.

WHO (World Health Organization). 2018. "Social Determinants of Health." http://www.who.int/social_determinants/en/.

Wilder Research. 2014. "A. H. Zeppa Family Foundation, Impacts and Opportunities: Results from a Discussion of the Fair Food Access Campaign's Work in the Lincoln Park Neighborhood of Duluth." Health Equity in Prevention Report. https://www.wilder.org/wilder-research/research-library/ah-zeppa-family-foundation-impacts -and-opportunities-results.

Wilhelm, Michelle, and Beate Ritz. 2005. "Local Variations in CO and Particulate Air Pollution and Adverse Birth Outcomes in Los Angeles County, California, USA." *Environmental Health Perspectives* 113 (9): 1212–1221. doi: 10.1289/ehp.7751.

Wilkinson, Richard G., and Kate Pickett. 2009. *The Spirit Level: Why More Equal Societies Almost Always Do Better*. New York: Bloomsbury Press.

Williams, Carol J. 2010. "Local Agencies Can't Limit Train Emissions, Court Rules." *Los Angeles Times*, September 16. http://articles.latimes.com/2010/sep/16/local/la -me-air-pollution-railroads-20100916.

Williams, David R. 2012. "Miles to Go before We Sleep: Racial Inequities in Health." *Journal of Health and Social Behavior* 53 (3): 279–295.

Williams, David R., Manuela V. Costa, Adebola O. Odunlami, and Selina A. Mohammed. 2008. "Moving Upstream: How Interventions That Address the Social Determinants of Health Can Improve Health and Reduce Disparities." *Journal of Public Health Management and Practice* 14 (6): S8–S17. doi: 10.1097/01. PHH.0000338382.36695.42.

Williams, Dennis C. 1993. "The Guardian: EPA's Formative Years, 1970–1973." U.S. Environmental Protection Agency.

Wilson, J., S. L. Dixon, D. E. Jacobs, J. Akoto, K. S. Korfmacher, and J. Breysse. 2015. "An Investigation into Porch Dust Lead Levels." *Environmental Research* 137: 129–135. doi: 10.1016/j.envres.2014.11.013.

Wilson, Sacoby, Malo Hutson, and Mahasin Mujahid. 2008. "How Planning and Zoning Contribute to Inequitable Development, Neighborhood Health, and Environmental Injustice." *Environmental Justice* 1 (4): 211–216.

Winneke, Gerhard. 2011. "Developmental Aspects of Environmental Neurotoxicology: Lessons from Lead and Polychlorinated Biphenyls." *Journal of the Neurological Sciences* 308 (1): 9–15.

Winslow, Charles-Edward Amory. (1923) 1984. *Evolution and Significance of the Modern Public Health Campaign*. Reprint, South Burlington, VT: Yale University Press.

Wondolleck, Julia Marie, and Steven Lewis Yaffee. 2000. *Making Collaboration Work: Lessons from Innovation in Natural Resource Management*. Washington, DC: Island Press.

Wu, Jun, Cizao Ren, Ralph J Delfino, Judith Chung, Michelle Wilhelm, and Beate Ritz. 2009. "Association between Local Traffic-Generated Air Pollution and Preeclampsia and Preterm Delivery in the South Coast Air Basin of California." *Environmental Health Perspectives* 117 (11): 1773.

Yaffee, Steven Lewis. 1996. *Ecosystem Management in the United States: An Assessment of Current Experience*. Washington, DC: Island Press.

Yeung, Bernice. 2012. "LA Freeway Expansion, the I-710 Corridor Project, Could Improve Public Health: Report." *HuffPost*, July 30. https://www.huffingtonpost.com /2012/07/30/la-freeway-expansion-the-_n_1719518.html.

Yin, Robert K. 1984. *Case Study Research: Design and Methods.* Beverly Hills: Sage Publication.

Zeitgeist Center for Arts and Community. 2018. "What We Do." https://zeitgeistarts .com/aboutus/.

Zhu, Yifang, William C. Hinds, Seongheon Kim, and Constantinos Sioutas. 2002. "Concentration and Size Distribution of Ultrafine Particles near a Major Highway." *Journal of the Air and Waste Management Association* 52 (9): 1032–1042.

Index

Urban and Industrial Environments

Series editor: Robert Gottlieb, Henry R. Luce Professor of Urban and Environmental Policy, Occidental College

Maureen Smith, *The U.S. Paper Industry and Sustainable Production: An Argument for Restructuring*

Keith Pezzoli, *Human Settlements and Planning for Ecological Sustainability: The Case of Mexico City*

Sarah Hammond Creighton, *Greening the Ivory Tower: Improving the Environmental Track Record of Universities, Colleges, and Other Institutions*

Jan Mazurek, *Making Microchips: Policy, Globalization, and Economic Restructuring in the Semiconductor Industry*

William A. Shutkin, *The Land That Could Be: Environmentalism and Democracy in the Twenty-First Century*

Richard Hofrichter, ed., *Reclaiming the Environmental Debate: The Politics of Health in a Toxic Culture*

Robert Gottlieb, *Environmentalism Unbound: Exploring New Pathways for Change*

Kenneth Geiser, *Materials Matter: Toward a Sustainable Materials Policy*

Thomas D. Beamish, *Silent Spill: The Organization of an Industrial Crisis*

Matthew Gandy, *Concrete and Clay: Reworking Nature in New York City*

David Naguib Pellow, *Garbage Wars: The Struggle for Environmental Justice in Chicago*

Julian Agyeman, Robert D. Bullard, and Bob Evans, eds., *Just Sustainabilities: Development in an Unequal World*

Barbara L. Allen, *Uneasy Alchemy: Citizens and Experts in Louisiana's Chemical Corridor Disputes*

Dara O'Rourke, *Community-Driven Regulation: Balancing Development and the Environment in Vietnam*

Brian K. Obach, *Labor and the Environmental Movement: The Quest for Common Ground*

Peggy F. Barlett and Geoffrey W. Chase, eds., *Sustainability on Campus: Stories and Strategies for Change*

Steve Lerner, *Diamond: A Struggle for Environmental Justice in Louisiana's Chemical Corridor*

Jason Corburn, *Street Science: Community Knowledge and Environmental Health Justice*

Peggy F. Barlett, ed., *Urban Place: Reconnecting with the Natural World*

David Naguib Pellow and Robert J. Brulle, eds., *Power, Justice, and the Environment: A Critical Appraisal of the Environmental Justice Movement*

Eran Ben-Joseph, *The Code of the City: Standards and the Hidden Language of Place Making*

Nancy J. Myers and Carolyn Raffensperger, eds., *Precautionary Tools for Reshaping Environmental Policy*

Kelly Sims Gallagher, *China Shifts Gears: Automakers, Oil, Pollution, and Development*

Kerry H. Whiteside, *Precautionary Politics: Principle and Practice in Confronting Environmental Risk*

Javiera Barandiarán, *From Empire to Umpire: Science and Environmental Conflict in Neoliberal Chile*

Benjamin Pauli, *Flint Fights Back: Environmental Justice and Democracy in the Flint Water Crisis*

Karen Chapple and Anastasia Loukaitou-Sideris, *Transit-Oriented Displacement or Community Dividends? Understanding the Effects of Smarter Growth on Communities*

Henrik Ernstson and Sverker Sörlin, eds., *Grounding Urban Natures: Histories and Futures of Urban Ecologies*

Katrina Smith Korfmacher, *Bridging Silos: Collaborating for Environmental Health and Justice in Urban Communities*